Neurology study guide

Neurology Study Guide
Oral Board Examination Review

Teresella Gondolo, MD

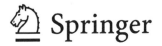 Springer

Library of Congress Cataloging-in-Publication Data

Gondolo, Teresella.
  Neurology study guide : oral board examination review / Teresella
Gondolo.
      p.   ;   cm.
  Includes bibliographical references and index.
  ISBN 0-387-95565-8 (s/c : alk. paper)
  1. Neurology—Examinations, questions, etc.   2.
Physicians—Licenses—United States—Examinations—Study guides.
  [DNLM: 1. Neurology—Examination Questions.   WL 18.2 G637n 2005]   I.
Title.
RC346.G655 2005
616.8′076—dc21

2002029449

ISBN 0-387-95565-8   Printed on acid-free paper.

Printed in the United States of America.   (APEX/EB)

9 8 7 6 5 4 3 2   SPIN 10890928

springeronline.com

Preface

The idea of a book to help neurologists prepare for the oral part of the Neurology Board Examination stemmed from numerous exchanges with colleagues on how they prepared for this important exam. Nobody seemed to have the magic formula to maximize their chances of passing and there were wide disparities of opinion on what they considered the best preparation. Some recommendations were based on often inaccurate impressions, others were the distorted product of their stressful experience while taking the test. On one thing everyone seemed to agree: There is not a single book available that systematically addresses the specifics of this crucially important test.

The task was daunting because the scope of knowledge required to pass the test is as wide as the field of clinical neurology itself. To make it relevant to the experience of the test it was clear that a good preparation needed to be based on practical advice on the technical aspects of the exam as well as on the proper attitude in taking it. Moreover, filling a void in the current neurology literature, an adequate preparation had to be based on cases and their discussion on evidence-based clinical literature.

Although primarily conceived for neurologists preparing for part 2 of the exam, this book intends to provide interesting case-based material to practicing adult and child neurologists, educators, academicians, supervisors, residents, and medical students.

The book is divided into two parts. Part 1 is devoted to practical tips on the exam's structure, its etiquette, and preparation. Particular emphasis is placed on reasons for failing the exam. Part 2 concerns itself with the adult and pediatric vignettes part of the oral Board. Each vignette is presented in a format similar to the one candidates find at the exam. The case is then comprehensively formulated with a differential diagnosis, most likely diagnosis, and treatment recommendations. Where relevant, potential pitfalls, dos and don'ts, musts and shoulds, and frequently asked questions complement the case discussion.

TERESELLA GONDOLO, MD

Foreword

What many Neurology residents do not realize is that they are preparing for the oral board examination every day. Presentations at rounds, at conferences, and even informal discussions regarding differential diagnosis and potential treatment plans are the "stuff" of the oral boards. Anxiety about the boards, however, is common to almost all trainees. And is doesn't seem to get better even with increasing clinical experience. One reason for this anxiety is that the Boards are shrouded by a veil of anecdotal experiences and myth, passed down with a variable degree of embellishment and probably a lot of inaccuracy. In fact, they are a highly structured and practical exercise in assuring the basic competence newly minted Neurologists.

There is no magic formula for passing—solid training, broad experience and clear thinking are all basic requirements. But a prescription for failure is a lack of preparation, which ideally includes not only knowledge of Neurology, but also an understanding of what is expected by the examiners. The exam structure provides relatively little time to present oneself (to a group of strangers, no less) as a competent and caring physician. Preparing for this interaction is essential. Many training programs have instituted mock oral board examination in order to better prepare trainees specifically for the exam. A formal syllabus for this exercise has been lacking.

In this book Dr. Gondolo provides that syllabus, with a clear description of what to expect when taking the boards, and practical guidelines for how (and how **not**) to approach the exam. Examinees should pay careful attention to Part I, the part not covered during clinical Neurology training. Here Dr. Gondolo outlines clearly the structure of the oral board exam, including information on the examiners themselves: who are they and what are their expectations? This is also a guidebook of "dos" and "don'ts" for the exam process that should be taken seriously. For example, dress in a businesslike fashion, get sufficient sleep before the exam, never argue with your examiner, and (when possible) focus your discussion on topics for which you have significant knowledge.

The section on "Reasons for Failing" provides useful test-taking tips even for the smartest and most accomplished Neurologists. Dr. Gondolo reminds us that the approach to a "case" in Neurology should always be structured and organized. Follow this path with each and every case: 1) localization, 2) differential diagnosis, 3) diagnostic workup, and 4) management plans. Straying from this path puts you at risk for overlooking essential information that could be important in convincing the examiner of your competence. Perhaps the most important function of the Boards is discussed under the heading of "The safety factor." First and foremost, the examiner is charged with the task of weeding out unsafe practitioners. Think carefully before suggesting a diagnostic test that may be risky, and never jump to a trivial diagnostic conclusion without first systematically excluding the more serious considerations.

Part II is a concise and sensible study guide of Neurologic disorders and treatments that serves as a review for board examinees, but also as a teaching tool and reference guide for more junior trainees and medical students. The case studies presented are typical of those that may be encountered during the Vignette portion of the exam, and thus are good tools for study.

What advice can I provide for the Neurologist about the take the oral board exams? Prepare well, play to your strengths, be considerate of your patients and your examiners, and get a good night's rest. You've trained long and hard for this moment—make the most of it!

JONATHAN D. GLASS, M.D.
Professor of Neurology and Pathology
Director, Neurology Residency Training Program
Emory University School of Medicine
Atlanta, Georgia

Contents

Part 1

1
General Information

Passing part 2 of the Neurology Board Exam depends on a variety of factors, circumstances and players. While it is true that one cannot control all the variables of this complex equation, it is possible to maximize the chances of success by becoming conversant with these variables and by acquiring the skills and attitudes appropriate to the task. The best preparation on books and clinical practice remains a necessary condition for passing, yet it may be a sadly insufficient one if it is not matched by a savvy understanding of the process. Candidates who come to the exam with a meticulous preparation on the players, the flow, and the overall choreography of the test are more likely to be able to deal with any unexpected circumstances and, at times, even turn obstacles or surprises to their advantage. Similarly to any tests, there are dos and don'ts, shoulds and musts. There is also the imponderable, the unexpected, the variable, for which there is no control. In spite of this inevitable uncertainty, the process has rules, some written, others unwritten, that give the exam an internal consistency and an overall fairness. We begin by looking at this process and its rules, illustrating along the way major pitfalls, misconceptions, errors to avoid, and suggestions that may help you make a favorable impression on the examiners.

The Candidate

Presenting Yourself

Presenting yourself appropriately is important for the outcome of the exam. First impressions may not "make you or break you" but, if they are favorable, they will certainly help you. Since you do not have much time to prove your competence, projecting a professional image is an opportunity, however slight, likely to help your cause. In some ways this process is very much like a job interview. As in most job interviews, you will not have much time to make a good impression and errors will cost you dearly.

Ask yourself: "Would your hire someone whose image does not meet professional standards?" The examiners are people who have never seen you before and will probably never see you again. Therefore, you have only one chance to affect the way they think about you. Here are some hints:

1. Dress appropriately, with business attire: Business suit with tie for men; business suit or appropriate dress for women.
2. Follow acceptable standards of grooming and hygiene; be neat in your appearance.
3. Be professional without being too formal, and cordial without being overly friendly. This may be hard at a time when anxiety may affect your every expression, but the rule of thumb should be: Do not overdo it and do not try too hard. Discretion and moderation should be your guide.
4. Be aware of your signs of nonverbal communication, such as posture or involuntary movements. Poise will go a long way toward projecting a confident image.

Overall you should try to present yourself as you would at your office with your patients and their families—professional, balanced, in control and able to tolerate the uncertainty and stress, without letting them affect your clinical judgment.

Good planning will maximize your chances of arriving for the exam sharp and focused instead of emotionally and physically drained. By the time you get to the Board, you have taken so many exams you may well be an expert. But this test is different and unique in so many ways. Therefore, you need to be extra careful on how you prepare for it from beginning to end. For example, if you are flying across time zones, make sure that you allow plenty of time to counteract any potential jet leg. There are no reasons to get anxious about having to fly across the country for your exam if you take the necessary precautions. Get abundant rest for several nights leading up to the exam, especially the night before. Do not overeat or drink alcohol in the days before the test. Do not "cram" the night before. What little information you will retain will not offset the effects that the loss of sleep will have on your performance. It is better to go to sleep at your regular time, making sure that you have taken the appropriate steps to wake up on time the next morning. In addition to setting an alarm, arrange to have a wake-up call, or for someone to wake you up. All the knowledge and preparation will not help you if you get to the exam burned out, overwhelmed and out of focus.

The Day You Arrive

You will get to your hotel the day before the test. After checking in, your next step is to proceed to the registration area, where you will receive a packet containing all the instructions on part 2, including a booklet, timetable, location of the exam, bus schedule, and name of the team leader who will administer your exam. It is absolutely essential that you familiarize yourself with the hotel's layout, and the place and time of departure of the buses. Although private transportation is certainly an option, it is less advisable than the official transportation, which is very efficient and certain to get to the destination on time. A general orientation will go over the details and logistics. Once you have taken care of registration and orientation you will have some time before you have dinner and retire. Spending the evening in the hotel lobby may not be the best idea. Examiners and examinees are accommodated in the same hotel. Therefore, it is likely to see examiners in the hotel lobby. They are easily recognizable for their red and white badges. It is best to avoid socialization between examiners and examinees, to avoid uncomfortable situations and any possible appearance of impropriety.

If you hook up with some colleagues for dinner, it is better to avoid the topic of the exam as much as possible. Beware of the anxiety-inducing doomsayers and obsessional types who may significantly reduce your chances of getting a good night's sleep.

The Examiners

Structure of the Examining Team

Since you will be evaluated by a team comprised of several people, it may be helpful to understand how this team is formed and which function each team person has. The American Board of Psychiatry and Neurology (ABPN) has a highly structured higherarchy consisting of eight teams headed by a Board Director.

The team leader works with four senior examiners who have considerable experience, sit in several exams at a time, and help settle scoring controversies between the two examiners, should they arise. The director himself may join the seniors during the evaluation to give the

examiners his attendance card and to assess the examiners. The exams themselves are administered by two examiners. Primary examiners are volunteers who have requested to be examiners and submitted their qualifications. In addition to their qualifications, examiners are selected for geographic criteria, which allows the Board to save on expenses. Examiners are paid a per diem and their expenses are reimbursed.

Training of Examiners

New examiners and old ones who have not examined for two years or more are trained the day before for half a day by experienced examiners and sometimes directors. During such training, examiners are instructed in detail about specific elements of the exams, minimum requirements for a passing grade, examples of conditional scores, and attitude to keep during the exam. Tapes and mock exams can also be part of the training. Fairness to the applicant in the examining process and its evaluation is stressed and examiners are taught to keep a neutral attitude throughout the experience to avoid giving candidates a false impression about their performance. Pitfalls are discussed: lecturing or teaching is discouraged, as is giving feedback to the candidate.

The examiners are also taught not to be hostile, sarcastic, or condescending, and not to dwell on what the candidate does not know. They are directed not to ask only questions pertaining to their area of expertise. Finally, they are reminded to be mindful of the anxiety factor during the examination, both on their approach to the candidate and to the grading.

How Examiners Plan for the Session

The two examiners agree in advance on who should take the lead in asking questions. Though often only a silent observer, the second examiner may ask questions as well. The Board takes great care to assure the highest standard of fairness during the exam. To that end, new examiners are coupled with more seasoned ones the during their first experience as examiners. Examiners are also given the opportunity of experiencing different partners as they are systematically rotated in their pairings during the two days of the exam. To further ensure unbiased and fair test conditions, examiners must report to the team leader the names of candidates they personally know. Similarly, information about the candidate's background and educational institution are purposely kept out of the process, again to avoid any undue influence on the course of the exam and evaluation.

In preparation for the exam, examiners spend a few hours going over the vignettes and discussing signs, symptoms, localization, and differential diagnosis, ensuring consensus on what the candidate will be expected to know.

Grading

The grading system is based on a form that contains grades on subcategories and a preliminary overall grade. Depending upon the importance the Board gives to each subcategory, the grading varies from pass/fail to pass/conditional/fail. The preliminary overall grade is pass-conditional or fail except when a candidate returns for one part only, when the choice is pass or fail. At the end of the grading conducted individually by each examiner, the two exchange their preliminary grading and after a brief discussion they attempt to come to a consensus grading. The condition grading can be upgraded to pass depending upon the discussion between the examiners about strengths and deficiencies of the candidate. The process is repeated for each of the three neurology tests, after which a final grade is given.

The criteria upon which the grading is based for the live patient test are the subcategories of

- Eliciting data and technique of the examination.
- Organization and presentation of data.
- Phenomenology, diagnosis, differential diagnosis and prognosis.
- Etiologic, pathogenic, and therapeutic issues.

For the vignette test and the child neurology case the first two categories above are replaced by the subcategory of observation of data. Otherewise, the subcategories are similar.

For each of the three tests, at the end of subcategory grading, the examiners give a grade of pass, conditional, or fail.

Examiners are instructed to give an overall evaluation of "pass" when, in their judgment, the candidate has shown to possess the minimum standards of neurological competence. "Conditional" is the grade by which the examiners express doubts or reservations about the candidate's performance/competence, precluding a pass grade. "High conditional" is closer to pass, while "low conditional" is closer to fail. A grade of "fail" in any of the three tests means that the candidate needs to repeat the failed part or parts.

The preliminary grading should reflect the subcategories. When there is wide difference on the grading by the two examiners, the senior examiner tries to have them arrive at a consensus grade. If consensus is not reached, the case is taken up by the director. The combination of one pass and one conditional is usually upgraded to a pass. Two conditionals are considered on the candidate's individual merits/deficiencies. A conditional/fail combination rarely gets converted to a pass.

By and large, however, strong disagreement among the examiners is rare. The senior examiners and directors base their final determination on clearly written evaluations with specific examples of deficiencies and assets. Because of this laborious process as well as the possibility that the candidate may appeal the final decision, examiners are told to be very careful and specific in their notes supporting their grades.

Your Interaction with the Examiners

During the first 30 minutes of the live patient examination your interaction with the examiners will be minimal. There may be examiners in and out of the room. Even though you may find that distracting, you need to make a conscious effort to ignore that process, as it is a normal occurrence in all the exams. In rare circumstances, the examiner will intervene to redirect a stalling process because the patient might not cooperate or the candidate might have crippling difficulties leading him to a dead end. Your interaction with the examiner will start when you present the case and your findings, and will peak during the 15-minute section with questions.

There are no hard and fast rules on how to interact with examiners, mostly because examiners themselves, like candidates, are different, have different styles and different views. However, there are some general rules which may maximize your chances of making a good impression:

- Be respectful.
- Be formal and professional. Excessive informality may sway your examiners in a negative fashion.
- Avoid sarcasm and arrogance.
- Listen carefully to their interventions/questions.
- Never interrupt the examiner in the middle of a sentence.
- Never argue with the examiners. Even if you disagree with some of the questions or the way an examiner redirects you, you should never lose your cool, get testy, or challenge the examiner. This is a cardinal rule to which there is virtually no exception.
- Do not split between the examiners. If you feel that one examiner is fairer than the other, act equally with both of them.
- Do not patronize/teach or correct an examiner (Example: "What you are saying is only partially true.").
- Excessive confidence is not advisable (Example: "I know that, of course.").
- If there is something you do not know, it is better to acknowledge it than to make it up: "I am sorry, but I don't remember. I will go back to the books and review it."
- If a question is not clear it is better to ask for clarification or repetition of the question than to give the wrong answer.

- Do not volunteer information that is not of consequence in the case, it may open a Pandora's box and you may end up grilled with all kinds of questions.
- If there is something you missed in your interview/ clinical examination because of lack of time or because you simply missed it, admit it or acknowledge it. Your examiners do not have any way of telling whether you did not think about it, did not know it, or did not have a chance to elicit it.
- If you think your examiners are too tough, do not lose your composure; stay the course, it will benefit you in the long run.
- If you feel you are not doing too well, do not fall apart; pull yourself together and do the best you can.
- Do not try to guess what the examiners are thinking; it will distract you and it will never help you.
- If you are looking for signs of approval, forget it. The examiners are trained to control them as much as they can.

The Anxiety Factor

The Board is the culmination of your training, what you have been working on for the past three years, perhaps longer. It provides the indication of what you know and how you present yourself professionally. Passing it confers affirmation of your work, study, and sacrifice; the prospect of a rewarding career; and recognition by your colleagues and mentors. In essence, it represents the closure of an important chapter of your career and the beginning of a new exciting one.

Conversely, failing the Board could be a blow to your self-esteem and a harsh judgment of the way you trained and studied. Failing the Board means more studying and financial sacrifices, forgetting about job offers for Board-certified neurologists only and the embarrassing feeling of telling your colleagues and supervisors about it. No wonder this is one of the most anxiety-provoking experiences of your life. Mishandled or excessive anxiety is also one of the main reasons why people fail the Board. Since anxiety does so many things to your cognition, including hampering your concentration and memory, it is important to recognize its effects on your performance and to take the appropriate steps to minimize its consequences. On the other hand, anxiety my be useful in channeling productive energy in the right direction and gearing up for what is coming. In other words, lack of anxiety and overconfidence may hurt you as much as being overanxious.

How anxious are you? You should have a good understanding about anxiety symptoms and how they affect your performance. Some people have good insight into how anxious they are and how anxiety affects their performance while others lack this awareness. A history of somatic symptoms, such as palpitation, excessive sweating, breathing irregularities, and restlessness, during previous exams or public performances should alert you to the possibility that excessive anxiety may affect your performance.

Hints for Dealing with Anxiety

As stated before, do not expect signs of approval or feedback from the examiners because they are instructed not to provide any. As much as it is not in human nature to ignore nonverbal signs in significant and emotionally charged interactions, remembering this simple fact throughout the exam should automatically decrease your anxiety.

Practice, practice, practice. Oral vignettes and examinations of live patients are invaluable reducers of anxiety as they build self-confidence and reduce the chances of error during the real exam. Seek out anxiety-provoking vignettes and discuss with examiners you do not know and ask them to zero in on your weaknesses.

Behavioral modification, biofeedback, and relaxation/ visualization techniques teach you ways to keep your anxiety in check.

Do not use alcohol, or benzodiazepines as they may considerably impair your cognition as well as your performance.

If you are unable to control your anxiety, propanolol is the most effective and safest choice. Taken appropriately (20–40 mg 45–90 minutes prior to the the anxiety-provoking situation), this drug acts on the physiological part of anxiety while keeping the psychological component intact. It is also wise to try its effects on yourself before the test. Propanolol may make a huge difference in your performance but it should be taken wisely, without exaggerating. High doses of Inderal may hamper your ability to adequately perform.

It also important to mention here that the Board discourages the use of any anxiety-controlling drug or substance.

Information on the Board

Any neurologist in training who has gotten this far will have plenty of information and more or less accurate news about part 2 of the Board. Although the ABPN also offers certification in child neurology and a double certification in psychiatry and neurology, we will deal only with the adult neurology certification. The ABPN itself is the best source of information. Its staff is professional and courteous and they will be more than happy to provide you with all the details you need, including the information booklet that contains all the essential information about the exam.

The Board itself is undergoing a massive process of

transformation dictated by a need to keep up with changing times. Therefore, one of the advantages of contacting the Board directly would be to have up-to-date information on recent changes.

The Board website www.abpn.org is well designed and exhaustive in dealing with the major questions and answers a prospective candidate might have. What follows is a summary of some of the most basic information a candidate needs.

Board eligibility—Although the Board does not use the term eligible, most applicants and prospective employers still do. The Board determines whether a candidate is admissible to take the examination based on requirements for certification. The four most important requirements are:

1. Graduation from an accredited medical school in the United States or Canada. For International Medical Graduates the requirement is graduation from a medical school listed by the World Health Organization. Accredited Doctor of Osteopathy schools leading to a D.O. degree are included.
2. Possession of a current license to practice medicine in a state, commonwealth, or territory of the United States or Canada.
3. Completion of neurology training in a program accredited by the Accreditation Council for Graduate Medical Education(ACGME), or by the Royal College of Physicians and Surgeons of Canada. The candidate may have the option of four years in neurology residency or a combination of a postgraduate year followed by three years in neurology. In the latter case, an internship year in medicine is acceptable. Alternatively, an internship year with at least six months of medicine and less than two months in neurology also meets the Board's qualifications
4. Pass Parts 1 (written) and 2 (oral) of the certification examination.

Transferring residents should have completed a minimum of two years of neurology in the same program to qualify. Exceptions are considered on an individual basis depending upon the type of rotations and appropriate documentation by the Training Director

While there is no limit to the number of times a candidate can apply for part 1 (written) of the exam, some limitations apply to part 2 (oral). A candidate who has passed part 1 has six years or three attempts (whichever comes first) to pass part 2. If six years pass or three attempts have been unsuccessful, the candidate is required to retake part 1. Since April 2000, unexcused absences count as one of the three chances to take the exam.

Depending upon space availability, the Board tries to schedule part 2 of the examination within one year of the passing of part 1.

Certificates issued after October 1, 1994, are valid for 10 years. Another exam is required prior to the expiration date to renew certification for 10 more years.

A detailed compendium of information about requirements and procedures, including applications forms, can be found in the Information for Applicants booklet which can be obtained from the Board or from its website.

Further info may be requested from
American Board of Psychiatry and Neurology, Inc.
500 Lake Cook Road, Suite 335
Deerfield, Ill 60015-5249

2
The Live Patient Examination

In interviews with candidates, lack of information about the structure of the exam clearly surfaces as the main reason for experiencing difficulties during part 2 of the Board. The oral part of the Neurology Board is divided into the following three parts:

1. The live patient examination.
2. The adult vignettes.
3. The pediatric vignettes.

This chapter focuses on the live patient examination and is supplemented by suggestions on how to address specific issues that might weigh on the examiners' grading.

The Board exam is not much different from a standard neurological examination. The purpose is to obtain all the information you need to arrive at a diagnosis and treatment plan through a carefully conducted neurological interview and a thoroughly performed neurological evaluation.

The live patient examination consists of three parts:

1. Neurological history and examination of the live patient (30 minutes).
2. Presentation and discussion of the case with the examiners (time varies).
3. Examiners' questions on the case as well as on general knowledge and competence in neurology (time varies).

The Room

The clinical interview takes place in a room with the two primary examiners, one senior and one junior. You will be standing in front of the patient while the examiners observe either by your side or behind you. In a corner, there is a table with a few chairs, where, when the examination is finished, the second part of the process will take place. The room does not have any clock, which brings us to the next point.

The Time Factor: 30-Minute History and Neurological Examination

It is absolutely essential that you adequately time yourself for the test. Good timing is the result of a combination of correct planning and practice. Keeping mental track of time also helps structure the examination, which in turn gives the examiners a sense of organization and command of the process. You have 30 minutes to collect information and perform a neurological evaluation. Five minutes before the end of your time, one of the examiners will alert you to the remaining time. The following are some suggestions about how to handle the time factor and things to avoid:

- Mentally divide the time you allocate for each part of the 30 minutes. There is no right or wrong way of doing this and you need to be flexible. One approach uses 15 minutes for history and 15 minutes for the neurological exam. Another approach is to spend 20 minutes on history taking and 10 minutes on the neurological examination.
- Glance sporadically at your watch without overdoing it, which would give the examiners the sense you are overly concerned with time.
- Follow the patient's leads and presentation of symptoms but redirect him or her if too much time is spent on information of limited importance.
- Do not panic if you feel you are running out of time.
- Use your last 5 minutes wisely without cramming in too many questions. The last few minutes should be used to wind down the interview/exam and to put the finishing touch to your test.

- Act like you are in charge of the time rather than the time being in charge of you.
- Make a mental note of the material you were not able to cover so that you can use it during your presentation.
- Remember not to rush when you present the case. The amount of time examiners allow you for presentation varies from examiner to examiner. Generally, you have between 10 and 15 minutes to present. Examiners greatly value well-organized and carefully assembled presentations.
- Be prepared to be interrupted during your presentation as the examiners may either want to redirect the flow of your presentation or ask you pointed questions on specific things you presented.
- Be direct in your responses to the questions. Dancing around the question with a circumstantial answer will not work in your favor. The examiners are as aware of the time factor as you are. They have the unenviable task of assessing a colleague's competence in a very limited time.
- Although strategizing about time is desirable, every exam is different. Things may come up that may force you to change course of action. Be flexible and ready to change your plan, but always keep your eye on the overall time structure. To use a musical analogy, the melody can have different variations but the background theme should remain the same.
- Never finish the examination before it is time. 30 minutes is considered not to be sufficient in some cases, and if you miss some information you will be called on it. Besides, if you finish too soon, you will give the impression of being less than thorough.

The Tool Box (Your Medical Instruments)

Here is a list of neurological tools you should bring to the exam:

- A vial of coffee to test olfaction (in patients with a history of head trauma or in patients with possible frontal lobe pathology).
- Vials of salt and sugar (testing taste).
- Ophtalmoscope/otoscope.
- Flashlight with rubber adapter.
- Strip to check nystagmus.
- Cotton wisp (corneal reflex and light touch).
- Reflex hammer.
- Tuning fork.
- Two stoppered tubes (testing hot and cold discrimination).
- Q-tips you can break for sensory pin prick (no needles or safety pins).

- Flexible steel measuring tape scored in metric system for measuring of occipitofrontal circumference (children).
- Stethoscope (auscultation of neck vessels, eyes, and cranium).
- Penny, nickel, dime, paperclip, and key (testing for stereognosis).

The Patient

The live patient generally is a neurology clinic outpatient and is the type of patient you usually see in your private office. You will not see a comatose or emergency patient.

Commonly found categories include movement disorders, primarily Parkinson's disease, occasionally parkinsonism, such as PSP (progressive supranuclear palsy), Huntington's chorea and tardive dyskinesia; demyelinating disorders and multiple sclerosis; headache, both migraine and cluster; and benign intracranial hypertension. Seizure disorders, both generalized and partial complex, cerebrovascular disorders, dementia, and neuromuscular disorders ranging from peripheral neuropathy to myasthenia gravis are frequently seen during the examinations.

Differential Diagnosis and Discussion of Treatment Options

Your Interaction with the Patient

Patients who participate in the Board exam are volunteers who are compensated with small amounts of money. They deserve our utmost respect because of their patience and willingness to cooperate with the testing procedure. The majority are happy to contribute to the process of certifying a professional and by-and-large have a good appreciation of the importance, as well as the anxiety, of the event. In that sense, they are very cooperative and in general less anxious than you are.

By the way your patient responds to your questions and cooperates with your neurological examinations, he or she will play an important part in the success of your live patient session. Moreover, your approach to the patient will be an important scoring factor in the final determination of your grade. This is the reason why you need to know the necessary steps in establishing a good rapport with the patient. Follow these guidelines for getting the patient's cooperation and making a professional impression with your examiners:

- Introduce yourself to the patient in a courteous and professional fashion.
- Although the patient knows the purpose of the examination, you may be better off explaining in your own words what is going to take place and why.

- Follow the patient's leads.
- Gently redirect the patient when necessary.
- Start with open-ended questions and narrow the focus as you go along.
- Even though you may have a mental list of symptoms you want to get to, do not rush the patient and do not ask them in a "menu" fashion.
- Do not abruptly interrupt the patient.
- Do not make demeaning, disparaging, or ethnically tinted comments to the patient.
- Never get angry with the patient.
- Respect the culture of the patient.
- Explain to the patient what you are doing every step of the way.
- Never act like a know-it-all; don't be condescending.
- Avoid comments and expressions that might sound too casual or informal.
- Respect the patient's space and reticence to share some information.
- In spite of this, do not neglect to ask about sensitive issues that have neurological implications (such as about AIDS, etc.).
- Avoid speaking in technical language that the patient may be unable to understand.
- Do not be afraid of asking for clarification if you did not understand the patient.
- Thank the patient and acknowledge him or her at the end of the process.
- Do not ask the patient his diagnosis.

The Difficult Patient

Candidates often talk about easy and difficult patients. Easy patients are those who are cooperative, verbal, follow the candidate's leads, and are easy to diagnose. Difficult patients respond in the opposite way. It is of utmost importance to realize, however, that this distinction sometimes proves to be a fallacy—a trap—as in the case of a seemingly easily diagnosable patient by a candidate who jumps to the sure diagnostic formulation and fails to formulate a comprehensive differential diagnosis. Nevertheless, a difficult patient generally presents more problems than an easy one. Your examiners know a difficult patient as well as you do, and will factor in the coefficient of difficulty in the final evaluation. Therefore you can be assured that fairness will be used in assessing your performance with a problematic patient.

When dealing with a difficult patient, maintain your composure and keep your anxiety to a minimum. If you practice dealing with difficult patients you may actually turn what appears to be a disadvantage into a plus when you present and discuss the case. Clearly, if you act prepared in the situation, you will project the winning image of a professional who is ready for any circumstance and case, no matter how tough.

The following are two examples of difficult patients and tips on how to handle the situation. Note, however, that these are not the only categories of difficult patients nor are the responses the only correct ones. Variables include your personal style in dealing with the patient, and the specific demeanor of the patient.

The Resisting Patient

Although most of the patients are cooperative, you occasionally may find patients who are vague, circumstantial, or outright oppositional. This may be due to a variety of reasons, such as

- The patient is in discomfort.
- The patient feels intimidated by you or the process.
- The patient feels that you have approached him or her the wrong way, or have established a bad rapport.
- The patient may have some significant psychiatric pathology, such as personality disorder or major depression, that accompanies the neurological disease and precludes the patient from fully cooperating with the process.
- The patient does not understand you.

Try to address the patient's resistance early in the process. Here are some suggestions:

- Ask if the patient is feeling any discomfort.
- Acknowledge that the patient might be having a hard time during the process.
- Ask the patient if there is anything you can do to help the patient along.
- Do not antagonize the patient.
- If you detect some psychopathology, do not highlight it but do mention it in your presentation.
- If the patient does not seem to understand you, repeat your question.

The Cognitively Impaired Patient

Patients with a history of cognitive impairment may be very difficult to interview and examine. Some patients can present with dysarthria, aphasia, or dementia. It is important to remember that the examiners are well aware of the difficulties you might have in obtaining a good history. Here are a few suggestions:

- Speak clearly and slowly, without shouting.
- Acknowledge the patient's frustration and be supportive.
- Perform a good, formal, cognitive testing.
- Do the best you can and mention your limitation in your exam.
- Do not get discouraged if you are unable to obtain enough information; proceed to perform your neurological exam regardless.

The 30-Minute Neurological History and Examination

The Art of History Taking

The neurological history includes four main parts that should be kept in chronological order:

1. The chief complaint and history of present illness.
2. The past medical history.
3. The family history.
4. The social history.

Chief Complaint. Some examples of chief complaint include headache, neck or low back pain, loss of consciousness, weakness, numbness, dyplopia, and dysarthria.

To find out more about these symptoms, inquire about them in the following manner:

- Time of onset.
- Mode of onset, acute or gradual.
- Character and severity.
- Location, extension, and radiation.
- Precipitating or exacerbating factors.
- Associated symptoms.
- Course: Progression or remission.

Past Medical History. This assumes particular importance in the setting in the list of disorders that can play a role as risk factors for neurological problems, such as diabetes, hypertension, heart disease, polio as a child, or alcohol/drug abuse.

Family History. Questions regarding other family members and relatives are particularly pertinent in the context of seizure disorders, headache, movement disorders, and muscle disease.

Social History. Social history is important in the context of alcohol and drug abuse and its complications, smoking, and other such factors.

Observation of the patient during history taking is important to pinpoint special features, for example, myopathic facies, such as myothonic dystrophy, facioscapular humeral muscular dystrophy, myasthenia gravis, or hypothyroidism; or skin abnormalities, such as adenoma sebaceum or café au lait spots.

Special History: Headache or Seizure Disorders

The complaint of headache is one of the commonest symptoms encountered in neurology and general practice. From the history alone, the nature of these headaches can be suspected in the great majority of cases. The characteristics that need to be emphasized when approaching the complaint of headache are

- Severity of pain.
- Temporal onset.
- Duration.
- Location.
- Quality.
- Associated symptoms, including physical changes.
- Presence of any warning minutes or hours before.
- Factors relieving or aggravating the pain.

Another topic that needs special consideration is the history of a patient with a seizure disorder, because an adequate history is of primary importance. It should include a description of the mode of onset of the generalized seizure and a careful description of the partial seizure. The patient should be questioned closely and required to define terms with as much care as possible. Too often the patient uses vague and generalized terms, such as dizziness, forgetful spells, little spells, etc. Warning symptoms and precipitating factors should clearly be emphasized.

The Neurological Examination

Each part of the neurological examination needs to be covered with particular emphasis and more time spent on the one relevant to the case that will help you make a diagnosis.

For example, in a case of peripheral nervous system involvement, such as radiculopathy, plexopathy, peripheral neuropathy, and myopathy, more time will be spent on the muscle, sensory testing, and reflex examination.

If you feel the need to repeat a part you are not sure about, you are allowed to do so during the time permitted.

The order of the neurological examination is fairly standard. Nevertheless, the amount of time and attention to details a candidate will devote to each section will depend in large part on the case. For example, in a patient presenting with obvious cognitive impairment, the candidate will need to perform a thorough mental status examination. Conversely, a suspected radiculopathy will require more attention to motor and sensory functions. Here following up on the symptoms and signs elicited in the history taking will serve as a guide. The most commonly followed general outline is

- Mental status evaluation.
- Cranial nerves.
- Motor examination
- Sensory examination.
- Coordination and gait.

Mental Status

After noticing appearance and general behavior, quickly check the main components of the mental status:

- Orientation with reference to time, place, and person.
- Immediate recall.
- Memory—recent and remote.
- Calculation, insight, and judgment (if indicated). Speech: naming, repetition, comprehension, reading/writing (if indicated).
- Ability to name, repeat, and follow commands.

Cranial Nerves

- Olfaction: Only if indicated. Smell does not need to be routinely tested, but the neurologist should have olfactory stimuli readily available. Examples of indications for testing the sense of smell are head injury, dementia, and unilateral gradual loss of vision in one eye.
- Vision: Visual fields; visual acuity (Snellen chart), if indicated; funduscopic examination.
- Pupillary light and accommodation, reflexes, and size of pupils.
- Eye movements.
- Facial sensation: corneal reflexes if indicated.
- Facial strength in muscles of mastication and muscles of facial expression.
- Hearing: threshold and acuity ability to hear a tuning fork or rustling of fingers; air-borne conduction test of Rinne and vertex lateralizing test of Weber (when indicated).
- Palatal movements.
- Shoulder elevation.
- Tongue inspection and movements.

Motor Examination

- Muscle tone and strength of individual muscles.
- DTR: check symmetrically: biceps (C5–6), triceps (C6–7), brachioradialis (C7–T1), knee-jerk (L2–4), ankle jerk (S1), jaw jerk (V).
- Plantar responses.
- Superficial reflexes (if indicated).
- Primitive reflexes (if indicated).

Sensory Examination

- Light touch, temperature, pain.
- Joint position sense.
- Vibration.
- Double simultaneous stimulation.
- Graphesthesia.
- Stereognosis.

Coordination Examination

- Finger to nose.
- Heel to shin.
- Gait.

The 30-Minute Case Discussion and Additional Questions

This part includes a discussion of the case you examined as well as other questions not necessarily pertinent to the case during the remaining time.

It is important to clearly summarize the history and neurological examination, highlighting the significant pertinent findings. A defective interview is an important reason for failure to arrive at a diagnosis.

The next point will be to try to localize the lesion. The most important information for localization comes from the neurological examination. Some symptoms and signs are quite specific for certain regions. Also, the distribution and combination of findings help localize a deficit.

Next in your mental order is to decide whether the lesion is focal, multifocal, or diffuse and the temporal profile (how the symptoms began and if they have changed over time). The next step is to categorize the lesion. Based on the anatomical and temporal profile of the neurologic problem, it is possible to formulate a hypothesis about the underlying etiology.

The categories of disorders are:

- Vascular.
- Inflammatory.
- Neoplastic.
- Toxic/metabolic.
- Degenerative.
- Traumatic.
- Hereditary/developmental.

Now you are ready to present a list of differential diagnoses and the one (or several) most likely. You will be expected to discuss the diagnostic and therapeutic issues.

During the first 30 minutes the examiners have observed how you obtain information from the patient and perform a neurological examination. The next 30 minutes are dedicated to your presentation of the case. The presentation is not different from any presentation you have done during the residency. It is based on a summary of the case that includes the most important elements of the history and neurological examination. The first step is therefore to summarize.

The last part (10 minutes or time left after the discussion of the case) is dedicated to more questions, depending on the availability of time. This could include clinical cases or neurological questions and can be unpredictable and difficult at times.

If you miss something and do not know the answer, do not panic. The most important factor is to admit it. On the other hand, not knowing certain topics is inexcusable and is listed in the reasons for failing.

Examples are provided below.

Example 1

"I just examined a 52-year-old male with a 6-month history of intermittent, fluctuating ptosis, diplopia, fatigue, and difficulty climbing stairs. His past history includes rheumatoid arthritis treated with penicillamine. His neurological examination shows mild bilateral ptosis, defect in medial and lateral eye duction and proximal muscle weakness in all four extremities."

This is a straightforward case, as are most of the live patient cases, considering the limited amount of time you have to make a differential diagnosis and possibly a best tentative diagnosis.

The second step is the localization of the lesion, as previously emphasized. You should have already formed an idea of localization and differential diagnosis while taking the history and performing the examination.

In this particular case, the history and neurological examination seem to localize a disorder of the motor unit, specifically the neuromuscular junction.

Disorders of neuromuscular transmission produce symptomatic weakness that predominates in certain muscle groups and typically fluctuates in response to effort and rest. The diagnosis is primarily based on clinical history and examination findings demonstrating the distinctive pattern of weakness.

The third step is to categorize the neuromuscular junction disorders and reach a good differential diagnosis.

Disorders of neuromuscular junction can be postsynaptic such as myasthenia gravis, or presynaptic such as Lambert-Eaton myasthenic syndrome, and botulism.

There are no clinical elements to support a presynaptic disorder and all the aspects indicate a postsynaptic disorder. Also, a very important element to formulate a differential diagnosis and a tentative diagnosis is the past medical history of rheumatoid arthritis treated with penicillamine.

This will elicit the most likely possibility of a drug-induced myasthenia gravis. In the case of D-penicillamine, symptoms usually start 4 to 9 months after beginning treatment. The most common symptoms and signs are ptosis, diplopia, dysphagia, dysarthria, and fatigue. In some patients weakness may also involve limbs.

Finally, although you may be interrupted, plan how you would work up the patient. However, if you state a conclusion without supporting data, you will not make a favorable impression, as most examiners will ask for the data that support your ideas. In this case you will probably be asked about drug-induced myasthenia, diagnosis and treatment.

Again, you should have a plan of action and avoid guessing the correct answer or disagreeing with the examiners.

If you don't understand a question, ask for clarification. If there is something you forgot to ask the patient or parts you did not cover, mention it to the examiners.

Never fake knowledge you do not possess. On the other hand, there are topics on which lack of knowledge is inexcusable. These topics are listed in the reasons for failing.

After the case discussion ends the candidate is expected to answer questions not necessarily related to the case. They may consist of simple questions with single answers, more complex questions, or vignettes. The main goal is to attempt to answer the questions as specifically as possible without volunteering much information, which may lead to probing questions on possible areas of weakness.

Example 2

Dr. G.Z. had just finished taking the history and examining a patient with clear cervical radiculopathy due to trauma. In the differential diagnosis of arm weakness and paresthesias, he mentioned the possibility of upper brachial plexus lesion which then led the examiner to inquire about the anatomy of the brachial plexus as well as etiology of brachial plexopathies. Although he felt at a loss since he was unable to answer specific anatomic questions on the anatomical division, he was able to maintain his composure and admitted he did not know the answer, adding that he would have to go back to the books and review the topic.

The examiner quickly changed the topic to the diagnosis and treatment of radiculopathies. In the end, the candidate's acknowledging his lack of knowledge on the topic allowed him not to be further questioned, shifting the focus of the test to a topic he was more familiar with. The examiners, in turn, did not consider his gap in knowledge serious enough to fail him.

Reference

Mayo Clinic and Mayo Clinic Foundation: Clinical Examination in Neurology, ed 5. Philadelphia: WB Saunders, 1981.

3
The Vignette

What is a vignette?

A vignette is a description of a neurological clinical case open for discussion. In the Neurology Board there are two types of vignettes, the adult vignette and the pediatric vignette. For the adult neurologist the live patient and the adult neurology case vignettes constitute the major portion of the exam, while the pediatric neurology case vignettes make up the minor part of the exam. The child neurologist candidate will be assigned a live pediatric patient (major), pediatric case vignettes (major) and adult neurology case vignettes (minor).

All major parts of the exam have to be a pass for a final grade of pass to be assigned for that part.

Adult and pediatric vignettes are contained in booklets. Each booklet is different and contains different vignettes.

Adult Vignettes

The adult vignette is a description of a clinical case concerning adult neurology open for discussion. It contains a neurological subject and it is the description of a neurological case. A vignette can vary in length and difficulty and can also contain elements that are not pertinent to the diagnosis as they can have one or more obvious correct answers or more than one pertinent answer. In a one-hour time frame, 50 minutes are dedicated to multiple adult vignettes and the last 10 minutes of the session are reserved for one or more questions and vignettes created by the examiners, usually concerning neurological emergencies.

After the candidate introduces himself or herself, he or she is given a booklet and is told to go to a certain case number.

The examiner then gives the candidate the choice of reading the case aloud or in silence, or having the case read aloud by the examiner.

The decision at this point may be an important one, as some people find themselves in trouble when they find out they made the wrong choice. My suggestion is to select the modality you are most comfortable with. Some people find reading to themselves more conducive to comprehension and concentration, while for others it does not appear to make a difference whether they read the vignettes or it is read to them.

Although some candidates have talked about a "feeling" that the examiners would prefer the case to be read, there is no clear evidence that this may be the case. Note taking is allowed, but in the interest of time and practicality one should avoid writing copious notes. Also, if after a first reading you have some doubts or, as it sometimes can happen, you have no clue, you can always request to read the vignette a second time.

How to Approach a Vignette

The approach to a vignette is

- Read.
- Think while you are reading, highlighting the most relevant signs and symptoms, which will be the basis for a differential diagnosis.
- Localize.

After the candidate reads the vignette the candidate is expected to briefly summarize the case, highlighting the most relevant signs and symptoms, which will be the basis for a differential diagnosis. The rule of thumb in doing this is not to jump to a definite diagnosis without building an argument, as this gives the examiners an idea of lack of in-depth understanding of neurological complexities.

The three main guiding principles that may help you organize your presentation are

- Localization.
- Categorization.
- Differentiation.

Localization

Localization is an essential step in generating a differential diagnosis. Recognizing the site of a lesion is the first step toward ruling in some illnesses and ruling out others. When localization is self-evident, it is advisable to state it anyway as a reminder to the examiners that the obvious was not overlooked. First comes a broader localization division that places the lesion in the

- Central nervous system.
- Peripheral nervous system.
- Both.

Next comes a narrower localization process. For example, in the central nervous system the level could be

- Supratentorial.
- Basal ganglia.
- Brainstem: Intrinsic and extrinsic.
- Cerebellum.
- Spinal cord.
- Motor unit:
    Anterior horn cells.
    Peripheral nerve.
    Neuromuscular junction.
    Muscle.

Categorization

The main categories of neurological disorders are

- Vascular.
- Neoplastic.
- Infectious/inflammatory.
- Toxic/metabolic.
- Degenerative.

    The lesion can also be divided into:

- Focal.
- Multifocal (spatial and/or temporal).

    Finally, the candidate should try to discuss the possible etiology of the case.

Differentiation

What the examiners are looking for is a well-organized and thought-out presentation on differential diagnosis on the case.

A few tips on organizing and presenting data may help

1. Do not rush to an obvious diagnosis; it gives the examiner an impression of lack of depth and critical analysis in your clinical judgment and it exposes you to unnecessary risks of further questioning by the examiners.
2. Be comprehensive in your including diagnosis but also pertinent to the case. In other words, it does not give a good impression to mention a potential diagnosis for which there is no clear-cut support in the symptoms/ signs or history.
3. Characterize the probability of your diagnostic classification in a way that is hierarchically clear. For example, you might want to say "I am considering . . . in the differential diagnosis because of. . . . However, because of,. . . this diagnosis would be less likely.
4. Provide all the supporting information (symptoms/ findings/history/laboratory data) to support your likely diagnosis.
5. When the picture of a probable diagnosis is not clear because of lack of data, mention what is missing, so as to prove that you know what it would take to get there.
6. Provide more details and supporting evidence for your most likely diagnosis.
7. Be prepared to be interrupted with questions. This should in no way be interpreted as negative, and you should be able to resume your discourse where you left off.

Adult Vignette Topics (Varies)

The topics of the adult vignette are those concerning the major categories of neurological disorders. Some very common topics are presented below.

First we will consider the disturbances of cerebrospinal fluid (CSF), normal pressure hydrocephalus (NPH), and pseudotumor cerebri. NPH is characterized by slow progressive gait disorder, impairment of mental functioning, and sphincteric incontinence.

Bening or idiopathic intracranial hypertension (pseudotumor cerebri) is a very popular topic. Diagnosis is made by the clinical presentation of headache and papilledema, elevated CSF pressure (>250 mm Hg) and normal cerebral imaging. Brain tumor and cerebral venous thrombosis in particular must be ruled out.

Cerebrovascular disorders, ischemic and hemorrhagic, thrombotic and embolic, are frequently found; particularly

- Amaurosis fugax (carotid).
- Vertebrobasilar insufficiency.
- Lacunar and large-vessel infarcts.

Middle cerebral artery and basilar artery occlusion, including the special top of the basilar artery are also frequently found.

Within the hemorrhagic disorders, basal ganglia and cerebellar hematoma are essential to recognize.

And last, subarachnoid hemorrhagic and sinus thrombosis need to be considered.

Intracranial neoplasms are the third category. They can be presented in cases of new-onset seizures or signs of increased intracranial pressure. Neoplasms as part of popular vignettes include:

- Acoustic neuroma.
- Pituitary adenoma.
- Tumors of the foramen magnum, etc.

Other popular topics in this category are

- Meningeal carcinomatosis.
- Paraneoplastic syndromes, particularly cerebellar degeneration and Lambert-Eaton myasthenic syndrome (LEMS).

The next category of disorders are the infections. Common topics include

- Viral infections, particularly
  Herpes encephalitis.
  Creutzfeldt-Jacob disease.
  HIV/HTLV myelopathy.
- Bacterial infections
  Tubercular meningitis.
  Lyme disease.
- Parasitic infections, particularly
  Neurocysticercosis

Within the category of traumatic disorders, it is important to keep in mind

- Chronic subdural hematoma.
- Carotid cavernous fistula.

Next comes the toxic/metabolic category, including:

- Complications of alcohol abuse, particularly Wernicke-Korsakoff syndrome and vitamin deficiencies, particularly B_{12}.
- Neuroleptic malignant syndrome, often recurring.

Another category is demyelinating disorders and multiple sclerosis with its various presentations (optic neuritis, transverse myelitis etc.).
Devic's disease should also be considered.
In the category of degenerative disorders, very popular topics are

- Parkinson's disease and parkinsonism, including progressive supranuclear palsy (PSP).
- Dementia, including Pick's disease and normal pressure hydrocephalus.
- Huntington's disease and other choreas.
- Ballism.
- Peripheral nerve disorders with different components are a very important source of vignettes. The topics vary from very simple entrapment neuropathy (medial, radial, peroneal) to brachial and lumbar plexopathies. Within the peripheral nerve disorders, acute and chronic inflammatory demyelinating polyradiculoneuropathy (AIDP and CIDP) are essential parts of very popular vignettes.

Neuromuscular function disorders include

- Myasthenia gravis.

- Lambert-Eaton myasthenic syndrome.
- Botulism.

Muscle disorders, particularly polymiositis, dermatomyositis, and, less likely inclusion body myositis are frequently included.
Motor neuron disease, particularly amyotrophic lateral sclerosis (ALS), is a very important topic and very popular in the Neurology Board Examinatiom.
Next to be considered are the headeache disorders, particularly migraine and clusters headaches, and seizure disorders, particularly temporal lobe and the partial complex seizures and then new-onset seizure secondary to neoplasm.

The Last Ten Minutes

The last 10 minutes of the hour are devoted to clinical cases generated by the examiners. These most likely concern neurological emergencies. Every well-trained neurologist should be able to recognize and treat emergency situations. Obviously, the inability to recognize an emergency, even if you had a previous good performance with the other vignettes, will cause you to fail this part.
Some of the most common emergencies that you need to recognize include

- Cerebellar hemorrage. This is a very important topic and a very popular, recurrent, clinical case presented in the oral Board.
- Myasthenic crisis.
- Neuromuscular disorder causing acute respiratory failure (other than myasthenic crisis).
- Convulsive status epilepticus.
- Acute spinal cord compression.
- Increased intracranial pressure.

Summary of the Most Important Findings in Some Neurological Emergencies

Cerebellar Hemorrhage (see also vignette in cerebrovascular disorders)

Establishing the diagnosis is important because of the potentially serious outcome if not treated and the contrasting surgical treatment. Important clues for the classical presentation include a patient brought to the ER

- Unable to stand or sit.
- Complaining of headache.
- Vertigo and vomiting also present.
- Signs of brainstem compression.

Treatment consists of urgent evacuation through a suboccipital craniectomy. Relief of brainstem compression may be life saving and operative morbidity is low.

Myasthenic Crisis

Typical patients known to have myasthenia develop significant respiratory insufficiency and oropharyingeal muscle weakness requiring mechanical ventilation. Therefore,

- Myasthenic patients with acute shortness of breath and dysphagia are in myasthenic crisis.

Precipitating factors include

- Infections.
- Surgery.
- Medications changes: Initiation or withdrawl of corticosteroids.
- Antibiotics
    Neomycin.
    Kanamycin.
    Gentamycin.
    Tetracycline.
    Colistins.
    Lincomycin.
    Polymyxin.
- Antirheumatic agents.
    D-penicillamine.
    Cloropine.
- Cardiac drugs.
    Procainamide.
    Verapamil.
- Menstrual cycle or pregnancy (especially first trimester).
- Alcohol.
- Emotional stress.

You are expected to know how to manage a myasthenic crisis:

- Assessment of a respiratory function.
    Forced vital capacity.
    Negative respiratory force.
- Intubate if VC < 12–15 ml/kg.
- Remove precipitating factors.
- Plasmapheresis is the best treatment for acute patients (Five exchange treatments of 3–4 liters each over a 1-week period is a typical program).
- If the patient has poor vascular access and there is concern about instituting plasmapheresis with cardiovascular instability, then IVG may be considered.
- Ventilated patients who have not previously been on steroids can be started on high doses of prednisone (60 mg daily).

Cholinergic Crisis

Cholinergic crisis occurs when an excessive amount of acetylcholine is present at the neuromuscular junction, desensitizing the acetylcholine receptors, leading to increasing weakness. These are patients with increased weakness after receiving cholinergic medications.

It can be suspected when the myasthenic patient presents with

- Diarrhea.
- Abdominal cramps.
- Nausea, vomiting, excessive secretions.
- Diaphoresis.
- Fasciculations.
- Weakness.
- Worsening of the weakness with edrophonium.

Treatment is based on withdrawal of anticholinesterase drugs, ventilatory support, plasmapheresis.

Convulsive Status Epilepticus

See vignette in Chapter 12.

The Candidate Without a Clue

The time may come when the examiners ask you a question that you are absolutely certain you cannot answer. This is an extremely unpleasant situation to be in, and a variety of thoughts may crowd your mind. You may feel like you have no option whatsoever. Yet you do, and being prepared for this circumstance may make the difference. Here are some hints:

- Ask for a little time to think about it. Your examiners will understand.
- Quickly make an assessment in your mind about whether this is a make-it or break-it issue. In other words, is this question related to a must in your knowledge. This is important, because if, for example, you have already answered all the questions about treatment of generalized seizures and you are asked about a latest development, you may feel more confident responding that you do not know.
- Even if you assess the essential nature of the topic, you may be better off conceding you do not know when the following circumstances occur:
    1. Trying to guess may make things worse. Examiners do not like candidates "winging it." These are seasoned clinicians who can see through deceitful attempts and will not forgive you for it.
    2. Trying to give an ambiguous or tentative answer may take you down a road you are unfamiliar with, a dangerous way of setting yourself up for further questions you may be unable to answer.

Overall, the strategy should be to minimize the losses in an honest way without giving the appearance of trying to manipulate the process.

In general, the candidate without a clue is usually the unprepared candidate who did not spend enough time in planning and pursuing a good preparation. However, there are exceptions. For example, in pediatric neurology, while reading a vignette, the candidate may feel so unfamiliar with the topic that the candidate may be unable to give an answer or discuss any differential diagnosis.

As indicated in the pediatric vignette part, it is acceptable to read the vignette one time and highlight in your mind the symptoms that may help you formulate a list of possible categories of disorders. Once you identify the category, you can at least provide a list of possible differential diagnoses. For example, when dealing with developmental delay or regression with multisystem involvement, high on your list of categories should be a neurometabolic disorder. Some combinations may also offer you clues. Examples include

Seizure + dementia = gray matter disorders.

Optic atrophy + long tract signs = white matter disorders.

Mental regression, neurological findings, orange skin or mucosa = think of adrenoleukodistrophy.

Seizures + pale patches on the skin + mental retardation = tuberous sclerosis.

Again, don't expect any help, additional information, or sympathy from the examiners.

The Pediatric Vignette

The pediatric vignette represents an entire hour of clinical pediatric cases.

It is anxiety-provoking for the adult neurologist, especially if the candidate did not get enough exposure to pediatric neurology during the residency. Pediatric neurology is different from adult neurology and many adult neurologists are not exposed to pediatric cases during their practice.

As with the adult vignette, the pediatric vignette is a clinical pediatric neurology case open to discussion. The approach is again, read, think, and try to localize. One of the differences between the pediatric vignette and the adult one is that in pediatric neurology they are age-specific, i.e., certain disorders are typical of different age groups.

To an adult neurology candidate, the pediatric vignette can be a great source of apprehension, particularly if the candidate lacks familiarity with pediatric cases or if the candidate had limited exposure to pediatric cases during pediatric neurology rotation. Nevertheless, the importance of this part should not be underestimated, as a passing grade is a requirement for Board certification.

It is important, therefore, that the candidate devote ample time to a comprehensive preparation based on sufficient knowledge of pediatric neurology topics as well as case-based practice. In this section, we will review the main categories of disorders in pediatric neurology, so that when you are presented with a case vignette you will be able to categorize it and formulate the most likely diagnosis. It is worth mentioning again that, by and large, candidates are not expected to make the right diagnosis, rather to identify the category of the disorder, its temporal profile, and age group.

Localization in pediatric cases may not be as clear as in adult ones. Nonetheless, the candidate needs to make an effort to localize the lesion. The examiners are aware that the adult neurology candidate is generally less adept with pediatric cases. However, that should not deceive candidates about the examiners' criteria for passing, which are based on the expectation of a basic knowledge of diagnostic and therapeutic issues in pediatric neurology.

The cases themselves tend to present basic diagnostic and therapeutic dilemmas, shying away from more complicated ones. Concerning suggesting ordering diagnostic tests or entertaining therapeutic options, it is generally advisable to maintain a cautious stance to avoid putting oneself into situations which may be difficult to resolve. One example would be to be sure to mention the necessity of performing a computed tomography (CT) scan of the head prior to proceeding to a lumbar puncture. Diagnostic and therapeutic issues raised should cover all the basic questions raised in the case. Finally, though the content of the case will by its very nature differ from the adult vignette case, its format is very similar. Therefore, the principles outlined for the adult vignette apply for the pediatric vignette. As mentioned previously, the candidate is expected to read, mentally highlight the most important findings, localize, categorize, differentiate, and reach a reasonable diagnosis.

Age Categories

In pediatric neurology there are several distinct age groups that the candidate will need to keep in mind when approaching the case. These are

- Newborn (including the first month to six weeks of life).
- Infantile.
- Early (up to the end of the first year).
- Late (from the second year to school age).
- Childhood (up to 10 years).
- Adolescence.

In each age category there are certain types of clinical presentations that help in the process of determining what diseases should be considered in the differential diagnosis.

4
How to Prepare for the Exam

The Board certification is an essential part of every neurologist's credit, particularly in view of the HMO and insurance companies' requirements.

From the standpoint of preparation, this exam is not different from any other exam, as your chances of passing will be much greater if you have done your homework in a thoughtful and reasonably organized fashion. Conversely, presenting yourself after a hurried and haphazard preparation sets the stage for a painful failure. Time after time, when candidates look back on what they could have done better, appropriate preparation is one of the most frequently mentioned responses. A good training and consistent studying throughout the residency do not guarantee you success either, considering all the variables that play a role in a positive outcome of the test.

While nobody has the magic formula for the Board preparation, a few steps and strategies have been known to be of use. But before we address them, we will briefly discuss getting information on the test from your colleagues who have already taken it. This is by all accounts a natural thing to do given the importance of the exam, the yearning for information to supplement what the Board gives and the mystique that the exam has acquired over the years as a terrifying rite of passage that has shattered countless reputations and self-esteem. Other than slightly and temporarily decreasing your anxiety about the test, however, the information you get from your colleagues may be less than useful, if not confusing, at times. This is due to a variety of reasons, such as:

1. The colleague giving you a distorted account of his or her perception of the exam or rationalizations for a poor performance.
2. The colleague may be reluctant to share much information and only provide conflicting and unhelpful bits and pieces of the experience. It is not unusual for people to hide having failed the Board once or more.
3. Every exam has a life of its own and it is hard to generalize.

4. Multiple variables, such as anxiety and poor preparation, may have contributed to the candidate's negative experience of the process.
5. Some of the stories you hear may have no factual basis at all (such as tales on where the exam is easier).

Thus, our advice is to take whatever your colleagues say about the Board with a grain of salt so that it will not influence your performance negatively, and focus on advice that can help build your preparation realistically.

As for when you should take this exam, the answer is simple: As soon as possible.

You should apply for the oral part as soon as you hear about the positive outcome of part 1. Waiting or procrastinating will only decrease your chances of getting to the exam optimally prepared, as it would further take you away from your residency, thus decreasing the impact of a good training on your preparedness. On the other hand, major events in one's life may distract from preparation and it would be counterproductive for you to present yourself for the exam with only limited preparation. This is a difficult decision as one has to balance one's assessed preparation against the risk of getting seriously burned after a resounding failure. If you have been out of the residency for a few years, your preparation might take a longer time and require a longer practice. This book is intended to help this group especially, since it may be problematic for these candidates to obtain accurate information.

Some of the tools candidates have used to prepare for the exam are discussed below.

Courses

Basically there are two types of courses:

1. The first type is a review of material in a lecture format with few hints about the oral part. Therefore, these courses are more geared toward the part 1 of the exam.

2. The second type tries to simulate the three sections of the oral Board, providing suggestions on presentation, preparation, and how to approach the different parts.

The ABPN does not recommend or recognize any preparation courses. There are, indeed, very few available and they have received mixed reviews from candidates as they are known to be expensive and not live up to expectations. Some candidates enthusiastically praise a course because it may contribute to lessening their anxiety about the exam itself. Here is what one candidate stated about a course he took:

> The course was very expensive and did not help my preparation. I was able to get a few hints about what the oral boards would be about. However I became gradually discouraged by hearing some stories of exams by other candidates. One disappointing aspect of the course was the pediatric part. It was poorly structured and the teachers seemed poorly informed about this section and did not seem to have significant information about it. In the end I passed this part, but I am unsure about how much of my passing was do to instructions I got from my taking the course.

This is only one opinion. So, our suggestion is, before you embark on a major expenditure of money, energy, and time, you should consider other methods of preparation, such as books and practice.

Books

By and large, what you are going to need is one book of general neurology, one book of differential diagnosis, one of treatment, and one of pediatric neurology. The best way to bring yourself up to date on the latest news in the field is by poring over the major neurology journals issued over the past three to four years. This is the best way to fill the gap in recent knowledge that most textbooks suffer from.

This is particularly valid for certain issues regarding treatment, such as

- Therapy of multiple sclerosis.
- Therapy of epilepsy with the new anticonvulsants and new treatment options, such as vagus nerve stimulation and surgical intervention.
- Therapy of Parkinson's disease.
- Headache treatment.
- Stroke therapy.

Below are some titles of books that can help in your preparation. Our suggestions do not mean that these book are necessary or sufficient to pass the test.

- Victor and Adams, *Textbook of Neurology.*
- J. Biller, *Practical Neurology.*
- G.M. Fenichel, *Clinical Pediatric Neurology: A Sign and Symptom Approach.*

- R.T. Johnson and J.W. Griffin, *Current Therapy in Neurologic Disease.*
- Some good review journals: *Seminars in neurology, Continuum,* etc.

In addition, many candidates find very helpful the courses on CD ROM by the American Academy of Neurology on the most recent meetings, where the most recent diagnostic and therapeutic options are presented.

The time spent on the review books is subjective, depending on your work and training schedule. Some candidates prefer to wait for the results of part 1 before committing to a new experience of studying for part 2. There are usually 45 days or more between knowing the results of part 1 and the part 2 exam. Therefore, if you know how to prepare and what your weak points are, it will save you a great deal of time.

Definitely, a large portion of this time needs to be spent on the pediatric neurology preparation.

Again the ABPN does not suggest any specific book.

Having passed part 1, candidates have already reviewed a great deal of clinical and theoretical material.

Practice

Practice is an excellent way to lessen your anxiety about the exam and to learn what your deficiencies are. Some residency training programs offer sessions that simulate the oral Board examination but often you will have to take the initiative and ask colleagues or teachers to be your examiner.

For the live patient examination, you can practice at the bedside or in your office on different neurological cases, timing yourself so that in 30 minutes you have completed a good history and neurological evaluation.

If you are fortunate, you will have a colleague or teacher supervising you on your history taking, neurological examination, summary, and differential diagnosis. The advantage in this case is to have someone who can give you feedback on your performance, highlighting weaknesses and strengths. If alone, practice standing in front of imaginary examiners while you present the case, keeping in mind the most important points related to history and neurological exam.

Practice at least once every day. If you do not have a patient, practice on a friend or family member while you become accustomed to the 30-minute time frame, which, over time, will become automatic.

Practice is an excellent way to lessen your anxiety about the exam and to learn where your deficiencies are. Some programs offer sessions for their residents but most often you will have to take the initiative and ask someone to be your examiner. By and large, a few general principles apply to planning for a productive session:

1. Select well-prepared examiners who might have taught courses on the topic or might be well known for interviewing and diagnostic skills. It also helps to be examined by colleagues who have recently passed the exam.

2. Unless you know they will be impartial, you should avoid selecting previous supervisors whom you know well and who have a tendency to be overly supportive.

3. You examiner should be someone who is completely free to highlight the areas you need to work on, without neglecting to mention the areas in which you demonstrated good preparation. Possibly, it should be someone you don't know very well.

4. Ask your examiner to elaborate on weaknesses and to offer suggestions on technique.

5. Do as many practicing sessions as possible, each time trying to work on the weaknesses your examiner addressed the previous time.

6. In addition to live patient examinations, you should do some dry runs with vignettes. Ask your colleagues to provide some vignettes or use some of the vignettes in this book.

7. It is important to choose patients and vignettes with a wide range of neurological problems so that you can be ready to deal with a variety of clinical and therapeutic situations.

5
Reasons for Failing

Understanding the reasons why candidates fail is an excellent way of recognizing and avoiding the most common pitfalls and traps. In interviews over the years, we gathered considerable insight into this important area. Some of the reasons are more obvious, while others are based on a global judgment by the examiners. By the same token, some candidates know they have failed as they walk out of the door, recognizing some fundamental flaw of their interview/test, while others are blissfully unaware of where they went wrong only to be dumbfounded when the notice comes in. In the event of a failing grade, the ABPN allows the candidate to request an explanation of reason for the failure determination, for a fee of $100, but not many who made such requests feel they received a satisfactory answer.

A Candidate's Story

Dr. CM volunteered to recount her failure to pass part 2.

I had had a good training and I felt I had kept up to date on the literature throughout the residency. I had spoken to some people who had passed them but did not find their suggestions very helpful. I felt I was as ready as I could ever be. Still I was very apprehensive about it. So, in spite of all my attempts the night before the test I had little if any sleep at all. My exam started at 8:30 AM with the pediatric session. Perhaps because of some Inderal I took before, I felt confident and relaxed, in control. I calmly went through the pediatric vignettes and I was able to discuss each case pointedly and comprehensively. Although I was told not to rely on the examiners' responses to my discussions, I couldn't help but notice what I interpreted as signs of approval. I walked out of the room thinking I had passed that part.

The next test, the live patient was scheduled for 1 PM in another hospital. I spent the four hours waiting for the time pacing around nervously. The patient was an easy case of radiculopathy. I did not feel pressured by the examiner and felt I had covered all the basics. I did not know the answers

to all the questions, but I felt that I had a good shot at passing.

The adult vignette was scheduled at 4 PM at yet another hospital. After four more hours of pacing, I was feeling tired and somewhat emotionally drained. I couldn't wait for the day to be over. From the outset, I felt the test was not going well. I felt intimidated by the examiners and thought my answers were not hitting the mark. I had the distinct perception from their nonverbal communication that they did not like my performance. I think I reached the bottom when the examiners were not satisfied with my answer on the localization of the lesion and although I had tried several answers they kept on asking me "Where, where?" After that I was very demoralized. I saw one of them leaving the room. I thought he did so because I had failed. The end of the exam came as a liberation. But for weeks after I obsessed about that third test, alternately blaming myself and my examiners for my dismal performance.

The candidate in this example failed the adult vignette and waited one year to repeat that single part.

This personal account can teach a few points:

1. Be prepared for a long day, although you may be luckier than the above candidate. During waits, do something to relax and take your mind off the exam, or else you will be physically and emotionally spent before the end of the exam.
2. Avoid scanning the examiners for signs. If you feel that the examiners are tough, continue doing what you know without losing it, getting anxious, or depressed. It will not help you.
3. Every exam has a story and a course of its own. You may be prepared, but you need to be flexible and ready to respond to unforeseen challenges.

Reasons for failing are a very important issue. In general, the examiners tend to be fair and impartial and to have solid and justified reasons for failing a candidate. Some of the reasons for failing are described below.

The Safety Factor

Perhaps a fundamental criterion used by the examiners in making a final decision is the determination of potential dangerousness to the patient. This domain can be divided into two categories:

1. Making dangerous decisions.
2. Not recognizing neurological emergencies.

A dangerous decision is a decision that can be life threatening for the patient. It can involve a dangerous diagnostic or therapeutic decision.

Here are some examples of dangerous diagnostic decisions:

- Performing a lumbar puncture in a patient with papilledema and focal signs because it may cause the risk of herniation (example, brain abscess).
- Not recognizing signs of impending spinal cord compression.
- Not recognizing impending myasthenic crisis or the difference between myasthenic and cholinergic crises.
- Not recognizing an acute cerebellar hemorrhage.
- Performing a Tensilon test without being in a special setting (Emergency Room) or without the necessary precaution (atropine sulfate has to be available due to the rare possibility of bradycardia).

Examples of dangerous therapeutic decisions include

- Giving the incorrect dose of medications to a child in status epilepticus.
- Lack of knowledge on how to treat status epilepticus.
- Giving the wrong dose of edrophonium chloride.

Obviously, not recognizing neurological life-threatening emergencies or being unable to intervene with the right treatment is as important as making unsafe decisions for the treatment of the patient.

The Information Factor

Another major factor in determination of failure is the information factor. An adequate fund of knowledge in clinical neurology is an essential prerequisite for taking and passing this exam.

The Board examination requires a deep and careful preparation which may require several months. This preparation is based on books and practice. All the major categories of neurological disorders need to be refreshed including diagnostic approach and treatment. Lack of information is a very essential reason for failing. This is particularly true for certain areas such as the pediatric part when the adult neurologist is involved. Pediatric neurology must not be underestimated, particularly because many disorders are different from the ones found in the adult population and have a different treatment.

The Differential Diagnosis Factor

During the live patient examination as well as the vignette, it is imperative to arrive at a sound differential diagnosis.

The perfect diagnosis is less important than a a comprehensive, pertinent, and well-thought-out differential diagnosis that takes into consideration all the symptoms and signs elicited in the test. You should be able to support every possible diagnosis with the appropriate findings as well as enumerate some of the diagnoses that are less likely and reasons why.

Localization of the Lesion

It is helpful to first place the signs and symptoms you have elicited though your interview into broad anatomical areas such as supratentorial, posterior fossa, spinal canal or vertebral column, peripheral neuromuscular system, or at several levels. Once the broad anatomical area is identified, a more narrow, focal and side localization may be hypothesized. Examples include focal on the right or left side of the nervous system, or focal in the midline area involving both areas of the nervous system. Obviously, the level of the lesion may also be characterized as nonfocal and diffuse. A question that needs to be answered is also the likely etiology of the lesion, i.e., inflammatory, vascular, neoplastic, traumatic, congenital, degenerative, or metabolic.

Determining the Temporal Factor

An essential element in the assessment of neurological signs and symptoms, as well as in the formulation of a differential diagnosis, is the temporal factor. Was the onset of the signs/symptoms acute, subacute, or chronic? Was the course/progression of the symptoms progressive or stepwise or chronic?

Poor Planning and Treatment

In dealing with treatment issues, there are therapies with which you need to be very familiar. This part can be a reason for failing, particularly if you do not know how to treat major illnessess such as status epilepticus or myasthenia gravis.

There is a difference between not remembering the latest medication for migraine headache treatment vs. the right management of acute cord compressions. It is also better to be honest than to give the wrong numbers.

The candidate is expected to know the best diagnostic procedures for the case as well as treatment options.

The Variability Factor

If you are well prepared and ready to appropriately react to unforeseen situations, you are likely to pass. Candidates who fail once or more than once often talk about a wide range of examiners, going from the toughest to the easiest.

Dr. MC failed the test the first time and passed the second. Here is an account of his experience.

> There was a huge difference between the examiners on my first exam and the second one. The first exam, the examiners seemed to react negatively to everything I said. I know they are trained not to react but I could tell. They asked me a lot of details which may or may not have been of consequence. I also felt I was interrupted too many times.
>
> The second time it was like night and day. They seemed to nod, never stopped me, and shook my hand like they meant it as I left. I knew I had passed.

While there could be a degree of variability in human nature, there is limited value in fixating yourself on how supposedly supportive the examiners are. The best idea is not to let your perception of the examiners influence your performance as it could cost you the exam. Just stay the course and do what you have trained for three years to do.

Part 2

6
Peripheral Nervous System Disorders

Motor Neuron Disease

Amyotrophic Lateral Sclerosis

Vignette

A 63-year-old TV producer started complaining of difficulty turning the car ignition key and twisting off jar caps with his right hand for six months. His general practitioner thought he had carpal tunnel syndrome, but also noticed wasting in the dorsum of his right hand. Two months later the patient was unable to take his customary one-hour walk because of fatigue and muscular tightness and stiffness. He had no prior medical problems and used to exercise frequently. The neurological examination showed weakness of the small right hand muscles and wrist extensor muscles. Hoffman's sign was present. In his lower extremity, he had great difficulty dorsiflexing his right ankle. There was wasting between the first two metacarpal bones on the right. The right toe was extensor. The left toe was equivocal.

Summary A 63-year-old man with progressive weakness, without sensory complaints. The clinical history and neurological examination help localize the lesion. The initial task is to determine whether the patient's weakness is caused by upper motor neuron dysfunction, characterized by increased deep tendon reflexes, increased tone, slowed rapid movements, and Babinski's sign, or by a lower motor neuron dysfunction, characterized by atrophy, decreased or loss of reflexes, and fasciculations. In
the vignette, we have signs of both upper and lower motor neuron involvement. Upper motor neuron signs include the following:

- Slowness, loss of dexterity.
- Weakness of antigravity muscles.
- Hoffman's sign (which consists of flexion and adduction of the thumb accompanied by flexion of the index and sometimes the other fingers after snapping the nail of the patient's middle finger).
- Leg stiffness (spasticity).
- Babinski's sign.

Lower motor neuron signs include wasting of the dorsum of the hand. It is important to notice that there are no sensory, sphincteric, or autonomic disturbances.

Localization

Upper and lower motor neurons.

   The first entity to be considered is a disease that involves both upper and lower motor neurons, specifically the anterior horn cells and the corticospinal tract. This disorder, amyotrophic lateral sclerosis (ALS), could explain the clinical findings described in the vignette. ALS is considered the most common form of motor neuron disease of undetermined cause in adults (Belsh and Schiffman).

   Spinal cord dysfunction needs great consideration in the differential diagnosis, particularly cervical spondylosis with associated myelopathy and radiculopathy. This disorder may manifest with signs of upper and lower motor neuron involvement, sometimes without apparent sensory symptoms. It is important to always rule out cervical cord dysfunction because it is a treatable disorder and does not carry the poor prognosis of ALS. Clinical findings that may suggest cervical spondylosis include the presence of pain localized in the neck or in a radicular distribution, the signs of upper motor neuron dysfunction with hyperreflexia below the level of compression, hyporeflexia at the level of the anatomical lesion, sensory findings such as paresthesias distributed along the nerve root, absence of widespread involvement including bulbar and respiratory system, and bladder or bowel dysfunction in some cases of cervical spondylotic myelopathy but never observed in ALS.

In the differential diagnosis, structural abnormalities such as spinal cord tumors, arteriovenous malformations, foramen magnum tumors, and syringomyelia need to be considered because they can manifest with signs of upper and lower motor neuron dysfunction.

Tumors of the spinal cord can simulate a progressive myelopathy or have a combination of signs of spinal cord compression and radicular symptoms. Extradural lesions cause early root symptoms of pain and paresthesias and usually a late involvement of the bladder. Intrinsic tumors, such as astrocytomas, ependymomas, and so on, produce motor dysfunction but also sensory abnormalities such as dissociate anesthesia and early bladder dysfunction. Dural arteriovenous malformation or fistula can also present with signs of upper and lower motor neuron dysfunction and need to be differentiated from ALS, but involvement of the sphincters and sensory abnormalities also occur.

Tumors of the foramen magnum can sometimes simulate ALS because they can present with signs of upper and lower motor neuron dysfunction and cranial nerve abnormalities causing dysphagia and dysartria but other important clinical features are prominent—occipital or posterior cervical pain, headache, paresthesias, dysfunction of the accessory nerve with weakness of the sternomastoid and trapezius muscles, and so on.

Syringomyelia that enters the differential diagnosis of upper and lower motor neuron involvement is associated with prominent sensory symptoms, such as dissociated sensory loss and neck pain, not present in the vignette.

With regard to disorders of peripheral nerves, multifocal motor neuropathy with conduction block needs to be carefully considered because of the possibility of treatment and more favorable prognosis compared with ALS. Multifocal motor neuropathy is a demyelinating disorder characterized by progressive asymmetrical weakness, atrophy, fasciculations, and cramps, without sensory involvement. It can also be excluded, because in this condition there are no signs of upper motor neuron involvement, and weakness and atrophy typically are in the distribution of individual peripheral nerves rather than the spinal segmental root distribution observed in ALS. Conduction block, which is defined as a decrease in amplitude or area of the compound muscle action potential

with proximal as compared with distal stimulation, is the hallmark of this disorder.

Disorders of the neuromuscular junction can be easily excluded. Myasthenia gravis characterized by fatigable weakness frequently involving the extraocular muscles does not include upper motor neuron signs or fasciculations. Lambert-Eaton myasthenic syndrome can occasionally simulate the progressive muscular atrophy variant of ALS. Muscle disorders such as polymyositis with the typical findings of progressive, predominantly proxymal, weakness usually associated with myalgia and without any upper motor neuron signs can be also easily excluded from the vignette.

Other entities that need to be mentioned for completion, but can be excluded by the vignette, are:

- Motor disorders associated with paraproteinemia, such as the peripheral neuropathy seen with osteosclerotic myeloma, usually manifest with signs of lower motor neuron involvement and may occasionally simulate progressive muscular atrophy. Upper motor neuron signs are never present.
- Polyglucosan body disease or type IV glycogenosis due to branching enzyme deficiency can manifest in adults with upper and lower motor neuron signs in an asymmetric distribution but other important features are sensory loss, neurogenic bladder, cerebellar ataxia, and dementia.
- The adult variant of hexosaminidase A enzyme deficiency can manifest with weakness and cramps in combination with cerebellar and extrapyramidal signs and cognitive impairment.
- Endocrine disorders, such as hyperparathyroidism and thyrotoxicosis, enter the differential diagnosis as well as tumors, such as lymphoma.

Progressive Muscular Atrophy

Vignette

A 70-year-old retired handyman complained for the last eight months that he has had difficulty buttoning his shirt, picking up small objects or turning the door's knob. He also developed neck stiffness and was treated by a physical therapist for several months without significant improvement. For the last four months he had experienced a tendency to fall, with difficulty getting back on his feet and mild right leg cramps. Thereafter, he began to experience several muscular twitches in his neck and arms and difficulty taking a deep breath. He had a 10-year history of diabetes treated with several oral agents. He stopped smoking seven years ago. The neurological examination showed that he had difficulty lift-

ing his arms above the shoulder and could be easily overcome. He could not spread his fingers apart. He had wasting of the muscles of the distal forearms and of the intrinsic hand muscles. There was moderate weakness of the right leg and wasting. DTRs were (⅕) in the upper extremities and trace in the lower, with an absent ankle jerk bilaterally. Vibration was decreased at both ankles.

Summary A 70-year-old man with progressive weakness of the upper and lower extremities, decreased reflexes, atrophy, fasciculations, and no significant sensory disturbances. (The decreased vibration at both ankles can be age-related.) He has a history of diabetes for 10 years.

Localization

The signs and symptoms of the vignette localize to the lower motor unit. It is important to differentiate which part of the motor unit is involved:

- Anterior horn cell.
- Nerve root.
- Peripheral nerve.
- Neuromuscular junction.
- Muscle fiber.

Disorders of the Anterior Horn Cells

Anterior horn cell disease causes involvement of motor neurons at multiple levels of the spinal cord. Different disorders can be identified in this category:

- Progressive muscular atrophy (PMA): ALS variant.
- Spinal muscular atrophy.
- Post-polio syndrome.
- Motor neuron syndrome associated with the remote effects of cancer.
- Adult-onset hexosaminidase A deficiency.

Progressive muscular atrophy is considered a variant of ALS with no signs of upper motor neuron involvement. It is characterized by progressive weakness and atrophy in an asymmetrical distribution, fatigue, muscle cramps, and fasciculations, affecting preferentially males and rarely with bulbar signs.

Many patients presenting with lower motor neuron dysfunction may later show signs of upper motor neuron involvement. The diagnosis of PMA is highly suggestive of the vignette where only lower motor neuron signs are demonstrated. The occurrence of lower motor neuron dysfunction in the absence of upper motor neuron signs may also indicate the possibility of an inherited motor neuron disorder such as adult-onset spinal muscular atrophy.

The adult-onset SMA is characterized by symmetrical, predominantly proximal muscle weakness and atrophy

with onset in the second or third decade of life and showing slow progression of symptoms. The clinical characteristics and absent family history clearly exclude this entity from the vignette.

Post-polio progressive muscular atrophy is responsible for fatigue, muscle pain, progressive asymmetrical weakness and atrophy, particularly in muscles previously affected by poliomyelitis.

Hexosaminidase A deficiency can have a motor-neuron-disease type of presentation with weakness, cramps, fasciculations, and hyporeflexia, but patients are usually younger, in the second or third decade of life. Other characteristics may include signs of cerebellar dysfunction, postural and action tremors, cognitive impairment, and laboratory abnormality showing a severe hexosaminidase A deficiency in serum or leukocytes.

Finally, motor neuron disease can be associated with remote effects of cancer, in particular, a lymphoproliferative disease. According to Dumitru et al., the most frequently associated lymphoproliferative disorders are Hodgkin's disease and non-Hodgkin's lymphoma.

Disorders of the Nerve Root

In a patient presenting with progressive weakness and atrophy, the possibility of cervical and lumbosacral radiculopathy needs to be considered. Radiculopathy, which can involve multiple roots, is usually characterized by sensory disturbances such as pain and paresthesias that may follow a radicular distribution, often with paraspinal muscle spasm and some motor weakness or reflex loss. In the above vignette, the patient presented with progressive muscle weakness and wasting, without sensory symptoms, which make the diagnosis of multiple radiculopathies an unlikely possibility. Plexus dysfunction that is usually caused by trauma, neoplasm, and radiation therapy usually presents with acute or subacute onset of motor paralysis and sensory loss.

Disease of the Peripheral Nerve

Among the pure motor neuropathies, multifocal motor neuropathy (MMN), which is a demyelinating disorder characterized by progressive asymmetrical distal weakness in combination with varying degrees of atrophy, cramps, and fasciculations, and without sensory symptoms, is an important consideration in the differential diagnosis of PMA. Multifocal motor neuropathy is a slowly progressive, potentially treatable disorder in which the asymmetrical weakness typically follows the distribution of individual peripheral nerves rather than the myotomal pattern of ALS. Bulbar involvement is rarely seen and there are no signs of upper motor neuron dysfunction. Important laboratory findings include the detection of antiGM1 antibodies in the serum and the electrophysiological evidence of conduction block in multiple upper and lower extremity nerves.

Diseases of the Neuromuscular Junction

Lambert-Eaton myasthenic syndrome in particular can occasionally simulate the lower motor neuron variant of ALS. LEMS, characterized by proximal muscle weakness that tends to improve after a brief period of contraction, does not include muscle fasciculations or prominent atrophy. Autonomic dysfunction (dry mouth, impotence, constipation, and so on) are important features of LEMS.

Diseases of the Muscle

The clinical characteristics of the muscle disorders polymiositis and dermatomyositis are not features of the vignette. Inclusion body myositis can sometimes enter the differential diagnosis of PMA. This disorder manifests in elderly patients with asymmetrical distal weakness and atrophy, particularly involving the wrist/finger flexor muscles associated with hyporeflexia. There are no fasciculations, and upper motor neuron signs are never seen.

Bulbar Palsy

Vignette

A 70-year-old female housekeeper and amateur singer started to notice some slurring of speech when singing during the past three months. Two months later she also began having difficulty drinking fluids often accompanied by coughing and the feeling that the fluid was stuck in her throat. On examination, she had mild dysartria, mild bilateral facial weakness, a positive snout reflex, and hyperactive jaw jerk. There was full strength in the limbs with symmetrical deep tendon reflexes and no evidence of atrophy. When reexamined one year later, dysartria and dysphagia had worsened. Deep tendon reflexes were hyperactive and fasciculations were noted in the shoulder girdle muscles.

Summary The vignette can be summarized as progressive bulbar dysfunction.

Localization

Multiple localization can be responsible for progressive bulbar palsy. Disorders to be considered are discussed below.

Cerebral Disorders

Patients with hypertension and multiinfarct dementia of vascular origin can present with pseudobulbar palsy caus-

ing dysphagia, dysartria, and emotional incontinence due to damage to the corticobulbar tracts. In the vignette there is no indication of any risk factor for stroke, and the evolution with the appearance of fasciculations indicates involvement of the lower motor neuron.

Structural brainstem abnormalities, either vascular or neoplastic, can manifest with signs of bulbar dysfunction but typically have other accompanying findings such as diplopia, gaze paralysis, nystagmus, cerebellar ataxia, dysmetria, dysarthria, and sensory involvement.

Syringobulbia can also present with signs of bulbar dysfunction such as dysphagia, dysarthria, and tongue atrophy, but other features include nystagmus, sensory loss involving the face, and so on.

Disorders of the Anterior Horn Cells

Anterior horn cell disease or ALS with bulbar onset followed by more widespread involvement can explain the symptoms described in the vignette. Abnormality of speech (dysarthria and dysphonia) due to UPM, LMN, or both, are the most common initial symptoms of bulbar muscle weakness in the ALS patient (Belsh and Schiffman). Dysphagia particularly for liquids is another characteristic finding as well as facial weakness. The examination usually discovers tongue atrophy and weakness of the soft palate. Eye movements are never involved. Patients initially presenting with the bulbar form eventually tend to manifest signs of widespread involvement typical of ALS.

Disorders of Peripheral Nerves

Among the neuropathies, in particular diphtheria can cause bulbar symptoms but usually in association with other typical findings such as blurry vision due to accommodation defect, distal paresthesias, and sensory loss.

Disorders of the Neuromuscular Junction

Myasthenia gravis (MG) can present with bulbar dysfunction as an initial symptom in 20 to 30 percent of the cases (Belsh and Schiffman). Typically, fatigable weakness is the hallmark of the disorder. Fasciculations and hyperreflexia are not signs of this disorder, but visual abnormalities, in particular diplopia, ptosis, and ophthalmoplegia, are characteristic findings of MG, as opposed to ALS.

Disorders of Muscle

Polymiositis and dermatomyositis can cause dysphagia, but are usually easily diagnosed and excluded by the vignette. Oculopharyngeal dystrophy can rarely be confused with the progressive bulbar palsy of ALS because the former is a hereditary disorder characterized by slowly progressive ptosis and dysphagia.

Kennedy's Syndrome

Vignette

A 56-year-old teacher had complained of mild difficulty swallowing and speech problems for the last five years. He had a long history of weakness, more marked in his legs, cramps, and twitching. His older brother had marked facial twitching and muscle cramps. On physical examination there was marked gynecomastia and muscle weakness more severe in a limb-girdle distribution. Prominent fasciculations were noted in the perioral facial muscles and the tongue with marked tongue atrophy."

Summary A 56-year-old man with progressive dysphagia and dysarthria, and a prior history of proximal upper extremity weakness and prominent fasciculations, particularly in the perioral area and the tongue associated with tongue atrophy. His older brother had facial fasciculations and muscle cramps.

Localization

There is clinical involvement of the lower motor neuron without upper motor neuron signs. Among the disorders of the motor unit, diseases affecting the motor neuron are considered first. Also, the slow progression of the disorder and the indication of an older brother with perioral twitching and cramps points to an inherited disorder. The disorders to be considered are

- Adult-onset spinal muscular atrophy.
- X-linked bulbospinal neuronopathy (Kennedy's syndrome).

Adult-onset spinal muscular atrophy, characterized by slowly progressive proximal muscle weakness and atrophy with onset in the third or fourth decade of life, can be excluded because bulbar involvement is unusual. X-linked bulbospinal neuronopathy or Kennedy's syndrome is an X-linked recessive disorder that affects males in the fourth and fifth decade of life and is characterized by progressive spinal muscular atrophy in a limb-girdle distribution, cramps, fasciculations, and typically facial and perioral fasciculations. Mild dysarthria and dysphagia are also present and there is no respiratory dysfunction. Several systemic clinical features include gynecomastia, diabetes, and testicular atrophy.

Laboratory findings that help confirm the diagnosis are

- Increased serum levels of creatine kinase (CK) and estrogen.
- Electrodiagnostic findings indicative of chronic denervation and sensory neuropathy.

- Genetic studies showing an expansion of the CAG repeat sequence(cytosine-adenine-guanine) in the androgen receptor gene.

Kennedy's syndrome has clinical features that help in making a distinction from ALS. In particular, the course of the disorder is slowly progressive with predominant involvement of the proximal muscles and mild bulbar findings in the absence of upper motor neuron involvement. A mild sensory polyneuropathy is usually present.

Diagnostic Tests That Help in Making the Diagnosis of Motor Neuron Disease

Neuroimaging studies are indicated in order to rule out structural pathology, particularly in cases of bulbar onset ALS, but also in order to exclude myelopathy or multiple radiculopathies. Electrodiagnostic tests are very important in confirming the diagnosis of motor neuron disease. Sensory nerve conduction studies are normal and motor nerve conduction studies can demonstrate normal findings, decreased amplitude, or decreased velocity related to the loss of faster conducting axons. It is important to perform an extensive study in order to demonstrate the possibility of conduction block or significant compound muscle action potential (CMAP) temporal dispersion, which are indicative of demyelination. Multifocal motor neuropathy with electrophysiologic evidence of conduction block can sometimes simulate ALS but is potentially treatable and carries a better prognosis.

The needle electromyogram (EMG) examination in ALS may reveal active denervation and reinnervation in widespread distribution that is unexplained by multiple mononeuropathies or radiculopathies (Preston and Shapiro).

Clinical laboratory studies are often obtained and include routine testing such as complete blood count, electrolytes, CK, serum VDRL, thyroid function tests, serum protein electrophoresis and antineural antigen testing (GMI, asialo-GMI). Special studies such as CSF, leukocyte hexosaminindase A assay, or test for cytosine-adenine-guanine repeat in androgen receptor gene (X chromosome) are reserved for selected cases.

Clinical Features and Diagnosis

ALS is the most common form of MND in adults with an incidence of 2 per 100,000 (Bromberg). Patients manifest symptoms related to dysfunction of the anterior horn cells and corticospinal tract. Progressive muscular atrophy, which is considered a variant of ALS and demonstrates only signs of lower motor neuron (LMN) involvement, is more common in men, and has a slower rate of progression.

Primary lateral sclerosis on the other hand only shows upper motor neuron (UMN) findings and like PMA carries a better prognosis with a slower progression. Patients who present with LMN or UMN signs only at onset and later develop ALS are considered to have LMN- or UMN-onset ALS.

Progressive bulbar palsy manifests with signs of bulbar dysfunction, particularly dysarthria and dysphagia, due to UMN or LMN dysfunction or both. This form may eventually progress to the more widespread ALS.

The El Escorial criteria for the diagnosis of ALS established a combination of upper and lower motor neuron signs and spread or progression of signs and symptoms within a body region and between regions over time. The four body regions established in the diagnosis of ALS are bulbar, cervical, thoracic, and lumbosacral. The diagnosis of definite ALS requires UMN and LMN signs present in the bulbar and at least two other spinal regions, or upper and lower motor neuron signs present in three spinal regions.

Limbs are the initial site of involvement in approximately 78 percent of patients and weakness present in an asymmetric pattern in approximately 60 percent of these patients (Bromberg). There can also be an onset with bulbar signs particularly dysartria and dysphagia.

Signs of upper motor neuron dysfunction include weakness, loss of dexterity, increased deep tendon reflexes, spasticity, Hoffman's sign, extensor plantar responses, clonus, pathologic spread, exaggerated jaw jerk and gag reflex, snout reflex, and emotional lability. Lower motor neuron signs include weakness, atrophy, fasciculations, and muscle cramps. Bulbar signs are represented by dysphagia, dysarthria, tongue atrophy, and weakness of the soft palate. Respiratory dysfunction due to weakness of the respiratory muscles may cause dyspnea related to exertion or at rest.

Etiology

The cause of these motor neuron diseases is unknown. However, possibilities include:

- Exogenous excitotoxins.
- Glutamate toxicity.
- Autoimmune hypothesis.
- Viral etiology.

Hereditary disorders include familial ALS and Kennedy's syndrome.

Peripheral Neuropathies

Guillain-Barré Syndrome (GBS)

Vignette

A 60-year-old businessman was in good health until three days earlier when he started to complain of a dull aching pain in his lower back and intermittent numbness of the soles of his feet. The day after the initial symptoms, he experienced increasing difficulty carrying his bags. One day he felt that his legs were heavy and his gait unsteady. He also noticed right facial numbness and difficulty eating and speaking. He had recently returned from a five-day business trip to Africa where he experienced some intestinal problems and a few bouts of diarrhea. He was a heavy smoker and had hypertension for two years and diabetes for 15 years. On examination he was alert and oriented with intact speech, memory, and calculation. Visual fields, optic disk and extraocular muscles were normal. There was right facial weakness and moderate weakness of neck flexion. He could barely elevate his arm from the horizontal position and his hand grip was very weak. He was unable to lift his legs against resistance and could not stand without support. Deep tendon reflexes could not be elicited, even with reinforcement.

Summary A 60-year-old man presenting with acute motor weakness of all four extremities and right facial muscles, associated with areflexia and some sensory complaints. The weakness involves both the proximal and distal muscles as well as the neck flexor and facial muscles. There is a history of a precedent gastrointestinal illness.

Localization and Differential Diagnosis

The pattern of weakness and diminished deep tendon reflexes obviously localize to the peripheral nervous system. Next it must be determined which segment of the motor unit is affected: the peripheral nerve, the neuromuscular junction, the muscle, or the motor neuron. The differential diagnosis of acute motor weakness needs particular attention, as it is a very important topic for the practicing neurologist, not just the Board candidate. In the differential diagnosis, diseases of the peripheral nerves and root need to be considered first.

Guillain-Barré syndrome (GBS) or acute inflammatory demyelinating polyneuropathy characterized by rapid onset of weakness, accompanied by sensory loss, and areflexia may correspond to the clinical picture presented in the vignette. Among the neuropathies and polyradiculoneuropathies responsible for acute motor weakness, infectious, inflammatory, metabolic, and toxic causes need to be ruled out.

Of the infectious processes, diphtheria may simulate GBS but the evolution of symptoms is longer and systemic manifestations such as fever, pharyngitis, headache, and nausea may dominate the initial picture. Blurry vision due to paralysis of accommodation common in diphtheria is rare in GBS (Ropper).

Cytomegalovirus can be responsible for the development of acute flaccid paralysis, areflexia, and sphincteric abnormalities in association with pain and paresthesias in the cauda equina distribution typically in severely immunosuppressed HIV patients.

An acute motor weakness simulating GBS may occur early during the HIV infection.

Lyme disease also enters the differential diagnosis of weakness, sensory loss, and areflexia. The peripheral neuropathy is generally not ascending and typically asymmetrical (Ropper).

Acute motor axonal neuropathy characterized by acute ascending weakness, areflexia, cranial nerve deficits, respiratory failure, and lack of sensory symptoms has been described as the most common variant of GBS in Northern China (Dumitru).

Vasculitic neuropathies are usually associated with polyarteritis nodosa, rheumatoid arthritis, systemic lupus erythematosus, and Wegener's granulomatosis. They need to be mentioned as part of the differential diagnosis of acute weakness. Several features distinguish them from GBS, and include the distribution of weakness usually asymmetric, uncommon respiratory or sphincter dysfunction, and involvement of multiple systems and organs.

Among the metabolic disorders causing acute weakness, hepatic porphyria with neuropathy needs to be considered. Acute intermittent porphyria due to porphobilinogen deaminase deficiency can manifest with acute ascending motor weakness simulating GBS. In addition, behavioral abnormalities, seizures, and psychosis can also occur as well as abdominal pain that usually initially predominates.

The periodic paralyses usually have episodic weakness and areflexia with no sensory, cranial nerve, or sphincteric disturbances.

Acute weakness can also be caused by exposure to certain toxins, including arsenic, thallium, dapsone, lead, exacarbon, neurotoxic fish, buckthorn, and tick paralysis.

Diseases of the neuromuscular junction, which can cause acute weakness and are differentiated from GBS, include botulism, myasthenia gravis, and organophosphate intoxication. Botulism results from a neurotoxin elaborated by *Clostridium botulinum* types A, B, and E (Ropper). It is characterized by the manifestation of nausea, vomiting, constipation, dysphagia, dry mouth, blurred vision, ptosis, and dysarthria over the course of 12 to 36 hours after the ingestion of contaminated food. Pupils can be dilated and nonreactive. Respiratory weakness is often marked, even when limb weakness is only mild or moderate, and DTR are frequently preserved even in the presence of significant limb weakness (Ropper).

Myasthenia gravis also enters the differential diagnosis of acute weakness but has certain characteristics such as fluctuation and fatigable weakness. Fatigable ptosis is an important finding of myasthenia gravis. Reflexes and sensory examination are normal.

Muscle disorders include the periodic paralyses as causes of acute weakness. Primary hypokalemic periodic paralysis, which is the most frequent form, is character-

ized by episodic weakness and areflexia that occur preferably at night, and is precipitated by meals rich in carbohydrates and strenuous exercise. Respiratory and cranial muscles are not involved.

Acute myopathies have been described with the administration of drugs such as clofibrate and lovastatin (Ropper) or after infections such as influenza, *Mycoplasma pneumoniae* and trichinosis. Sensory function and reflexes are normal, CPK levels are elevated: all factors that should help in making the right diagnosis.

Diseases of the anterior horn cells causing acute weakness include poliomyelitis which has an asymmetrical distribution of muscle weakness and is accompanied by systemic symptoms. Among CNS disorders causing acute weakness, transverse myelitis needs to be mentioned but the distinction from GBS should be obvious. Transverse myelitis presents with symptoms and signs of spinal cord dysfunction, such as weakness, increased DTR, Babinski's sign, sensory level, and sphincteric dysfunction.

Etiology

Specific agents are not identified, but GBS has been linked to viral infection cytomegalovirus, Epstein-Barr virus, and HIV, or to bacterial infections such as *Mycoplasma pneumoniae* and Lyme disease. *Campylobacter jejuni* enteritis may be the most common bacterial organism associated with GBS, particularly its axonal forms preceding the disease in approximately 25 to 38 percent of patients (Barohn).

Clinical Features

Acute inflammatory demyelinating polyneuropathy manifests with rapid progressive weakness, sensory loss and areflexia. GBS is the most common cause of acute generalized weakness with an incidence of 1 to 2 per 100,000 people (Barohn and Saperstein). An antecedent infection related to the gastrointestinal or respiratory system is recognized one to four weeks prior to the neurological symptoms, but other factors include prior surgery or immunization.

The characteristic clinical features include progressive relatively symmetrical weakness of more than one limb associated with areflexia or hyporeflexia evolving over the course of four weeks. Other findings are represented by mild sensory symptoms, cranial nerve involvement in particular the seventh nerve that can be affected bilaterally, signs of autonomic dysfunction, elevated CSF proteins, evidence of a demyelinating neuropathy on electrodiagnostic studies and recovery that usually starts 2 to 4 weeks after plateau phase.

The pattern of weakness is an ascending paralysis with onset in the lower extremities but occasionally a descending presentation characterized by neck, face, and pharyngeal involvement and then progression to the arms and legs can also occur. The weakness tends to be symmetrical and to involve proximal and distal muscles. Sensory symptoms such as numbness and paresthesias can be prominent as well as pain in the back and limbs and may represent the initial symptoms.

Cranial nerve dysfunction, particularly facial diplegia and oropharyingeal weakness, are seen in 50 percent of patients but ophthalmoparesis is rarely observed (Bosch). Autonomic abnormalities include cardiovascular complications due to tachyarrhythmia, bradycardia, asystole, sustained hypertension, orthostatic hypotension, and so on. Other manifestations of autonomic dysfunction are urinary retention, impotence, constipation, anhydrosis, pupillary abnormalities, and so on. Respiratory complications requiring mechanical ventilation occur in about one third of cases.

The majority of patients reach the nadir by by four weeks, then a variable plateau phase occurs before the onset of recovery, which can last up to 24 months (in 82 percent of patients according to Bosch).

GBS Variants

Several clinical variants of GBS have been described. Acute motor axonal neuropathy (AMAN), characterized by rapidly progressive motor weakness and areflexia without sensory loss, has electrophysiological findings of primarily axonal degeneration and normal sensory nerve action potentials. Antecedent *Campylobacter jejuni* infection was found in 76 percent of AMAN patients from northern China (Bosch). Serum antibodies, mainly of the immunoglobulin G (IgG) class, to several glycolipids, notably GM1 and GD1a, are found in a greater proportion of GBS patients with axonal features (Bosch).

Acute motor-sensory axonal neuropathy is another primarily axonal form that involves motor and sensory axons. Miller Fisher syndrome, characterized by ophthalmoplegia, ataxia, and areflexia, is another variant and is discussed later in this chapter. A pure sensory form with ataxia but no ophthalmoplegia is also described. The pharyngeal cervicobrachial variant is characterized by marked cervical, facial, and pharyngeal weakness in the early stages with later involvement of the limbs. Autonomic variants have also been described.

Diagnosis

The examination of the cerebrospinal fluid after the first week demonstrates increased protein level and normal cell count in most cases. A mild to moderate increase in cell count in the CSF is typically found in GBS associated with HIV infection.

Electrodiagnostic tests in AIDP show evidence of multifocal demyelination. Early findings are prolonged or absent F waves and H responses, an indication of proximal demyelination at the root level. Slow conduction velocities, prolonged distal latencies, conduction block, and temporal dispersion are the important electrophysiologi-

cal features supportive of demyelination. A secondary axonal loss is suggested by the presence of fibrillation potentials on needle EMG that appear in two to five weeks during the course of the process. The axonal variant demonstrates low amplitude or unobtainable compound motor action potential.

The EMG can represent an important prognostic factor. In particular, the mean amplitude of the CMAP can indicate poor outcome if its value is less than 20 percent of the lower limit of normal recorded 3 to 5 weeks after the onset of symptoms (Katirji).

Several antibodies to various gangliosides (GM_1, GM_1-b, GD_1-b) have been documented in patients diagnosed with GBS. The majority of patients presenting with the Miller Fisher variant have serum GQ1b antibodies.

Treatment

Supportive care with particular attention to respiratory support and correction of autonomic dysfunction is an important part of the treatment. Elective intubation is required when forced vital capacity (FVC) decreases to less than 15 to 20 ml/kg.

Immunotherapies, in particular plasma exchange (PE) and intravenous human immunoglobulin (IVIG), have shown efficacy in the treatmant of AIDP and should be initiated within the first week of symptoms. The dose of PE is 200 to 250 ml/kg of body weight over 14 days. Complications include hypotension, anemia or low platelet count, pneumothorax, pulmonary embolism, and so on. Intravenous immunoglobulin should be given with an infusion of 0.4 g/kg per day for five days (total dose 2.0 g/kg). IVIG side effects include flu-like symptoms, nausea, vomiting, headache, renal failure, hepatitis C, and so on.

Barohn has described factors implicated in the prognosis. In particular, a poor outcome is related to advanced age of the patient, rapid evolution of symptoms, necessity of ventilatory support, low CMAP amplitude, and prior gastrointestinal infection with *C. jejuni*.

Chronic Inflammatory Demyelinating Polyradiculoneuropathy

Vignette

A 32-year-old lawyer had been in excellent health until six months ago when he noticed some difficulty climbing a flight of stairs. He also experienced hypersensitivity on the soles of his feet, low back pain, and numbness and stiffness of both hands that slowly worsened. His balance was poor, especially with the eyes closed. There was no dysphagia, dysartria, urinary or bladder dysfunction. No history of weight loss or rash. He was particu-

larly concerned because his father had ALS. On neurological examination, cranial nerves were intact. Neck flexors, deltoid, biceps, triceps, and distal muscles were 4/5 in the upper extremities. In the lower extremities, proximal muscle strength was 3/5 and distal was 4/5. DTR were 1+ in the upper extremities, trace at the knees, and absent at both ankles. Sensory examination revealed decreased vibratory sensation, joint position, and pinprick below the knees. A bilateral postural tremor was noted in the arms.

Summary A 32-year-old man with progressive proximal and distal weakness, sensory loss, hyporeflexia, and postural tremor.

Localization

The clinical findings described in the vignette localize to the peripheral nerves. The pattern of progressive weakness, sensory loss, and hyporeflexia evolving within six months are typically suggestive of a chronic neuropathic process.

The vignette therefore describes a chronic progressive symmetric sensory and motor deficit that includes distal and proximal weakness, sensory loss, paresthesias and hyporeflexia. Symmetrical weakness that involves proximal and distal muscles associated with sensory loss and hyporeflexia or areflexia is highly suggestive of a demyelinating neuropathy, particularly acute/and chronic acquired inflammatory demyelinating polyneuropathy (CIDP). The sensory findings described also point to involvement of the large myelinated sensory fibers. The demyelinating neuropathies can be distinguished into acquired and inherited processes.

Clinically, the vignette fits the diagnostic criteria for CIDP, which are characterized by progressive stepwise or relapsing symmetrical proximal and distal weakness of the upper and lower extremities of at least two months' duration associated with sensory findings and hyporeflexia or areflexia. The involvement of neck flexor and facial muscles can occur, but the extraocular muscles are rarely affected. Sensory complaints can be prominent and usually include distal numbness and paresthesias. Autonomic dysfunction is not frequent particularly compared to GBS and respiratory compromise is rare.

The differential diagnosis includes disorders of the peripheral nerves that can be acquired or inherited. Chronic progressive polyneuropathy with clinical, laboratory, and electrophysiological criteria similar to CIDP can be sometimes associated with an underlying systemic disorder. These cases have been defined by Barohn as "CIDP with" concurrent illnesses such as AIDS, connective tissue disease, monoclonal gammopathy, lymphoma, chronic active hepatitis, and so on.

The polyneuropathies associated with paraproteinemias should be well considered because monoclonal gammopathy occurs in approximately 10 percent of all patients with idiopathic polyneuropathy (Mendell). The paraproteinemias associated with polyneuropathy include multiple myeloma, osteosclerotic myeloma, macroglobulinemia, primary amyloidosis, cryoglobulinemia, and benign monoclonal gammopathy.

Osteosclerotic myeloma occurs in only 3 percent of patients with myeloma (Mendell) and may be associated with the presence of a neuropathy in over half of the cases. The neuropathy that manifests with osteosclerotic myeloma can be clinically indistinguishable from CIDP, presenting with symmetrical weakness of the proximal and distal muscles, sensory loss preferably of the large fiber type, and hyporeflexia or areflexia, and can occur as an early manifestation or even initially during the disease. Other systemic abnormalities can be associated with osteosclerotic myeloma and involve multiple organs representing the POEMS syndrome (polyneuropathy, organomegaly [hepatomegaly, splenomegaly, cardiomegaly], endocrinopathy [diabetes, gynecomastia, amenorrhea], monoclonal gammopathy, and skin lesions (thickening, increased pigmentation, hypertrichosis) (Mendell).

(MMN)

Multifocal motor neuropathy with conduction block also enters into the differential diagnosis of acquired chronic demyelinating neuropathy and in the differential diagnosis of CIDP. Typical clinical manifestations of MMN include progressive, asymmetrical predominantly distal weakness, associated with cramps and fasciculations and without sensory symptoms. Atrophy can occur but less than expected with the degree of weakness that characteristically follows a peripheral nerve distribution. Therefore, MMN can clinically be distinguished from CIDP, which typically presents with progressive predominantly symmetrical and proximal but also distal weakness associated with sensory deficit and characteristic laboratory findings. The patient in the vignette does not have symptoms suggestive of MMN. (Obviously, we don't have laboratory and electrodiagnostic studies to help us with the diagnosis.)

Inherited demyelinating neuropathies, particularly hereditary sensory-motor neuropathies type I or Charcot-Marie-Tooth disease, are the most common form of hereditary chronic polyneuropathies. The absence of family history of this disorder, which has an autosomic dominant pattern of inheritance, and the lack of characteristic features (marked distal weakness and atrophy in the legs; foot deformities such as pes cavus or equinovarus and hammer toes in some cases) make the diagnosis unlikely in this vignette.

Refsum's disease, which is an autosomic recessive disorder due to abnormalities of phytanic acid metabolism, is also associated with a chronic progressive demyelinating neuropathy. But other characteristic clinical features are retinitis pigmentosa manifesting with night blindness, cerebellar ataxia, neurogenic deafness, and so on.

Disorders of other parts of the motor unit, which are differentiated from CIDP (but clinically excluded in the vignette) are presented below.

Anterior horn cell disorders
• ALS: Upper and lower motor neuron signs in the absence of sensory symptoms.
• Spinal muscular atrophy type 3: Hereditary disorder characterized by proximal muscle weakness and atrophy with intact sensation to all modalities, affecting individuals in the third or fourth decade of life.
Disorders of muscle
• Polymiositis: Proximal muscle weakness, normo-hyporeflexia, normal sensation, myalgia.
• Inclusion body myositis: Slowly progressive asymmetrical proxymal and distal weakness and atrophy, preferentially affecting knee extensor muscles and wrist and finger flexors.
Disorders of the neuromuscular junction
• Myasthenia gravis: Fatigable weakness often affecting the extraocular muscles without sensory findings.
• Lambert-Eaton myasthenic syndrome: Progressive proximal weakness and hyporeflexia that improves with brief muscle contraction associated with autonomic findings.

Clinical Features

CIDP is characterized by progressive, stepwise or relapsing muscle weakness of varying severity and of at least two months' duration, predominantly symmetrical and proximal but also distal, associated with hyporeflexia or areflexia. Facial and neck muscles can also be involved but autonomic and respiratory compromise are rare, particularly compared with GBS. Sensory symptoms can include paresthesias and numbness and can cause severe sensory ataxia or pseudoathetosis due to proprioceptive loss (Small and Lovelace).

Diagnosis

Examination of the CSF shows characteristic albumino-cytologic dissociation with markedly elevated protein content (CSF protein >45 mg/dl; cell count <10/mm^3). Electrodiagnostic studies demonstrate evidence of demyelination with its characteristic findings of decreased nerve conduction velocity in distal nerve segments to at least 60 percent of normal, absent or prolonged F wave latencies and H reflex latencies, prolonged distal motor latencies, conduction block or temporal dispersion in one or more motor nerves. Nerve biopsy demonstrates predominant features of demyelination

Blood tests that are usually obtained in patients diagnosed with chronic demyelinating neuropathy include

• Serum paraprotein: Serum and urine immunofixation, electrophoresis, quantitative immunoglobulins, cryoglobulins
• Fasting glucose.
• Thyroid function test.
• HIV and hepatitis serology.
• Antinuclear antibody, rheumatic factor, ESR.
• Antibodies to GM$_1$ and asialo-GM$_1$.
• MAG (myelin-associated glycoproteins) and sulfated acidic glycoproteins).
• Other studies, such as phytanic acid long-chain fatty acids, and so on, are indicated in selected cases.

Treatment

Corticosteroids remain the first line of therapy. Prednisone can be initiated at an oral dose of 80 to 100 mg a day for four to six weeks and then slowly tapered and changed to alternate-day dosing. The duration of treatment is six months or longer. The side effects are well known. Plasmapheresis is indicated if patients have marked weakness or if they are not fully controlled on a prednisone regimen because of side effects or contraindications. IVIG has also been considered, but is more costly and requires maintenance therapy every 6 or 12 weeks.

Miller Fisher Syndrome

Vignette

A 26-year-old art student, while vacationing in Spain, woke up experiencing double vision, particularly when looking to the right, that worsened toward the end of the day. He began to stagger when walking. The following day while in a local emergency room, a neurologist noted that the student had bilateral incomplete abducens paralysis, ptosis, and mild hyporeflexia. His gait was wide-based and he could only walk with assistance. His past medical history was unremarkable except for some gastrointestinal complaints and bouts of diarrhea after eating fish in the beginning of his vacation. His father had hypertension and his mother had a mild form of multiple sclerosis.

Summary A 26-year-old man with sudden onset of diplopia and unsteady gait. The neurological examination shows bilateral partial sixth and third nerve involvement, hyporeflexia, and ataxia.

Localization

First, it is important to localize the lesion and determine if the pathology involves the central or the peripheral nervous system. Considering the central nervous system the localization more appropriate is in the brainstem and the cause may be attributed to a vascular event, infectious process, nutritional deficiency, space-occupying lesion, or demyelinating process.

Brainstem ischemia due to vertebrobasilar artery occlusion will be unlikely in a 26-year-old without significant risk factors for stroke. The student was in good health prior to the event and did not have any history of heart disease, vasculopathy or coagulopathy, or any predisposing factor for a cerebrovascular accident to occur. Therefore, this possibility does not represent a primary concern. Wernicke encephalopathy due to nutritional deficiency can manifest with ataxia and ophthalmoplegia, but typically includes a severe memory dysfunction as well as mental status changes with a global confusional state. Brainstem encephalitis can also be excluded by the lack of other signs and symptoms as well as fever, headache, and altered sensorium. Posterior fossa tumors other than metastasis are rare in adults and manifest with signs of progressive brainstem dysfunction. Ectasia of the basilar artery, which is a rare condition, can also cause signs of progressive brainstem involvement. Demyelinating disorders, such as multiple sclerosis, may involve the brainstem causing ophthalmoplegia and ataxia but hyporeflexia is not found.

Localizing to the peripheral nervous system, the part of the motor unit that is involved must be determined. The discussion can certainly be limited to disorders of the peripheral nerves and disorders of the neuromuscular junction. Miller Fisher syndrome, characterized by ophthalmoplegia, ataxia, and areflexia, is a very important diagnostic consideration in the vignette and also represents a clinical variant of GBS. Other neuropathies also featuring external ophthalmoplegia include infectious processes such as diphtheria, nutritional disorders such as hypophosphatemia, Whipple disease, diabetes, toxic causes such as thallium intoxication, and so on. Diphtheria has particular clinical features, such as longer evolution of symptoms, that also include systemic manifestations such as fever, sore throat, and myalgia, in addition to palatal paralysis and paralysis of accommodation. Hypophosphatemia can cause a subacute sensorimotor peripheral neuropathy. Weakness, ataxia, and hyporeflexia can also be noted. Whipple disease, which can be complicated by peripheral neuropathy and supranuclear ophthalmoparesis rather than external ophtalmoplegia, has prominent abdominal symptoms and weight loss. Diabetes can manifest with sudden ophthalmoplegia, particularly involving the third nerve, due to a vascular mechanism in association with signs of peripheral neuropathy usually in older patients with long-standing diabetes. Thallium neuropathy manifests with gastrointestinal symptoms such as nausea and abdominal pain,

painful paresthesias, relative preservation of DTR, psychotic behavior, alopecia, and so on.

Disorders of neuromuscular transmission, such as botulism, myasthenia gravis, and tick paralysis, are an important consideration in the differential diagnosis and can manifest with external ophthalmoplegia and, except for myasthenia, hyporeflexia and ataxia. Botulism in particular is characterized by acute onset of diplopia, dysphagia, and dysarthria often preceded by gastrointestinal symptoms. Respiratory distress and weakness of the upper and lower extremities create a dramatic picture. Deep tendon reflexes may be normal or diminished. Autonomic abnormalities include constipation, dry mouth, and abnormal pupils. Myasthenia gravis can present acutely but fatigable weakness that improves with rest is an important characteristic. Ataxia and hyporeflexia are not found. Tick paralysis can manifest with acute weakness, ophthalmoplegia, hyporeflexia, and respiratory compromise.

Clinical Features

Miller Fisher syndrome typically manifests with ophthalmoplegia, gait ataxia, and hyporeflexia or areflexia. Ophthalmoplegia can be asymmetrical and accompanied by ptosis but pupillary involvement is rare. Other symptoms include paresthesias and mild loss of sensation in the distal limbs, and mild oropharyngeal and facial weakness. The ataxia has the features of cerebellar disease (Mendell et al.).

Ropper has established some diagnostic criteria for Miller Fisher syndrome that include the following clinical features

- Bilateral and relatively symmetrical ophthalmoparesis associated with ptosis, limb and gait ataxia with cerebellar tremor, and areflexia. The progression of the symptoms is over three weeks.
- Facial or oropharyngeal weakness or paresthesias are minimal or absent, and the mental status is normal. Signs of upper motor neuron dysfunction or cerebellar dysartria are never observed.

Diagnosis

Laboratory findings include

- CSF shows increased protein content without significant pleocytosis.
- Electrodiagnostic studies demonstrate decreased amplitudes of the sensory nerve action potentials with a return of these responses during recovery, suggestive of a demyelinating sensory neuropathy (Mendell et al.).
- Serum anti-GQ1b antibodies are seen in the majority of patients with Miller Fisher syndrome (95% according to Mendell).

Treatment

The treatment is similar to that for typical GBS with IVIG or PE.

Disorders of the Neuromuscular Junction

Botulism

Vignette

A 45-year-old Chinese waiter woke up with blurry vision and bilateral ptosis. He felt nauseated and vomited several times. The next day he had complete ophthalmoplegia, dysarthria, difficulty swallowing, and shortness of breath. Neurological examination showed marked limitation of horizontal gaze and upgaze, ptosis, facial diplegia, and a weak tongue, with no fasciculations. Pupils were dilated and not reactive. Neck flexors and extensor and proximal limb muscles were weak. Deep tendon reflexes were diminished and sensation was normal.

Summary A 45-year-old man presenting with the acute onset of rapidly progressive bulbofacial, extraocular, respiratory and neck muscle weakness, accompanied by poor pupillary responses and hyporeflexia.

Localization

It is important to determine which component of the motor unit is involved: anterior horn cell, peripheral nerve, neuromuscular junction, or muscle.

Among the disorders of the peripheral nerve causing acute weakness, the entities to consider are Guillain-Barré syndrome, diphtheric polyneuropathy, and porphyric polyneuropathy. Guillain-Barré syndrome is characterized by rapidly progressive, relatively symmetrical weakness involving the proximal and distal muscles, usually with an ascending pattern that tends to involve the lower extremities first and is associated with hyporeflexia or areflexia. Sensory symptoms such as numbness, paresthesias, and even moderate or severe pain involving the limbs and lower back can also occur. A rare descending presentation that can simulate botulism or diphtheria is the pharyngeal-cervical-brachial variant described by Ropper with involvement of the facial, oropharyngeal, neck, and upper extremity muscles, which can create some diagnostic difficulties. Diphtheria, which also enters the differential diagnosis of the case presented in the vignette is characterized initially by fever, nausea, headache, pharyngitis, and other systemic symptoms as well

as a longer evolution of symptoms. Weakness of the extraocular muscles and the face are not as prominent as with botulism. Pupillary responses to light and convergence are often normal on examination (Ropper).

The acute porphyrias are hereditary disorders presenting with acute neurological symptoms. Acute intermittent porphyria due to porphobilinogen deaminase deficiency is characterized by neurological manifestations usually preceded by gastrointestinal signs such as nausea, vomiting, and abdominal pain. Behavioral abnormalities, psychosis, and seizures are also seen. The distribution weakness involve the facial, oropharyngeal, and proximal limb muscles often resembling GBS. Deep tendon reflexes can be decreased or not elicitable. Sensory loss may be prominent in a proximal distribution with a shield-like or bathing trunk pattern. Other characteristic features of the acute intermittent porphyrias include autonomic abnormalities, particularly tachycardia, hypertension, postural hypotension, urinary retention, and so on.

After discussing diseases of the peripheral nerves that may explain the symptoms described in the vignette, neuromuscular junction disorders need to be considered, in particular botulism, myasthenia gravis, and organophosphate poisoning. Botulism (food-borne botulism) is the most likely diagnosis. The clinical manifestations start 12 to 36 hours after consumption of the contamined food. Gastrointestinal symptoms include nausea, diarrhea, vomiting, and abdominal pain. Blurred vision and diplopia can be experienced acutely in combination with dysphagia, dysarthria, dysphonia, and dry mouth. Large, poorly reactive pupils are a typical finding but this varies in different cases. Weakness of the upper and lower extremities also occurs together with disturbances of autonomic function with hypotension, tachycardia, and urinary retention. Weakness of respiratory muscles may require ventilatory support and deep tendon reflexes are usually retained but may be diminished in case of severe weakness.

Myasthenia gravis can be excluded because it typically presents with fatigable weakness often affecting the extraocular muscles in an asymmetric pattern and always sparing the pupils.

Organophosphate poisoning manifests with limb weakness and respiratory distress in combination with other signs, such as altered consciousness, seizures, fasciculations, nausea, vomiting, bradycardia, salivation, and so on.

Disorders of the anterior horn cells causing acute weakness include acute polio, which is mentioned for completion. Polymyelitis is responsible for an asymmetrical flaccid paralysis that usually involves the lower extremities. The IX and X nuclei can be involved withh resultant dysphagia and dysarthria. Other symptoms that may precede the neurological signs are fever, vomiting, fatigue, abdominal pain, and headache.

Clinical Features

Clostridium botulinum is responsible for the production of neurotoxin that has been divided into eight immunologically distinct subtypes of which A, B, and E are the most common. Several clinical forms are identified, particularly

- The classic food-borne botulism, which is the most severe.
- Infantile botulism, which is the most common form of botulism in the United States and affects infants younger than one year of age.
- Wound botulism, which is very rare.
- Hidden botulism, which may be the adult equivalent of infant botulism (Dumitru et al.).

The onset of the manifestations may occur 12 to 36 hours after the consumption of food contaminated with the toxin and are characterized by nausea, vomiting, diarrhea, or constipation. The neurological symptoms can be dramatic with rapidly progressive ophthalmoplegia, often with pupillary dilatation, bulbar weakness causing dysphagia, dysarthria, and dysphonia, and weakness of the extremities. Autonomic dysfunction may cause orthostatic hypotension, urinary retention, impairment of lacrimation, and so on. Deep tendon reflexes are normal but hyporeflexia or areflexia may be observed in severe cases. Respiratory muscle weakness is responsible for reduced forced vital capacity and ventilatory support may be necessary.

Diagnosis

The diagnosis of botulism requires a high index of suspicion, particularly when there is a history of ingestion of contaminated food, a wound's infection, or severe constipation in infants. The botulinus toxin acts primarily at the level of the neuromuscular junction, more specifically on the presynaptic endings.

Electrophysiologic studies are important and may demonstrate a decreased amplitude of the CMAP in the affected muscles and a modest increment between 30 and 100 percent of the CMAP with rapid repetitive stimulation. Other confirmatory studies include the identification of the toxin in serum, stool, and wound cultures.

Treatment

The treatment is supportive, particularly for pulmonary care, and also based on the prompt use of the trivalent antitoxin.

Lambert-Eaton Myasthenic Syndrome

Vignette

A 60-year-old x-ray technician had difficulty climbing stairs and getting up from the toilet seat for the last five months, particularly in the morning on waking up, which seemed to slightly improve a short time thereafter. He also complained of dry mouth and fatigue. There was no dysphagia or dysarthria. He had borderline diet-controlled diabetes and angina. He had smoked two packs of cigarettes per day for 30 years, but had discontinued six years ago. He consumed several alcoholic drinks a day. The neurological examination showed that the cranial nerves were intact except for questionable sluggish pupils. Neck flexion was weak. Deltoids were 4/5. Hip flexion was 3/5. He could hardly walk on his heels and toes. DTR were trace with an absent ankle jerk bilaterally. His gait was cautious and slightly wide-based.

Summary 60-year-old man with progressive weakness predominantly proximal. Other important information given in the vignette includes dry mouth, sluggish pupils, hypoflexia and areflexia, and a long history of heavy smoking.

Localization

There is no doubt that the localization is the peripheral nervous system, indicated by the progressive weakness, hyporeflexia, and absent long tract signs. It is important to determine which part of the motor unit is involved:

- Anterior horn cell
- Peripheral nerve
- Neuromuscular junction
- Muscle

Disorders of the anterior horn cells to be considered are ALS and spinal muscular atrophy. ALS usually presents with progressive asymmetrical weakness and atrophy in combination with upper motor signs such as hyperreflexia, pathological reflexes, and spasticity. The PMA variant does not have signs of upper motor neuron involvement. Dry mouth and autonomic disturbances (represented also by the sluggish pupils in the case described) are not part of the clinical features of MND. Instead, drooling of the saliva if dysphagia is present invariably occurs in ALS. Spinal muscular atrophy is a hereditary autosomal recessive disorder characterized by predominantly symmetrical proximal weakness accompanied by atrophy that manifests in a younger age group, usually in the third decade of life.

Disorders of peripheral nerves are considered next and can be easily excluded by the vignette. Subacute or chronic sensory motor polyneuropathy is characterized by prominent sensory symptoms, distal weakness, and decreased deep tendon reflexes. Particular consideration needs to be given to chronic inflammatory demyelinating polyneuropathy (CIDP) as part of the differential diagnosis. This disorder is characterized by chronic progressive, stepwise or relapsing, relatively symmetrical motor and sensory deficits including distal and proximal weakness, sensory loss, paresthesia, and hyporeflexia (which are not among the symptoms of the patient described in the vignette). Pure motor neuropathies, such as multifocal motor neuropathy, can be also clinically excluded, being characterized by progressive, asymmetrical predominantly distal limb atrophy and weakness that follow a peripheral nerve distribution.

Next are disorders of the neuromuscular junction, typically myasthenia gravis and Lambert-Eaton myasthenic syndrome. The clinical case does not suggest myasthenia gravis, characterized by fatigable weakness often affecting the extraocular muscles with an asymmetric pattern of distribution and always sparing the pupils. Proximal limb weakness as well as weakness of the diaphragm and neck extensors muscles can also be seen. The weakness is typically fatigable, therefore tends to increase with repeated exercise and improve with rest or sleep (just the opposite of what the patient in the vignette is experiencing: he had difficulty climbing stairs and getting up from the toilet seat in the morning on waking up that seemed to improve shortly thereafter). Isolated weakness of the extremities is not very common in myasthenic patients, and dry mouth and other autonomic abnormalities are not seen.

The symptoms described in the vignette clearly reflect Lambert-Eaton myasthenic syndrome. This presynaptic neuromuscular junction disorder is characterized by proximal limb weakness, preferentially involving the lower extremities, and fatigability. Hyporeflexia or areflexia is also observed. Autonomic nervous system abnormalities, in particular dry mouth but also pupillary abnormalities, decreased sweat and lacrimation, impotence, and so on, are other important characteristics. The weakness as well as hyporeflexia tend to improve temporarily with brief repeated muscle contractions. Therefore LEMS is the best tentative diagnosis.

Finally, the last part of the differential diagnosis involves muscle disorders, such as polymiositis, dermatomyositis and inclusion body myositis. Polymiositis is characterized by progressive, relatively symmetrical proximal weakness of the upper and lower extremities and neck flexor muscles. Deep tendon reflexes are normal or decreased in severe cases. Myalgia, tenderness, and systemic symptoms may also occur. Dermatomyositis has the characteristic rash that may manifest before or after the discovery of the weakness. Inclusion body myositis typically presents with slowly progressive, asymmetrical proximal and distal weakness and atrophy that preferentially affects the quadriceps and wrist and finger flexor muscles.

Clinical Features

LEMS is a presynaptic disorder of the neuromuscular junction caused by antibodies directed against the voltage-gated calcium channels. Men are affected more than women and the onset of symptoms is usually after the fourth decade of life. LEMS is considered a paraneoplastic disorder in the majority of the cases with a strong association with small-cell lung carcinoma and less frequently with lymphoma, and breast and ovarian carcinoma. It can also rarely represent an idiopathic autoimmune disorder without further evidence of cancer. The weakness involves the proximal muscles, particularly of the lower extremities, and may transiently improve with brief contractions (muscle facilitation). Hyporeflexia/areflexia is another feature, but typically the DTR may normalize immediately after brief exercise of those muscles activated by the reflex.

Autonomic symptoms include

- Dry mouth (the most common).
- Decreased lacrimation and sweating.
- Abnormal pupillary responses.
- Impotence.
- Orthostatic hypotension.

Diagnosis

Laboratory studies demonstrate IgG antibodies directed against the voltage-gated calcium channel on the presynaptic nerve terminal. Electrophysiological tests of particular importance are based on repetitive nerve stimulations that when performed at slow rate (3Hz) show a decremental response similar to MG. After rapid RNS (30 to 50 HZ) or brief (10 sec) intense contractions, a marked increase of the CMAP amplitude by more than 200 percent is demonstrated (postexercise facilitation). Single-fiber EMG may show increased jitter with blocking and improvement at high rate of stimulation. Imaging studies such as X-ray or CT of the chest are important in ruling out an underlying malignancy. LEMS symptoms usually precede tumor diagnosis by about 10 months (Dumitru et al.). Broncoscopy can also be performed in selected cases.

Treatment

The treatment is directed primarily to an aggressive search and treatment of a possible underlying malignancy, particularly in older patients with a long-standing history of smoking, because the symptoms may significantly ameliorate with the appropriate cancer therapy.

Immunotherapy is particularly indicated in patients with LEMS who do not have cancer. Steroid treatment is based on the use of oral prednisone or prednisolone at 1.0 to 1.5 mg/kg every other day that may cause marked improvement of the weakness and is administered over several months until the desired benefits are obtained and than slowly tapered toward the minimal effective dose. Azathioprine is also used sometimes in combination with the steroids, with an effective dose of 2 to 3 mg/kg/day and cautious consideration of the adverse effects, such as leukopenia, liver toxicity, bone marrow suppression, and so on. Another important consideration involves the fact that beneficial effects may take several months to appear. Cyclosporine can be administered in patients who have not responded to azathioprine. Plasmapheresis or high-dose intravenous immunoglobulin has also been beneficial.

Other therapies include guanidine hydrochloride, which causes an increase in the amount of Ach release at the nerve terminal. Adverse effects include bone marrow depression, renal tubular acidosis, hepatotoxicity, chronic interstitial nephritis, and so on. The aminopyridines tend to facilitate Ach release at the nerve terminal by blocking voltage-dependent potassium channels. 3,4-Diaminopyridine in particular may cause improvement in strength and autonomic functions in most patients with LEMS. Adverse effects consist of transitory perioral and acral paresthesias. The dose is usually 20 mg three times a day. Most patients experience beneficial effects with this therapy, which last as long as the drug is administered. 4-Aminopyridine carries risks of inducing seizures due to the central nervous system toxicity.

Myasthenia Gravis

Vignette

A 21-year-old homemaker started complaining of double vision, speech difficulty, and dysphagia. For the last month she had tended to slur her speech, dribble saliva while talking, and occasionally choke on food. She had been aware of double vision while watching television in the evening. Her husband had noticed that her left eyelid at times seemed droopy, especially under sunlight. On examination there was bilateral ptosis, worse on the left, and bilateral horizontal gaze limitation. On the right, adduction was complete, but abduction was decreased 60 percent. There was upward gaze limitation and bilateral facial weakness with diminished gag reflex. Motor strength in the limbs, as well as DTR and sensation were normal.

Summary A 21-year-old woman with history of diplopia, dysarthria, and dysphagia, and neurological findings of ptosis, ophthalmoparesis, facial weakness, and diminished gag reflex.

Localization

The first step is to determine whether the lesion involves the peripheral or the central nervous system, and in the latter case, if it is intrinsic or extrinsic to the brainstem.

Brainstem intrinsic pathology that involves the medulla, pons, and mesencephalus are characterized by signs of involvement of the long sensory and motor tracts often realizing a crossed pattern of weakness and sensory loss. Extrinsic brainstem lesions often cause painful involvement of adjacent cranial nerves with minimal involvement of motor or sensory tracts.

Considering peripheral nervous system, lesions, disorders of the different parts of the motor unit can be discussed in order to reach the best tentative diagnosis (peripheral nerves, neuromuscular junction, muscle, anterior horn cell). Among the disorders of peripheral nerves, Miller Fisher syndrome (GBS variant) can cause external ophthalmoplegia associated with dysphagia and dysarthria, but clinical findings important for the diagnosis are also ataxia and hyporeflexia/areflexia, features that do not occur in the vignette.

Disorders of the neuromuscular junction, in particular myasthenia gravis, can explain the symptoms presented in the vignette, characterized by ocular findings of external ophthalmoplegia that spares the pupils and bulbar signs of dysphagia and dysarthria. The phenomenon of fatigability is also implicated in the vignette when it is mentioned that the patient experiences diplopia in the evening when she watches television. Another sign is the intermittent ptosis aggravated by direct sunlight. Other disorders of the neuromuscular transmission, such as LEMS, are clinically differentiated from myasthenia gravis by the weakness predominantly affecting the proximal lower limb muscles and only mild involvement of the ocular and bulbar muscles. There is hyporeflexia or areflexia, but strength and reflexes can be improved by brief period of contraction (muscle facilitation). Autonomic abnormalities, in particular dry mouth, are other important features of LEMS.

In botulism, symptoms usually occur 12 to 36 hours after the ingestion of the contaminated food, with nausea, vomiting, diarrhea, and rapid progressive neurological dysfunction including ophthalmoplegia with unreactive pupils, bulbar paralysis, weakness of muscles of neck, trunk, and limbs, and respiratory compromise.

Muscle disorders that enter in the differential diagnosis include oculopharyngeal muscular dystrophy and mitochondrial myopathies. Oculopharyngeal muscular dystrophy is a hereditary disorder with onset during the fourth to sixth decades of life and characterized by progressive ptosis dysphagia and dysarthria. Fatigability or fluctuations of the weakness, are not features of this disorder and the pupils are also spared. Mitochondrial myopathies such as Kearns-Sayre syndrome (KSS) and progressive external ophthalmoplegia usually have signs of involvement of multiple organ systems (KSS for example has associated retinitis pigmentosa and heart block) that address the correct diagnosis.

Disorders of the anterior horn cells, such as ALS, poliomyelitis, or spinal muscular atrophy, are clearly not represented in the vignette.

Clinical Features

Myasthenia gravis is an autoimmune postsynaptic disorder of the neuromuscular junction characterized by fluctuating weakness and fatigability. The weakness typically affects ocular, facial, oropharyngeal, and limb muscles. Ptosis and ophthalmoparesis are the most common symptoms and are often asymmetrical. Other symptoms include dysphagia, dysphonia, and dysarthria due to weakness of the facial and bulbar muscles. Proximal limb and neck weaknesss is the presenting sign in 20 to 30 percent of patients (Dumitru et al.). Weakness of the diaphragm and respiratory muscles can also occur. The weakness is fatigable and typically worsens with sustained physical activity or during the course of the day, but improves with rest. Exposure to bright light may also worsen the ocular abnormalities. Deep tendon reflexes are usually normal and sensation is intact. MG is an autoimmune disorder caused by an antibody-mediated autoimmune attack directed against acetylcholine receptors at the postsynaptic portion of the neuromuscular junction. Three types of Ach receptor antibodies are detected: binding, modulating, and blocking (AchR binding antibodies are the most frequent subtype) (Dumitru et al.).

Diagnosis

The history of fatigable and fluctuating weakness is characteristic of MG. Pharmacological tests such as the Tensilon (edrophonium) test is important in demonstrating transitory improvement of symptoms, particularly ptosis, within few minutes of injection. Edrophonium chloride, which is a short-acting inhibitor of acetylcholinesterase, is administered in incremental doses, intravenously, with an initial dose of 2 mg (0.2 ml), followed by two more doses of 3 mg and 5 mg, if no untoward side effects occur and if no improvement is observed with a previous dose. A positive test is obtained when objective improvement is noted in some sign, such as ptosis, ophthalmoparesis, muscle strength, or respiratory function. This result is compared with what was obtained from a previous placebo injection of saline or atropine, the latter to block the muscarinic effects of this short-acting anticholinesterase. Hypotension and bradycardia can occur even if they are uncommon and atropine sulfate (0.6 mg intramuscular or

intravenously) should be always available for a prompt intervention.

Laboratory studies are based on the detection of AchR antibodies.

Elecrophysiological studies are performed to confirm a deficit in neuromuscular transmission and include routine nerve conduction studies, repetitive nerve stimulation, exercise testing, and, in selected cases, single-fiber EMG. Repetitive nerve stimulation (RNS) can show normal results, particularly in patients with the restricted ocular form of MG. When abnormal, the typical findings observed in MG with repetitive nerve stimulation at 2 to 5 Hz is a progressive decrement of the second through the fourth or fifth response with some return toward the initial CMAP size during the subsequent responses to a train of 9 to 10 stimuli, the so-called U-shaped pattern. A decrement greater than 10 percent is considered abnormal. If RNS shows negative results at rest, the muscle is activated for one minute and then RNS is performed immediately after exercise and once per minute for the next 5 minutes. Single-fiber EMG is used in selected cases when there is clinical suspicion but routine electrophysiologic studies are not conclusive in order to measure the relative firing of adjacent single muscle fibers from the same motor unit and can demonstrate both prolonged jitter as well as blocking of muscle fibers.

CT scan or MRI of the mediastinum is considered to exclude thymoma.

Treatment

Cholinesterase Inhibitors

Anticholinesterase medications are considered the first line of treatment in myasthenic patients. Pyridostigmine (Mestinon) has been used in a dosage of 60 mg every 4 hours if tolerated. Muscarinic side effects include abdominal cramps and diarrhea, which are dose related.

Thymectomy

Thymectomy is usually recommended in all patients with thymoma or in myasthenics younger than age 60 with generalized weakness (Massey). Thymectomy has been discouraged in patients over age 60 because of increased morbidity as well as evidence of atrophy of the involved gland and has also been discouraged in children. The degree of improvement and the time before improvement is noted are variable and may require several years for demonstrated efficacy.

Immunosuppressive Therapy

Corticosteroids have been particularly effective in generalized or ocular MG when symptoms are disabling and not controlled with cholinesterase inhibitors. Patients can be started at relatively high doses (60 to 80 mg) for rapid improvement, or with low, gradually increasing doses in order to avoid a possible exacerbation of symptoms that may occur one to two weeks after the high-dose steroid regimen is initiated. When there is maximal improvement, which may sometimes take 6 to 12 months, the dose is gradually reduced at a rate of 10 mg every one or two months. Many patients need long-term maintenance on low-dose steroid therapy to prevent relapses. Complications of steroid therapy include weight gain, cushingoid features, cataract, aseptic meningitis, gastrointestinal symptoms, psychiatric symptoms, and increased susceptibility to hypertension, diabetes, and infections.

Azathioprine (Imuran) has been used particularly in patients in whom steroid use is contraindicated. The dose is usually 2 to 3 mg per kg per day, with careful monitoring of liver enzymes and blood counts. An improvement may not be noted for 12 to 24 months. Adverse effects consist of increased susceptibility to opportunistic infections, anemia, leukopenia, trombocytopenia, hepatic toxicity, and possible increased risk of malignancy. Cyclosporine is used for severe MG in patients refractory to other therapies and shows a more rapid beneficial effect than azathioprine that varies from 2 weeks to 6 months. The starting dose is 2 to 5 mg per kg per day and adverse effects include nephrotoxicity, hypertension, headache, and hirsutism. Cyclophosphamide is also a potent immunosuppressive drug and can also be used in intractable patients. The dose is 3 to 5 mg per kg per day orally in divided doses or 200 mg intravenously weekly. Side effects include leukopenia, hemorrhagic cystitis, anorexia, nausea and vomiting, and alopecia.

Plasma exchange or IVIG may also be used in some patients. These treatments are particularly indicated in the settings of acute exacerbations, such as impending myasthenic crisis or actual crisis, exacerbation due to steroids, or prior to thymectomy.

Brachial Plexopathy

Vignette

A 65-year-old retired teacher has been complaining, for the last three months, of severe left upper extremity pain, particularly at night when lying in bed. She felt some weakness when trying to open a jar and tingling and numbness radiating down the medial arm and forearm into the little and ring fingers. On examination there was weakness and atrophy of the left abductor pollicis brevis and first dorsal interosseus. The flexor pollicis longus was quite weak. Hypoesthesia was present in the left fifth finger and medial aspect of the fourth finger and forearm. Five years ago she underwent left mastectomy, followed by radiation and chemotherapy.

Summary A 65-year-old woman experiencing progressive left upper extremity pain as well as left hand weakness, atrophy, numbness, and paresthesias. Past medical history is significant for breast cancer treated by mastectomy, radiation, and chemotherapy.

Localization

This patient presented with weakness of muscles innervated by the C_8–T_1 roots via the lower trunk and medial cord of the brachial plexus. The sensory findings do not suggest an ulnar nerve lesion because there is also involvement of the medial forearm indicating pathology of the plexus or nerve roots. The medial antebrachial cutaneous sensory nerve, which supplies sensation to the medial forearm, originates from the medial cord of the brachial plexus. The patient has a history of breast cancer treated with radiotherapy. This may underlie the possibility of a metastatic process because brachial plexus involvement by breast but also lung carcinoma, melanoma, lymphoma, and sarcoma is well documented. Spread of breast cancer to the lateral group of axillary lymph nodes causes compression or invasion of the lower brachial plexus carrying nerve fibers of the C_8–T_1 roots (Stubgen and Elliot).

Since the patient in the vignette received radiation therapy to treat the neoplasm, it is extremely important to distinguish between metastatic and radiation plexopathy. Brachial plexopathy related to radiation therapy or metastatic cancer may both manifest months to years after the initial treatment. Malignant brachial plexopathy is usually characterized by severe pain and tends to affect the lower trunk in the majority of patients. Therefore, since the lower trunk is formed from the C_8–T_1 roots, all ulnar muscles and the median C_8–T_1 muscles are involved. The area of sensory loss and paresthesias includes the medial arm, medial forearm, medial hand, and fourth and fifth fingers. Horner's syndrome can also develop more commonly in malignant plexopathy due to invasion of the sympathetic trunk. Radiation plexopathy is related to the dose of radiation received and can sometimes be difficult to differentiate from malignant plexopathy. Malignant brachial plexopathy as stated, usually presents with severe pain, preferential involvement of the lower brachial plexus, and Horner's syndrome. In contrast, in radiation plexopathy, which usually occurs months to years after the exposure to doses greater than 6000 rads, pain is mild to moderate and lymphedema can be prominent. Horner's syndrome is not common and myothymic discharges can frequently be found.

Diagnosis

The diagnosis is based on neuroimaging studies that in cases of tumor invasion may demonstrate a hyperintense mass on T_2-weighted images that may enhance with gadolinium. In cases of radiation fibrosis, a nonenhancing low intense signal mass on T_2 will be seen. Electrodiagnostic studies may show prominent myothymic discharges and fasciculations in radiation plexopathy.

Electrodiagnostic studies help distinguish plexopathy from radiculopathy. A brachial plexus lesion characteristically demonstrates abnormal sensory nerve action potential (SNAP) amplitudes, as opposed to a lesion at the root level where they remain normal (sensory nerve action potential remains normal in lesions proximal to the dorsal root ganglion). Needle EMG shows normal paraspinal muscles as well as rhomboids and serratus anterior muscles in lesions of the plexus.

Treatment

The treatment of malignant plexopathy is based on management of tumor invasion with chemotherapy or radiation therapy and pain management.

Femoral Neuropathy

Vignette

A 72-year-old diabetic woman started complaining of left leg pain and weakness 10 days after undergoing total hip replacement. Following the operation she developed deep vein thrombosis and was placed on anticoagulant therapy with an INR of 3. On examination, right knee extension and hip flexion were weak (MRC 3/5), with normal thigh adduction and ankle dorsiflexion. There was decreased sensation in the right anterior thigh and medial leg. Right knee jerk could not be elicited. Plantar responses were flexor.

Summary A 72-year-old woman complaining of left leg pain, weakness of left knee extension and hip flexion, hypoesthesia in the area of left anterior thigh and medial leg, and absent left knee jerk. The past medical history is significant for total hip replacement and deep vein thrombosis treated with anticoagulants.

Localization

The distribution of weakness and sensory loss points to left femoral nerve involvement. The weakness typically affects the left quadriceps and ileopsoas muscles with paralysis of left knee extension and left hip flexion. The distribution of sensory loss involves the left anterior thigh and medial leg. Left knee jerk is also absent. The involvement of the ileopsoas muscle causing hip flexion weakness localizes the lesion proximal to the inguinal ligament. Femoral neuropathy needs to be differentiated from lumbar plexopathy and L2–L4 radiculopathy. Typically a plexus lesion causes weakness, sensory loss, and reflex loss that are not limited to the territory of a simple root or nerve. Lumbar plexopathies affect particularly the L_2–L_4 fibers, resulting in weakness of the quadriceps and ileopsoas muscles (innervated by the femoral nerve) and thigh adductors muscles (innervated by the obturator nerves). The knee jerk can be decreased or absent. Sensory loss may extend over the lateral, anterior, and medial thigh and sometimes the medial calf. L2–L4 radiculopathies are characterized by weakness that also involves hip adductors and ankle dorsiflexors muscles, which are spared in cases of femoral neuropathy.

Assuming that this patient has a femoral neuropathy, several important causes need to be discussed:

- Acute retroperitoneal hemorrhage, particularly in patients undergoing anticoagulation or in cases of coagulopathy, should be ruled out promptly by computed tomography (CT) or magnetic resonance imaging (MRI) of the pelvis. This may be the situation that occurred in the patient in the vignette who was treated with anticoagulants after developing deep vein thrombosis (DVT).
- Femoral nerve compression can occur after abdominal aneurysm rupture or femoral artery catheterization complicated by hemorrhage.
- Pelvic masses, such as neoplasm, abscess, cyst, or lymphoadenopathy, as well as abdominal or pelvic surgery may also cause femoral nerve dysfunction.
- Compression of the femoral nerve at the inguinal ligament has been observed after prolonged lithotomy position during laparoscopy, vaginal hysterectomy, and so on.
- Stretch injury or diabetes complicated by nerve infarction can also cause a femoral neuropathy.

Diagnosis

Electrodiagnosis is often useful in differentiating a femoral neuropathy from plexopathy and radiculopathy. Ultrasound and MRI are effective measures for diagnosing iliacus hematoma. Management depends on the etiology.

Postpartum Plexopathy

Vignette

A 28-year-old woman started complaining of difficulty walking and right foot numbness one day after the delivery of her baby. Labor was prolonged and complicated by fetal distress, therefore a decision to perform a cesarean section was made. On examination there was marked weakness of right ankle dorsiflexion, eversion, and inversion and moderate weakness of hip extension and internal rotation. Hip flexion and knee extension were normal. There was an area of hypoesthesia to pinprick in the right lateral leg and dorsum of the foot. Deep tendon reflexes including ankle jerk were normal and symmetrical.

Summary A 28-year-old woman with acute onset of right lower extremity weakness and numbness one day postpartum. Labor was prolonged and difficult, and complicated by fetal distress.

Localization

In order to localize, we need to consider the weak muscles and the area of sensory loss. Weakness involving the ankle dorsiflexors and evertors of the foot placed the lesion in the territory of the peroneal nerve. Foot inversion due to tibialis posterior muscle has a predominant tibial nerve innervation. Hip extension and internal rotation are gluteal innervated muscles and their involvement indicates a lesion that is not confined only to the peroneal territory. Therefore the pathological process should be placed at the level of the lumbosacral trunk or the L5 root. The lumbosacral trunk consists primarily of the L5 root with an additional component from the L4 root.

When the lumbosacral trunk is affected the weakness includes ankle and toe dorsiflexion eversion, inversion and toe flexion.The gluteus muscles (gluteus medius and minimus and tensor fascia lata which abduct and rotate the thigh internally, and the gluteus maximus which extends, abducts, and rotates the thigh externally) as well as the hamstrings (flexion of the leg at the knee) can also be involved. Plantar flexion and ankle jerk are usually normal. The area of sensory abnormality commonly extends in the L5 dermatomal distribution. It is not always easy to differentiate a lumbosacral trunk lesion from L5 radiculopathy, because the weakness in both conditions involves the L5 myotome. Labor and delivery can be complicated by a lesion compressing the lumbosacral trunk, particularly in prolonged and difficult labor and if other factors such as abnormal presentation, a large fetal head, and a small maternal pelvis are present. The prognosis is usually good with full recovery.

Mononeuritis Multiplex

Vignette

A 65-year-old man had a three-week history of left foot pain and numbness, followed by the abrupt onset of left foot drop. The following week, right wrist drop developed as well as weakness of the left hand grip and numbness involving the ring and the little fingers of the left hand. On examination there was moderate weakness of the right wrist extensors, all finger extensors, and the brachioradialis, and decreased pain and touch on the dorsum of the right hand. On the left upper extremity, first dorsal interossens, abductor digiti minimi and flexor digitorum profundus to digits 4 and 5 were markedly weak, and there was diminished sensation in the left hypothenar region and digits 4 and 5. The left foot had weakness of toe and ankle dorsiflexion and there was diminished sensation below both knees. Past medical history included several months of fatigue, progressive weight loss, and low-grade fever.

Summary A 65-year-old man with history of left foot drop, right wrist drop, and bilateral weakness and sensory involvement associated with systemic signs (fever, weight loss, fatigue).

Localization

There is involvement of multiple peripheral nerves (right radial, left ulnar, and left peroneal) in an asymmetrical pattern typical of mononeuritis multiplex. Mononeuropathy multiplex is characterized by asymmetrical, stepwise progression of individual cranial or peripheral neuropathies (Preston and Shapiro). Specific etiological factors need to be investigated, in particular the possibility of vasculitis and vasculitic neuropathy. Many disorders are described among the vasculitic syndromes but the peripheral nerve is most frequently involved in polyarteritis nodosa, Wegener's granulomatosis, and the allergic angiitis and the granulomatosis syndromes. Mononeuropathy multiplex has long been considered the hallmark of peripheral nerve involvement in systemic necrotizing vasculitis (Aminoff). The symptoms can develop acutely or insidiously and may be accompanied by severe neuritic pain. Cranial neuropathies tend to preferentially involve the trigeminal, facial, and vestibuloacoustic nerves (Aminoff).

Aside from vasculitis, other disorders can present with a multifocal picture. These include chronic inflammatory demyelinating polyradiculoneuropathy; infectious processes such as leprosy; Lyme disease, HIV, HTLV-1, herpes zoster, and hepatitis A. Mononeuritis multiplex can occur in association with cancer and granulomatous disorders due to infiltration of peripheral nerves. Diabetes can also be complicated by multiple focal neuropathies occurring as a result of ischemia or as a result of pressure or entrapment. Other disorders to be mentioned are genetic neuropathies (hereditary neuropathy with liability to pressure palsies).

Vasculitis Neuropathies

Vasculitis characterized by inflammation and necrosis of the vessel wall with subsequent ischemia may involve the peripheral nerves. The peripheral neuropathy is an early manifestation of vasculitis and can have different presentations, such as features typical of mononeuritis multiplex; overlapping (extensive) multiple mononeuropathies; or distal symmetrical polyneuropathy. Mononeuritis multiplex is characterized by dysesthesia, sensory loss, and weakness along multiple peripheral nerves, cranial nerves, or both. Symptoms may be acute or indolent, and the neuropathy can occur in isolation or as part of systemic involvement with multiorgan failure or connective tissue disorders.

Diagnosis

The diagnosis is based on serological studies, electrodiagnostic studies, and nerve biopsy. Laboratory tests include standard tests, such as complete blood count and chemistry panel, as well immunological tests such as antinuclear antigen, rheumatoid factor, serum complement levels, and so on. Other immunological tests are indicated selectively (e.g., ANCA [antineurophil cytoplasmic antibodies], serum cytokines, antibodies to endothelial cell antigens). Also HIV, HTVL-1, Lyme, hepatitis B and C, and glycosylated hemoglobin can be sought in selective cases.

Electrophysiological studies may demonstrate low amplitude or absent response of the sensory or motor action potential. Conduction block occurs in some patients. Needle EMG shows signs of denervation. Nerve biopsy may demonstrate inflammation and necrosis of the vessel wall in the acute stages and later intimal proliferation and hyperplasia.

Treatment

The treatment of vasculitic neuropathy is based on immunosuppresive therapy, particularly in patients with underlying systemic necrotizing vasculitis. The approach is a combination of agents, including prednisone and a cytotoxic agent (usually cyclophosphamide).

Differential Diagnosis of Mononeuritis Multiplex

- Vasculitis
    Polyarteritis nodosa
    Wegener's granulomatosis
    Churg-Strauss syndrome
    Lymphomatoid granulomatosis
    Cryoglobulinemia
    Sjögren syndrome
    Systemic lupus erythematosus
    Rheumatoid arthritis
- Infections
    Leprosy
    Lyme disease
    HIV, HTLV-1
    Herpes zoster
    Hepatitis
    Cytomegalovirus
- Infiltration
    Granulomatous disease: Sarcoidosis
    Neoplastic disorders: Leukemia, lymphoma
- Multiple entrapment
    Hereditary neuropathy with lability to pressure palsies
    Acquired multiple entrapment neuropathies
- Diabetes
- Multifocal demyelinating neuropathy with persistent conduction block

Inflammatory Myopathies

Polymyositis

Vignette

A 65-year-old housewife began complaining of weakness, fatigue, and shortness of breath after brief physical exercise. She could not exactly tell when her symptoms started, but could recall that less than one year ago she first noticed fatigue on walking long distances and some trouble climbing stairs. Six month ago she developed some difficulty swallowing solid food. Her leg weakness worsened and she needed a cane for support. She also noticed some pain in her shoulders and could not lift her grocery bags from the supermarket. She denied any sensory complaints, as well as diplopia, dysarthria, or visual disturbances. There was no family history of neuromuscular disorders. On examination she had difficulty lifting her arms against resistance and the neck flexors seemed to be weak. She was barely able to flex her hips against gravity. DTR were reduced, plantar responses were flexor, and sensory examination was normal.

Summary A 65-year-old woman with progressive proximal weakness, dysphagia, fatigue, and shortness of breath on exertion. The neurological examination shows proximal and neck flexor weakness, reduced DTR, and normal sensation.

Localization

The localization points to a disorder of the motor unit, which has several components: anterior horn cell, motor axon, neuromuscular junction, and muscle fibers. The case as summarized describes a patient with progressive symmetrical weakness and hyporeflexia in the absence of sensory symptoms, therefore we can narrow the diagnosis to specific pathology. Considering the muscle disorders first, the pattern of progressive subacute symmetrical proximal weakness points to the possibility of an idiopathic inflammatory myopathy, typically polymyositis, particularly if metabolic, toxic, endocrine, and familiar disorders are excluded (Dalakas). Features supporting the diagnosis and present in the vignette are the distribution of the weakness which is proximal and symmetrical, the lack of dermatological findings such as a rash, as well as lack of ocular or facial dysfunction. Dysphagia can also be part of the clinical manifestation. Muscle pain and tenderness is usually an early finding. Hyporeflexia and areflexia can be observed particularly in cases of severe weakness and atrophy. The absence of sensory symptoms and the presence of myalgia support a myopathic process but lack of sensory abnormalities is also associated with motor neuropathies and anterior horn cell disorders. The dyspnea on exertion can be explained by interstitial lung disease, which occurs in approximately 10 percent of patients affected with polymyositis, at least half of whom have Jo-1 antibodies (Amato and Barohn).

Other inflammatory myopathies, such as dermatomyositis and inclusion body myositis, need to be excluded before confirming the diagnosis. Dermatomyositis is accompanied or preceded by the characteristic rash characterized by a purplish discoloration of the eyelids (Amato and Barohn) often accompanied by periorbital edema. Inclusion body myositis, which affects predominantly older men, is characterized by early weakness and atrophy and preferential involvement of certain groups of muscles, such as the quadriceps, wrist and finger flexors, and foot extensors muscles.

Muscular dystrophies such as facioscapulohumeral dystrophy (FSH) and myotonic dystrophy need to be considered in the differential diagnosis. FSH is an autosomic dominant disorder characterized by marked facial weakness and scapular winging. The tibialis anterior muscle is usually the earliest affected muscle in the lower extremities (Dumitru et al.). Patients with myotonic dystrophy have a characteristic facial appearance due to weakness and atrophy of the facial and masseter/temporalis muscles (Dumitru et al.). Frontal balding is also observed. The distribution of weakness in the lower extremities is predominantly distal. Myotonia characterized by a delayed muscle relaxation after contraction is very important for the diagnosis.

In the differential diagnosis of polymyositis, systemic etiologies need to be excluded, in particular infectious processes, and endocrine and toxic disorders. Viral, parasitic and fungal infections (HIV, HTLV-1, echovirus, coxsackievirus, trichinosis, toxoplasmosis, etc.) can all cause a myopathy usually associated with other systemic symptoms.

Endocrinopathies are frequently associated with myopathies, in particular thyroid disorders (hypothyroidism, hyperthyroidism, hyperparathyroidism), Cushing's syndrome, and pituitary disorders. Myopathies associated with electrolyte disturbances include, in particular, hypokalemia, hyperkalemia, hypophosphatemia, and hypermagnesemia. Toxic myopathies are numerous and the best known is the steroid myopathy. Other drug-induced myopathies are associated with the use of cimetidine, procainamide, levodopa, phenytoin, colchicine, vincristine, and so on. Toxic myopathies are associated with chronic alcohol abuse, toluene inhalation, and so on.

Other systemic disorders that can cause muscle disease are diabetes, amyloidosis, neoplastic and paraneoplastic disorders, and sarcoidosis.

Considering the neuromuscular junction disorders, myasthenia gravis and Lambert-Eaton myasthenic syndrome enter the differential diagnosis. There is nothing in the vignette to suggest a neuromuscular junction defect. Patients with generalized myasthenia gravis can manifest with proximal weakness, but fatigability and fluctuation of the symptoms that frequently involves the extraocular and bulbar muscles are important characteristics. LEMS typically presents with proximal weakness and hyporeflexia that improves with brief muscular contractions. Autonomic symptoms, in particular dry mouth, are also an important part of the diagnosis.

Anterior horn cell disorders include ALS and spinal muscular atrophy. ALS has signs of upper and lower motor neuron dysfunction and is unlikely to be mistaken for a myopathy. Spinal muscular atrophy characterized by proximal weakness and marked atrophy associated with hyporeflexia or areflexia is a hereditary disorder that manifests in the third decade of life and can be easily excluded by the vignette.

Considering disorders of the peripheral nerves, chronic inflammatory demyelinating polyneuropathy (CIDP) characterized by progressive, stepwise or relapsing muscle weakness, predominantly proximal, also enters the differential diagnosis. Sensory symptoms are an important part of this disorder and can be prominent, and manifesting different degrees of severity from mild distal numbness and paresthesias to severe sensory involvement and even sensory ataxia (Mendell et al.).

Clinical Features

Polymyositis is an inflammatory disorder of muscles more prevalent in women characterized by progressive symmetrical weakness of the upper and lower extremities and neck muscles. The distribution of weakness is predominantly proximal but distal muscles can be affected in more advanced stages of the disease. Deep tendon reflexes are usually normal but can be diminished or absent in cases of severe weakness and atrophy. Sensation is always intact. Extraocular muscles are normal and facial muscles are only rarely and mildly affected. Frequent complaints are muscle pain, tenderness, and fatigue. Due to the proximal weakness, affected patients notice difficulty climbing stairs, blow drying and combing their hair, and getting up from a low seat.

Polymyositis is defined by Dalakas as a diagnosis of exclusion. Characteristic features that exclude this disorder are the presence of a rash, extraocular or facial muscle weakness, family history significant for neuromuscular disorders, endocrine disorder, toxic or drug-related myopathy, inclusion body myositis, neurogenic disease, dystrophy or biochemically defined muscle disease. Dysphagia can also occur and can vary in severity due to pharyngeal and esophageal muscle weakness and impaired motility. Systemic complications are due to cardiac involvement manifesting with pericarditis, congestive heart failure, dilated cardiomyopathy, pulmonary hypertension and so on. Interstitial lung disease, which affects at least 10 percent of patients, at least half of whom have Jo-1 antibodies (Amato and Barohn), manifests with nonproductive cough and dyspnea. Connective tissue disorders, such as systemic lupus erythematosus, rheumatoid arthritis, and Sjögren's syndrome, can also be associated with polymyositis. According to Dalakas, the risk of malignancy, which is increased in dermatomyositis, is not frequently associated with polymyositis or inclusion body myositis (Dalakas).

Diagnosis

The laboratory studies in polymyositis include primarily the determination of serum CK level, which may be increased up to 50 times the upper limit of normal. However, it does not consistently correlate with disease activity or severity and can be normal in some cases. Other enzymes, including SGOT, SGPT, and LDH, may also be elevated. Myositic specific autoantibodies (MSA) to nuclear and cytoplasmatic antigens involved in protein synthesis may be found in polymyositis, in particular anti-Jo-1, which is detected in 20 percent of patients and is associated with interstitial lung disease (Dumitru).

Electrodiagnostic studies may demonstrate normal motor and sensory nerve conduction and profuse spontaneous activity on needle EMG. The fibrillation potentials are more commonly seen in the paraspinal muscles (thoracic), followed by the proximal shoulder and hip muscles (Shapiro and Preston). In acute and subacute cases MUAPS are short in duration, low in amplitude, and polyphasic with early recruitment (myopathic units). In chronic polymyositis (lasting longer than one year) MUAPS become long in duration with many components, but the early recruitment points to the myopathic process.

Muscle biopsy demonstrates endomysial inflammation with invasion of nonnecrotic muscle fibers, variability in fiber size, and so on.

Treatment

Corticosteroids are the first line of treatment. A single, high daily dose of 80 to 100 mg can be given for four weeks and than changed to an alternate-day regimen for four to six months which is thereafter tapered at a rate of 5 mg every two to three weeks until the lowest effective dose is reached. Adverse effects of corticosteroids include weight gain, hyperglycemia, menstrual irregularities, hypertension, edema, osteoporosis, hypertension, and psychosis.

Nonsteroidal immunosuppressive therapy is indicated if patients do not respond to the use of steroids, relapse during taper, or have intolerable side effects. Azathioprine is given at a dose of 2 to 3mg per kg per day but has the disadvantage of taking several months in order to show its efficacy. Adverse effects include bone marrow suppression, pancytopenia, nausea, anorexia, abdominal pain, liver toxicity, and pancreatitis. Methotrexate can be tried intravenously at weekly dose of up to 0.8 mg/kg, or orally up to a total of 25 mg weekly. Adverse effects include alopecia, pneumonitis, stomatitis, renaltoxicity, hepatotoxicity, and malignancies. Cyclophosphamide is given intravenously or orally at 1 to 2 mg/kg. Side effects include nausea, vomiting, alopecia, hemorrhagic cystitis, and bone marrow toxicity.

Plasmapheresis did not show efficacy in several studies. IVIG can be used if steroids and nonsteroidal immunosuppressive therapies have failed. When the treatment of polymyositis is ineffective, other possible diagnoses should be considered (inclusion body myositis or other diseases).

Dermatomyositis

Dermatomyositis, which affects children in the first decade of life and adults, preferentially women, is characterized by the typical rash that can accompany or precede the onset of muscle weakness. The skin manifestations are characterized by a bluish discoloration of the eyelids often associated with periorbital edema and a flat, erythematous rash involving the face, neck, anterior chest, shoulders, and upper back. Subcutaneous calcifications of different sizes over pressure points can be observed in children with severe disorder and inadequate treatment, but are rare in adults. Muscle weakness is subacute and progressive, and involves the proximal muscles, often accompanied by myalgia, fatigue, low-grade fever, dysphagia, and dysarthria.

Systemic complications are common and tend to involve the heart and lungs. The association with cancer is increased in patients with dermatomyositis. Ovarian cancer is most frequent, followed by intestinal, breast, lung, and liver cancer (Dalakas). Muscle biopsy reveals the characteristic perifascicular atrophy.

Inclusion Body Myositis

Vignette

A 62-year-old banker complained of difficulty walking for the last five years, with occasional tripping and falling. His left leg was especially bothersome when climbing stairs. He also noticed some difficulties using his right hand, particularly when opening cans. He claims that all his problems started after his left knee replacement surgery. No other medical history could be found. On examination, he had mild weakness of the neck flexor muscles and right wrist and finger flexors. There was also moderate weakness and atrophy of bilateral knee extension and ankle dorsiflexion worse on the left. DTR were symmetrically present and plantar responses were flexor. No sensory abnormalities were noted.

Summary 62-year-old man with a history of slowly progressive (five years) weakness of neck and right upper and both lower extremities with atrophy. Weakness mainly involved neck flexor, right wrist and finger flexors, bilateral knee extensors, and ankle dorsiflexors. No sensory or reflex abnormalities.

Key words: Asymmetrical pure motor weakness.

Localization

There is no doubt that the localization in this difficult vignette is the motor unit. The element involved (anterior horn cell, motor axon, neuromuscular junction, or muscle) must be decided. Progressive asymmetrical muscle weakness can be caused by disorders of the anterior horn cells, polyradiculopathies, multiple mononeuropathies, polyneuropathies, and myopathies. Clinical consideration in the differential diagnosis of this vignette should be given to motor neuron disease/motor neuropathy or myopathy. There are definitely no elements suggesting a neuromuscular junction defect. Considering first a motor neuron disease, ALS can initially present with signs of lower motor neuron involvement characterized by weakness, atrophy, cramps, and fasciculations. In the majority of patients, later on signs of upper motor neuron involvement usually appear with spasticity, hyperreflexia, and pathological reflexes. Only a minority of patients (8 to 10 percent) diagnosed with the clinical variant of ALS, progressive muscular atrophy, have pure lower motor neuron signs.

Disorders of peripheral nerves, such as multifocal motor neuropathy, can present with progressive asymmetrical distal weakness and atrophy in the distribution of individual peripheral nerves. Cramps, fasciculations, and hyporeflexia also occur and sensation is intact. A demyelinating neuropathy with conduction block in multiple upper and lower limb nerves is the hallmark of this disorder. Therefore, even if MMN should be part of the differential diagnosis, it does not explain all the findings of the vignette.

Considering myopathic processes, inclusion body myositis (IBM) may clearly explain the findings in the vignette, especially the typical distribution of weakness, which preferentially involves the quadriceps, wrist and finger flexors, and ankle dorsiflexors; the age of the patient; and the long evolution of the process.

Clinical Features and Diagnosis

Inclusion body myositis, which tend to affect older males after the fifth decade of life, is characterized by insidious, slowly progressive asymmetrical weakness that involves proximal and distal muscles. Some muscle groups are preferentially involved, particularly the quadriceps, wrist and finger flexors, and ankle dorsiflexors. Dysphagia is also common. Extraocular muscles are never affected. Chronic progressive asymmetrical quadriceps and wrist/finger flexor weakness that occur in a patient over age 50 strongly suggests the diagnosis of IBM. IBM is not complicated by cardiac or pulmonary dysfunction, and is not associated with increased risk of malignancy. Laboratory studies show minimal to mild elevation of the serum CK. EMG shows motor units of different amplitude and duration, prominent fibrillations, and positive sharp waves. Muscle biopsy shows rimmed vacuoles in muscle fibers and endomysial inflammatory cells invading nonnecrotic fibers. Amyloid deposition can be demonstrated using Congo red staining.

Treatment

There is no definitive treatment. Steroid therapy and immunosuppressive treatments as well as high doses of intravenous immunoglobulin infusion only show a modest and transitory beneficial effect.

References

Motor Neuron Disease

ALS: Misdiagnosis and diagnostic dilemmas. American Academy of Neurology, 49th annual meeting, Boston, April 12–19, 1997.

Belsh, J.M. and Schiffman, P.L. Amyotrophic lateral sclerosis: Diagnosis and management for the clinician. New York: Futura, 1996.

Bromberg, M. Accelerating the diagnosis of amyotrophic lateral sclerosis. Neurologist 5:63–74, March 1999.

Case records of the Massachusetts General Hospital. Case 21. N. Engl. J. Med. 1326–1335, 1987.

Case records of the Massachusetts General Hospital. Case 36. N. Engl. J. Med. 1406–1411, 1995.

Dumitru, D. et al. Electrodiagnostic Medicine, ed. 2. Philadelphia: Hanley and Belfus, 2002.

Engel, A.C. and Armstrong, C.F. Myology, ed 2. New York: McGraw-Hill, 1854–1869, 1994.

Jackson, C.E. and Bryan, W.W. Amyotrophic lateral sclerosis. Semin. Neurol. 18:27–39, 1998.

Mitsumoto, H. et al. Amyotrophic Lateral Sclerosis. Contemporary neurology series. Philadelphia: F.A. Davis, 1998.

Preston, D.C. and Shapiro, B.E. Electromyography and Neuromuscular Disorders. Boston: Butterworth-Heineman, 1998.

Pryse-Phillips, Murray T.J. Essential Neurology. New York: Medical Examination Publishing, 1986.

Vinken, P.J., et al. Handbook of Clinical Neurology. Vol. 59, Diseases of the motor system. Amsterdam: Elsevier Science, 1991.

Williams, R.G. and Polin, R.S. Cervical Spondylotic Myelopathy MedLink. Arbor Publishing, 1993–2001.

Guillain-Barré Syndrome and CIDP

Barohn, R.J. Approach to peripheral neuropathy and neuronopathy. Semin. Neurol. 18:7–18, 1998.

Barohn, R.J. and Saperstein, D.S. Guillain-Barré syndrome and chronic inflammatory demyelinating polyneuropathy (abstract). Semin. Neurol. 18:49–61, 1998.

Bosch, E.P. Guillain-Barré syndrome: An update of acute immune-mediated polyradiculoneuropathies. Neurologist 4:212–226, 1998.

Case Records of the Massachusetts General Hospital, Case 39. N. Engl. J. Med. Vol. 323, No. 13, 1990.

Case Records of the Massachusetts General Hospital. Case 13. N. Engl. J. Med. April 23, 1212–1218, 1998.

Griffin, J.W. The Guillain-Barré syndrome and CIDP. American Acadamy of Neurology, 51st Annual Meeting, Toronto, 1999.

Johnson, R.T. and Griffin J.W. Peripheral nerve disorders. In: Current Therapy in Neurologic Disease, ed. 5. St. Louis: Mosby, 359–363, 1997.

Katirji B. Electromyography in Clinical Practice. St. Louis: Mosby, 1998.

Latov, N. et al. (eds.). Immunological and Infectious Diseases of the Peripheral Nerves. Cambridge: Cambridge University Press, 1998.

Mendell, J.R. et al. Peripheral neuropathy. Continuum 1:A22–67, 1994.

Mendell, J. R. et al. Diagnosis and Management of Peripheral Nerve Disorders. Oxford University Press, 2001.

Ropper, A.H. et al. Guillain-Barré Syndrome. Philadelphia: F.A. Davis, 1991.

Small, G.A. and Lovelace, R.E. Chronic inflammatory demyelinating polyneuronopathy. Semin. Neurol. 13:305–312, 1993.

Botulism

Bella, I., and Chad D.A. Neuromuscular disorders and acute respiratory failure. Neurol. Clin. North Am. 16:391–417, 1998.

Katirji, B. Electromyography in Clinical Practice. St. Louis: Mosby, 233–244, 265–275, 1998.

Ropper, A.H. et al. Guillain-Barré Syndrome. Philadelphia: F.A. Davis, 201–204, 1991.

Lambert-Eaton Myasthenic Syndrome

Case records of the Massachussetts General Hospital. Case 32. N. Engl. J. Med. 528–535, 1994.

Engel, A. and Amstrong, C.F. Myology. ed. 2. New York: McGraw-Hill, 1798–1806, 1994.

Johnson, R., and Griffin J.W. Current Therapy in Neurologic Disease, ed. 5. St Louis: Mosby, 399–400, 1997.

Katirji, B. Electromyography in Clinical Practice. St. Louis: Mosby, 233–244, 1998.

Preston, D.C. and Shapiro, B.E. Electromyography and Neuromuscular Disorders. Boston: Butterworth-Heinemann, 503–524, 1998.

Sanders, D.B. Lambert-Eaton myasthenic syndrome (LEMS). American Academy of Neurology, 52nd Annual Meeting, San Diego, 2000.

Myasthenia Gravis

Bella, I. and Chad, D.A. Neurologic emergencies: Neuromuscular disorders and acute respiratory failure. Neurol. Clin. North Am. 16:391–416, 1998.

Case records of the Massachussets General Hospital. Case 15. N. Engl. J. Med. 343:1508–1514, 2000.

Drachman, D.B. Myasthenia gravis (review article). N. Engl. J. Med. 330:1797–1810, 1994.

Dumitru, D. et al. Electrodiagnostic Medicine, ed. 2. Philadelphia: Hanley and Belfus, 2002.

Engel, A. Myasthenia gravis. Neurology MedLink. Arbor Publishing, 1993–2001.

Gooch, C.L. Myasthenia gravis and Lambert-Eaton myasthenic syndrome. In: Rolak, L.A. (ed.). Neuroimmunology for the Clinician. Boston: Butterworth-Heinemann, 263–298, 1997.

Hopkins, L.C. Clinical features of myasthenia gravis. In: Myasthenia Gravis and Myasthenic Syndromes. Neurol. Clin. North Am. 12:243–261, 1994.

Keesey, J. Six steps to manage myasthenia gravis: A treatment. Advan. Neuroimmunol. 6:3–14, 1999.

Massey, J.M. Autoimmune myasthenia and myasthenic syndromes. American Academy of Neurology, 51st Annual Meeting, Toronto, April 17–24, 1999.

Pascuzzi, R. Neuromuscular junction disorders. American Academy of Neurology, 53rd Annual Meeting, May 5–11, Philadelphia, 2001.

Brachial Plexopathy

Aminoff, M. Clinical EMG. American Academy of Neurology, 49th Annual Meeting, Boston, April 12–19, 1997.

Preston, D.C. and Shapiro, B.E. Electromyography and Neuromuscular Disorders. Boston: Butterworth-Heinemann, 433–454, 471–489, 355–389, 1998.

Stubgen, J.P. and Elliot, K.J. Malignant radiculopathy and plexopathy. In: Handbook of Clinical Neurology. Vol. 25, Neurooncology. New York: Elsevier, 71–103, 1997.

Femoral Neuropathy/Postpartum Plexopathy

Abrams, B.M. Entrapment and compressive neuropathies: Lower extremities. In: Progr. Neurol. Sept. 2000.

Katirji, B. Electromyography in Clinical Practice. St. Louis: Mosby, 39–54, 47–54, 1998.

Preston, D.C. and Shapiro B.E. Electromyography and Neuromuscular Disorders Boston: Butterworth-Heinemann, 319–327, 471–489, 1998.

Mononeuritis Multiplex

Aminoff, M. Neurology and General Medicine. New York: Churchill Livingstone, 389–412, 1989.

Mendell, J. R., et al. Peripheral neuropathy. Continuum. 1:A22–67, 1994.

Mendell, J.R., et al. Diagnosis and Management of Peripheral Nerve Disorders. Oxford: Oxford University Press, 202–232, 2001.

Preston, D.C. and Shapiro, B.E. Electromyography and Neuromuscular Disorders. Boston: Butterworth-Heinemann, 358–359, 1998.

Stewart, J.D. Focal Peripheral Neuropathies, Ed 2. New York: Raven Press, 431–450, 1993.

Inflammatory Myopathies

Amato, A. and Barohn, R.J. Idiopathic inflammatory myopathies. Neurol. Clin. 15:615–148. 1997.

Amato, A. and Barohn, R.J. Evaluation and treatment of inflammatory myopathies. American Academy of Neurology, 53rd Annual Meeting, May 5–11, Philadelphia, 2001.

Case Records of the Massachusetts General Hospital. Case 40. N. Engl. J. Med. 1026–1035, 1991.

Dalakas M. Strategy in immunotherapy: Case studies in autoimmune peripheral neuropathies. In: Advances in Neuroimmunology 5:1, 1998.

Dalakas, M.C. Polymyositis "inflammatory myopathies." MedLink Arbor Publishing, 1993–2001.

Dalakas, M.C. How to diagnose and treat the inflammatory myopathies. Semin. Neurol. 14:137–145, 1994.

Dumitru, D. et al. Electrodiagnostic Medicine, ed. 2. Philadelphia: Hanley and Belfus, 2002.

Engel, A.C. and Armstrong, C.F. Myology. ed. 2. New York: McGraw-Hill, 1335–1383, 1994.

Karpati, G. Inclusion body myositis. Neurologist 3:201–208. 1997.

Mendell, J.R. et al. Diagnosis and Management of Peripheral Nerve Disorders. Oxford: Oxford University Press, 192–201, 2001.

7
Cerebrovascular Disorders in Adults

Sinus Thrombosis

Sagittal Sinus Thrombosis

Vignette

A 30-year-old woman, three days after the delivery of her baby, started complaining of severe generalized headache. She was brought to a local emergency room by her concerned husband and discharged on ibuprofen with the diagnosis of tension headache. The headache persisted, accompanied by transient blurriness of vision especially when stooping down. She then experienced a generalized tonic-clonic seizure. In the emergency room she was drowsy and uncooperative. A bilateral papilledema was noted. She could move her arms but had moderate weakness of both lower extremities. A bilateral Babinski's sign was also noted. She was too uncooperative for the sensory examination.

Summary A 30-year-old woman, three days postpartum, experiencing headache, blurriness of vision and a generalized tonic-clonic seizure. Neurological examination shows evidence of papilledema, paraparesis, and bilateral Babinski's sign.

> **Key words:** Postpartum, headache, seizure.

Localization

The vignette includes signs of intracranial hypertension represented by headache and papilledema and focal cerebral signs characterized by paraparesis and bilateral Babinski's signs. Focal symptoms and signs and generalized seizures indicate unilateral or bilateral cerebral hemispheric involvement.

Differential Diagnosis

The differential diagnosis includes

- Cerebrovascular disorders.
- Space-occupying lesions.
- Infectious and inflammatory disorders.

The fact that the vignette indicates the puerperium makes it important to consider all the possible causes that can create this neurological picture in the postpartum period. Considering first the cerebrovascular disorders, arterial and venous occlusive disorders and subarachnoid hemorrhage must be distinguished. It may be difficult to determine if the etiology of an acute cerebrovascular event is due to an arterial or venous occlusion.

The clinical characteristics described, such as prominent headache, papilledema and seizures, and the situation in which they occurred, may point to the possibility of venous thrombosis. Imaging studies, which were unavailable, may demonstrate in this case bilateral hemorrhagic infarction in the high parasagittal convexities or hemorrhagic infarction, which does not follow a specific arterial distribution (Broderick).

1. Occlusive arterial disease that occurs during pregnancy or the postpartum period can be attributed to various etiologies such as cardiac disorders causing cerebral embolization, coagulopathies, vasculitis, hypercoagulable states, atheromatous thrombosis, and so on. Predisposing factors during pregnancy and the puerperium include hormonal changes, coagulation factors, abnormalities and hypertension.

2. Subarachnoid hemorrhage (SAH) may occur during pregnancy and cause an acute vascular event. Causes include aneurysmal rupture, cerebral arteriovenous malformations accompanied by hemorrhage, placental abruption with diffuse intravascular coagulation, mycotic aneurysm rupture, cerebral vasculitis complicated by hemorrhage, and so on. Symptoms of SAH

may include severe headache, seizures, focal signs, changes in mental status, stupor and coma.

3. Other conditions such as neoplastic (tumor), infectious (meningitis, encephalitis abscess) and inflammatory (vasculitis) processes also enter the differential diagnosis of an acute neurological event with headache, seizures, and focal signs. The possibility of pituitary apoplexy, which increases in a pregnant woman during the time of delivery, and is characterized by headache, visual abnormalities, and altered consciousness, is an important consideration.

4. Occlusive venous disease is the preferred diagnosis. Cerebral venous thrombosis (CVT) during pregnancy or the puerperium is the etiological factor most commonly identified in cerebral venous thrombosis and occurs in about 20 percent of patients (Bousser and Russell). CVT should be suspected in any woman manifesting neurological symptoms in the postpartum period since nearly 15 percent of cases occur in the first two days after a normal childbirth (Cantu). CVT is particularly significant in underdeveloped countries, and an hypercoagulable state is the main cause. During the puerperium, hematological changes include elevated levels of procoagulant proteins, decreased protein S levels, and inhibition of fibrinolysis (Bousser and Russell 1997). Systemic or localized infections such as bacterial sepsis, otitis, sinusitis, orbital cellulitis, and so on, as well as inflammatory disorders such as systemic lupus erythematosus and Behçet's disease can also be the causative factor of CVT. Hematological disorders can predispose to the occurrence of CVT, particularly polycythaemia, sickle cell disease, leukemia, primary trombocytopenia, and paroxysmal nocturnal hemoglobinuria. Also, coagulopathies such as protein C, S deficiency and antithrombin III deficiency may increase the risk of CVT. Venous thrombosis can complicate cancer, nephrotic syndrome, and marked dehydration.

Clinical Features

Cerebral venous thrombosis can manifest with various modes of presentation that can be acute, subacute, or chronic depending upon the onset of the symptoms—respectively, less than 48 hours, less than 30 days, or more than 30 days. Headache is the presenting manifestation in most patients (at least 80 percent of cases with CVT according to Bousser and Russell). Papilledema, which is seen more frequently in association with CVT that occurs in the postpartum period, is another frequent finding in at least half of patients (Bousser and Russell) and can be accompanied by bilateral visual obscurations.

Seizures are also a frequent manifestation and can be focal, generalized, or both. Focal neurological deficits are seen in over half the patients and consist of hemiparesis, paraparesis, aphasia, sensory loss, and cerebellar dysfunction. The focal findings often help in localizing the lesion; for example, cavernous sinus thrombosis usually manifests with complete ophthalmoplegia; sagittal sinus thrombosis may be characterized by paraparesis, tetraparesis, or alternating hemiparesis; jugular venous thrombosis may involve the ninth and tenth cranial nerves.

Transient ischemic attacks or migraine-like phenomena (Ameri and Bousser) are also described.

Diagnosis

CAT scan of the brain may demonstrate some suggestive findings:

- The cord sign on unenhanced CT indicating a thrombosed cortical vein has a picture of a linear increased density.
- The dense triangle sign suggests acute thrombus in the superior sagittal sinus.
- The empty delta sign on enhanced CT scan indicates a defect in the contrast-filled sagittal sinus.

Magnetic resonance imaging (MRI) is more sensitive than CT in discovering parenchymal abnormalities. In the first stages, absence of flow void is noted and the occluded vessel remains isointense on T_1- and hypointense on T_2-weighted images. The intermediate changes are demonstrated by high intense signal of the thrombus initially on T_1- and then on T_2-weighted images. Later, there will be hyperintensity on T_1 and isointensity or hyperintensity on T_2.

Angiography remains the definitive diagnostic test, particularly when there is a high index of suspicion and MRI is not available. It will show absence of opacification of veins or sinuses.

CSF studies may show elevated opening pressure and increase protein level and cells.

Prognosis

The mortality rates of CVT varies from 6 to 38 percent (Bousser and Russell). A poor outcome is associated with the type of involvement, particularly if there is evidence of a massive hemorrhagic infarct. Important factors that complicate the prognosis are intractable seizures, sepsis, pulmonary embolism, and underlying conditions, such as cancer or infection (Bousser and Russell). Prognosis is worse in infants and the elderly, or in patients with severe altered level of consciousness and focal neurological findings (Bousser and Russell). According to these authors, thrombosis of the deep venous system and cerebellar veins also may be a poor prognostic factor.

Treatment

The treatment is based on two important aspects:

- Symptomatic: For appropriate control of seizure and to reduce intracranial pressure.
- Antithrombotic: Heparin followed by warfarin.

There is clear agreement on the beneficial effect of heparin in patients with CVT, but there is disagreement on the best indications and duration of treatment.

After a few days of heparin, warfarin is administered, monitoring the INR on a range between 2 and 3.

Subarachnoid Hemorrhage

Vignette

A 33-year-old legal secretary was brought to the emergency room by her sister because of headache, generalized weakness, and decreased level of consciousness. One day prior to this event, after lifting a heavy box of books, the patient developed severe left temple and orbital pain that quickly radiated to her neck. She vomited several times before finding her way to bed, where she thought she might have lost consciousness momentarily. Her sister discovered her sleepy and difficult to arouse. Two weeks earlier, while visiting her parents, she experienced sudden sharp headache and nausea. She visited a local hospital and was diagnosed with tension headache. The headache persisted for three days during which time she remained in bed too sick to do her usual activities. In the emergency room she was lethargic. Bilateral retinal hemorrhages were noted around the optic discs (subhyaloid). She was able to move her upper extremities and withdraw her lower extremities to pain. Babinski's signs could be elicited on both sides.

Summary A 33-year-old woman with chief complaints of severe headache and decreased level of consciousness. Two previous episodes of severe headache and vomiting (one with neck pain) and loss of consciousness after strenuous exercise were reported one day and two weeks prior to admission. The neurological examination shows a lethargic patient with retinal hemorrhages, lower extremities weakness, and bilateral Babinski's signs. In conclusion: Sudden onset of headache, mental status changes, and focal findings.

Localization

The vignette presents a patient with signs of increased intracranial pressure and signs of meningeal irritation.

Differential Diagnosis

The differential diagnosis includes vascular disorders, tumors, infectious, and inflammatory processes.

Acute Vascular Event

The sudden onset of severe headache should suggest the possibility of subarachnoid hemorrhage (SAH). The radiation to the neck may indicate meningeal involvement and irritation. Heavy lifting which in the patient described triggered the headache suggests the Valsalva's maneuver, which also occurs with straining, squatting, sneezing, and so on, and may precipitate aneurysmal rupture and SAH. Another characteristic clinical finding is loss of consciousness of varying duration, brief or protracted, that according to Adams may be an associated or presenting feature of aneurysmal rupture in 45 percent of patients (Adams). Other symptoms include nausea, vomiting, and intraocular hemorrhages (seen in approximately 20 percent of patients with recent SAH (Adams)). Retinal subhyaloid hemorrhages indicative of increased intracranial pressure may also be observed during ophthalmoscopic examination, particularly with SAH due to aneurysmal rupture and less commonly with other causes of SAH (Caplan 1996).

Intracranial aneurysms often manifest with a warning leak or so-called sentinel hemorrhage, characterized by severe occipital headache of varying duration but that usually resolves within 48 hours. Sentinel headaches are often misdiagnosed as migraine, tension headache, flu, aseptic meningitis, or other disorders (Caplan 1993).

Focal neurological findings also occur, such as transient paraparesis, that may be observed in cases of anterior communicating–anterior cerebral artery aneurysms (Adams). Mental status changes are described with such aneurysms.

Neoplasms and Other Space-Occupying Lesions

The headache associated with chronic increased intracranial pressure caused by brain tumors does not present acutely or with the intensity and severity of the headache related to SAH. Hemorrhage that occurs within a pituitary tumor may be as intense as the headache that accompanies aneurysmal rupture.

Infectious/Inflammatory Processes

Meningitis, meningoencephalitis, and vasculitis are included in the differential diagnosis but can be clinically ruled out by the absence of fever and other systemic symptoms and organ involvement.

Headache represents the main feature of SAH; therefore, disorders characterized by headache as a primary complaint need to be considered and ruled out, such as migraine, tension headache, meningeal infection, and so on, which are common misdiagnoses. Thunderclap headache (crash migraine) may simulate aneurysmal subarachnoid hemorrhage headache with the intensity of the pain but neuroimaging studies do not reveal any evidence of hemorrhage. A lumbar puncture should always be performed in controversial cases.

Any patient experiencing the worst headache of their life should be treated cautiously and SAH should always be considered until proven otherwise.

Etiology of SAH

The incidence of SAH has been reported to be between 6 and 16 cases per 100,000 in the United States (Bendock et al.). SAH due to aneurysmal rupture represents approximately 25 percent of cerebrovascular deaths, 8 percent of all strokes, and 80 percent of all SAH (Bendock et al.). The most common cause of SAH is trauma. Other etiologies include hemorrhage due to aneurysm rupture and vascular malformations, such as arteriovenous malformations and Moya Moya syndrome; intracerebral hematoma with invasion of the subarachnoid space; coagulation disorders; perimesencephalic hemorrhage; venous thrombosis; drugs, such as cocaine and amphetamines; and meningeal infections.

Aneurysmal SAH

Saccular aneurysms characteristically form at the arterial bifurcations. The majority according to Weir involve the anterior circulation 85 to 95 percent. The anterior circulation has seven main locations of aneurysm formation. The most common is the anterior communicating artery region, followed by the posterior communicating artery origin, and the middle cerebral artery bifurcation (Weir). The presence of cerebral saccular aneurysm can accompany other disorders, such as coarctation of the aorta, polycystic kidney disease, fibromuscular dysplasia, Marfan's syndrome, and Ehlers-Danlos syndrome.

Warning Symptoms

Headache is the most common complaint indicated by patients with ruptured aneurysms and according to Weir one third of patients have a history of headache in the weeks or months preceding the acute event (Weir).

Sentinel bleeds (caused by intermittent leakage of small amounts of blood) may precede large hemorrhage. Sudden onset of severe headache with or without neurological signs should always be aggressively investigated for the possibility of SAH.

Clinical Features

Sudden onset of severe headache is the most significant clinical symptom in SAH, and is present in 85 to 95 per-cent of patients (Adams). Patients complain of the worst headache of their life, described as excruciating, terrifying, and agonizing. Decreased level of consciousness can also occur, sometimes as the initial manifestation. The cause can be attributed to a sudden increase in intracranial pressure with subsequent cerebral hypoperfusion. Neck pain, nuchal rigidity, and other meningeal signs can accompany the headache, as well as nausea, vomiting, photophobia, and low-grade fever.

Ocular abnormalities include subhyaloid or preretinal hemorrhages and intravitreous hemorrhages. Intraocular hemorrhages in a comatose patient are strongly suggestive of intracranial bleeding (Adams).

Focal neurological findings can also be present and have a localizing value in suggesting the location of the aneurysmal rupture:

- Involvement of the third cranial nerve may localize to an internal carotid–posterior communicating artery aneurysm.
- Paraparesis, bilateral Babinski signs, and changes in mental status are suggestive of an anterior cerebral–anterior communicating artery aneurysm.
- Transient hemiparesis can be present in middle cerebral or internal carotid artery aneurysms.
- Transitory loss of vision can occur in ophthalmic artery aneurysm.

According to the Hunt and Hess classification of SAH, there are five grades of severity varying from grade I (asymptomatic or minimal headache and slight nuchal rigidity) to grade V (comatose decerebrate patient).

Diagnosis

If the patient presents with symptoms suggestive of SAH, the neurosurgical unit should be alerted and promptly consulted. A CT scan of the brain should be obtained as soon as possible because of the high sensitivity of a CT scan for demonstrating subarachnoid blood during the first 24 hours. In case of a negative study, a lumbar puncture needs to be performed.

The CSF usually shows a bloody specimen due to the large numbers of red blood cells, without clearing of cells in sequential tubes. Glucose is normal and protein slightly elevated. Unlike SAH, a traumatic tap shows clearing of the red cells between the first and last tube and does not demonstrate the persistent xanthochromia in the supernatant.

Cerebral angiography is the most important diagnostic tool, particularly in order to detect the source of bleeding.

Prognosis and Complications

The neurological complications associated with SAH include:

- Rebleeding.
- Vasospasm.
- Hydrocephalus.
- Seizures.

The crucial time for the risk of rebleeding is during the first 24 hours after SAH. Early aneurysmal rebleeding carries the worst prognosis with a mortality rate over 50 percent. Symptoms that suggest rebleeding are worsening of the headache, seizures, changes in the level of the sensorium, stupor, coma, or the occurrence of a new neurological deficit.

Vasospasm carries significant morbidity and mortality. Vasospasm can be defined clinically but also based on the angiographic studies. Over 50 percent of patients develop angiographic vasospasm and half of them are symptomatic. Symptoms indicative of vasospasm are decreased level of sensorium, worsening of the headache, focal neurological deficits, and so on. Vasospasm does not manifest for three or four days after the initial SAH but usually has its peak timing from days 7 to 10 after the event.

Hydrocephalus can be due to acute intraventricular obstruction with symptoms of headache, nausea, vomiting, drowsiness, ocular palsies, papilledema, and so on, or it can be communicating (late hydrocephalus).

Seizures can also complicate SAH.

The medical complications include

- Hyponatremia
- Pulmonary edema
- Cardiopulmonary complications (ECG changes, enzyme elevation, rhythm abnormalities).

Treatment

Surgical clipping of the aneurysm is the treatment of choice. Opinions differ between early or late surgery. Patients with nonaneurysmal SAH should be treated according to the causes.

Cerebellar Hemorrhage

Vignette

A 50-year-old high school teacher started complaining of headache and dizziness after a confrontation with a student. For the last two years he had experienced occasional pounding headaches and was found to have borderline hypertension. The day of the confrontation he felt ill and unsteady when trying to walk, falling to the right side. He vomited twice and complained that his vision was foggy and the room was spinning. In the emergency room, pupils were 2.5 mm and reactive. The eyes were de-viated to the left. There was right facial weakness. He could move all four extremities, but was unable to sit in bed without assistance. Plantar responses were flexor. Eight hours later he was lethargic. The pupils were 1.5 mm and not reactive. Corneal reflexes were sluggish; the plantar responses extensor.

Summary A 50-year-old man with sudden onset of headache, vertigo, unsteady gait. Neurological examination shows left eye deviation and truncal ataxia in absence of motor weakness. Subsequently the symptoms worsened with the occurrence of lethargy, small nonreactive pupils, right facial paralysis, sluggish corneal reflexes, and extensor plantar responses.

Localization: Right Cerebellum

The patient's history and symptoms are strongly suggestive of an acute cerebellar vascular event that could be a hemorrhage or an infarction. The cerebellar involvement is indicated by the ipsilateral appendicular ataxia presenting as inability to walk or stand and by truncal ataxia presenting as inability to sit. In fact, the patient of the vignette felt ill and unsteady, falling toward the right side (which is the side ipsilateral to the lesion) and in the ER was unable to sit without support. In addition, there are clinical signs indicative of lateral pontine tegmental involvement, such as ipsilateral horizontal gaze palsy and facial palsy. The progressive decline in level of alertness and the extensor plantar responses suggest clinical deterioration with brainstem compression. Headache and vomiting are due to increased intracranial pressure in the ventricular system.

Management

Emergency CT scan and neurosurgical unit alert are immediately obtained. In case of large hemorrhage and signs of brainstem compression, there is indication for immediate ventriculostomy while preparations are being made for posterior fossa craniotomy and drainage of hematoma.

Etiology and Clinical Features

Cerebellar hemorrhages represent 10 percent of parenchymal intracranial hemorrhages (Caplan 1993) and can be responsible for severe neurological complications, such as brainstem compression and obstructive hydrocephalus. There is approximately one patient with cerebellar hemorrhage for every nine with cerebellar infarcts (Amarenco).

Hypertension remains the main cause of cerebellar hemorrhage in the majority of patients (80 percent of the cases according to Amarenco). Other etiological factors are trauma, vascular malformations, aneurysm, use of anticoagulant medications, coagulopathies, hemorrhagic transformation into a tumor, vasculitis, amyloid angiopathy, and hemorrhagic infarction (Amarenco).

Hemorrhages in hypertensive patients mainly involve the region of the dentate nucleus, arising from distal branches of the superior cerebellar artery and the posterior inferior cerebellar artery (Caplan 1993). Those coming from angiomas tend to lie more superficially. Hemorrhages can extend into the subarachnoid space or fourth ventricle leading to brainstem compression and coma.

Signs and Symptoms

The most common presenting symptoms are disturbance of gait with inability to walk and vomiting (Caplan 1993). The inability to stand and walk can be significant. Other symptoms include headache localized in the occipital or frontal area and vertigo. Altered level of consciousness is not usually an initial symptom. Ocular abnormalities are characterized by conjugate lateral gaze, paresis to the side of the hematoma, forced deviation of the eyes to the opposite side, or an ipsilateral abducens nerve paresis (Adams and Victor).

Life-threatening complications include brainstem compression caused by large hemorrhages. Also, if there is lateral extension toward the pons, signs of cerebellopontine angle dysfunction can be observed with the occurrence of facial paralysis, loss of corneal reflex, hearing loss, and tinnitus.

Hemorrhages in the vermis can simulate a primary pontine hematoma with rapid neurological deterioration and coma, unless emergent posterior fossa decompression is obtained (Caplan 1996).

A prompt diagnosis of cerebellar hematoma is necessary in order to avoid fatal complications

Treatment

The treatment is based on the size of the hematoma. If it is small (less than 3 cm), without signs of hydrocephalus or decreased level of sensorium, treatment can consist of medical management in an intensive care unit. In the case of a large hematoma, surgical intervention is necessary, particularly when complications have occurred such as hydrocephalus and altered consciousness, stupor and coma, that may indicate brainstem compression. Emergency surgical treatment includes ventriculostomy if hydrocephalus is present and posterior fossa craniotomy for evacuation of the hematoma.

Cerebral (Lobar) Hemorrhage

Vignette

A 70-year-old retired teacher started experiencing episodes of numbness in her left fingers that spread over 1 to 2 minutes to involve the arm and face, lasting 20 minutes before complete recovery. Two similar spells were associated with clumsiness and weakness. She had a history of migraine and, according to her husband, lately she had experienced more frequent and severe headaches and had been anxious, unable to sleep, forgetful, and depressed for quite some time. Neurological examination showed left side weakness associated with left hemianopia and hemineglect.

Summary A 70-year-old woman with recurrent transitory episodes of neurological dysfunction that spread along contiguous parts of the body over a period of minutes. There is also a history of increasing headache and forgetfulness. The neurological examination shows focal findings: left hemiparesis, hemineglect, and hemianopia.

Localization

The examination indicates a cortical localization, particularly right frontoparietal and occipital, including the motor, sensory, and visual areas.

Diagnosis

The transitory episodes of neurological dysfunction can represent transitory ischemic attacks, partial seizure, or aura phenomenon of migraine.

Several possible etiologies need to be considered in the differential diagnosis:

- Vascular abnormalities
  Lobar hemorrhages
  Cerebral emboli
- Other structural lesions
  Neoplasm or hemorrhagic transformation into a tumor
- Infectious/inflammatory processes
  Abscess
  Vasculitis
- Other possibilities
  Migraine with aura
  Migrainous stroke

Vascular lesions, particularly lobar hemorrhages, should be considered first and rank high in the list of the differential diagnosis. The etiology of lobar hemorrhages includes trauma, cerebral vascular malformations, coagulopathies, anticoagulant therapy, tumors, in particular metastatic tumor complicated by hemorrhage, and cerebral amyloid angiopathy. Cerebral amyloid angiopathy is an important cause of lobar hemorrhage in the elderly. Patients are typically over age 60 and normotensive (Feldmann). A presentation with transitory focal neurological deficits spreading to contiguous parts has been described (Greenberg).

Almost half of the cases with CAA-related parenchymal brain hemorrhage demonstrate mental status changes indicative of some degree of dementia during life and neuropathological features of Alzheimer's disease at necropsy (Barnett et al.).

Considering the other causes of lobar hemorrhage, vascular malformations are unlikely to manifest symptoms for the first time in a woman of this age. Also, in the patient presented, there is no history of trauma, coagulopathy, or use of anticoagulants or other substances. Lobar hemorrhage can be the result of metastatic tumor, but there is a lack of manifestations of systemic cancer in the vignette and no indication of this possibility. Cerebral abscess and vasculitis are also accompanied by systemic manifestations not described in the vignette.

Migraine with aura (classical migraine) typically manifests in younger patients, usually with a strong family history of migraine. A migrainous stroke is a diagnosis of exclusion only when no other causes can be demonstrated and often manifests with a visual field deficit.

Cerebral Amyloid Angiopathy

Cerebral amyloid angiopathy is considered a significant cause of lobar hemorrhage in older patients. The hemorrhage typically occurs in superficial, "subcortical" or lobar locations, since the angiopathy selectively involves arteries of the cortical surface and leptomeninges (Kase). This disorder is caused by accumulation of amyloid in the media and adventitia of small- and medium-sized arteries of the cerebral hemispheres and is not consistent with generalized amyloidosis.

The parietal and occipital areas are preferentially affected and the hemorrhages can occur again over periods of months or years, and sometimes can manifest simultaneously in different brain areas.

Symptoms of dementia are present in at least half of the patients presenting with hemorrhages related to CAA and in an equal proportion of cases histopathological features consistent with Alzheimer's disease can be demonstrated (Barnett).

CAA-related brain parenchymal hemorrhage tends to affect older normotensive patients who usually have some symptoms of dementia, such as forgetfullness or disorientation, and may involve mutiple lobes, often of both hemispheres.

Cerebral amyloid angiopathy can have other clinical manifestations besides acute lobar hemorrhage, such as insidious progressive dementia and episodes of transitory neurological dysfunction, such as weakness, numbness, and paresthesia, with possible spreading of the symptoms in different body areas possibly due to transient ischemia.

The pathology of CAA is based on the presence of amyloid beta protein that infiltrates the cortical vessels.

This component is also found in senile plaques of patients with Alzheimer's disease.

Cerebral-amyloid-angiopathy–related hemorrhages tend to recur and this pattern increases the risk of disability and mortality. Specific treatments based on prevention of recurrent hemorrhage in patients with cerebral amyloid angiopathy is not available.

Posterior Circulation Syndromes

Wallenberg's Syndrome

Vignette

A 56-year-old waitress began complaining two weeks ago of dizziness and nausea. During this time, she once was noted veering to the left and had to hold on to a wall in order not to fall. She recovered after 10 minutes. This morning while bending to pick up heavy dishes, she felt a sharp burning pain in her left eye and face as if salt and pepper had been thrown in her eye. She felt the room was upside down. In the emergency room the waitress staggered to the left and had rotatory nystagmus, worse on looking to the left. Her speech was fluent but slightly hoarse. Her pupils were both reactive, but the left seemed smaller. Her left corneal reflex was not present. She was unable to walk and fell to the left when attempting to stand. Her right leg sensation was diminished. She had a history of borderline hypertension and a heart murmur. She has been smoking a pack of cigarettes a day since the age of 15.

Summary A 56-year-old woman with a history of one episode of transitory neurological dysfunction, preceding one sudden event of left facial pain, environmental tilt ("room upside down"), and unsteadiness with veering to the left. Neurological examination findings were rotatory nystagmus, hoarse voice, absent left corneal reflex, pupillary anisocoria, unsteady gait, right leg hypoesthesia.

Localization

The combination of symptoms presented by this patient can be easily explained by localization in the lateral tegmentum of the brainstem: precisely, the left lateral medulla. The lateral medulla includes several anatomical structures, and lesions in this area cause a wide variety of neurological symptoms and signs:

- Ipsilateral facial and eye pain is due to involvement of the spinal tract and nucleus of the fifth nerve. The pain is often described as sharp, jabbing, or burning (Caplan

1993). A feeling of salt and pepper on the face has been described in acute lateral medullary syndrome (Caplan and Gorelick). Ipsilateral facial numbness is also present with hypoesthesia to pain and temperature sensation and diminished or absent corneal reflex.

- Nausea, vomiting, vertigo, nystagmus, and lateropulsion of eye movements are due to involvement of the vestibular nuclei and their connections. A special mention of ocular motor abnormalities in lateral medullary syndrome should be made. In the vignette, the patient felt that the room was upside down. Visual abnormalities are a common symptom in Wallenberg's syndrome. They include blurriness; difficulty focusing; and vertical, horizontal, or oblique diplopia. The occasional tilt of the visual field is suggestive of lateral medullary infarction (Sacco et al.). Patients with Wallenberg's syndrome may experience the sensation of environmental tilt in which the entire room is tilted on its side or even upside down (floor-on-ceiling phenomenon). This syndrome is also probably caused by a disturbance of the vestibular otolith central connections (Brazis). Nystagmus is usually positional and can be horizontal, torsional, or mixed, with torsional, vertical, or horizontal components (Brazis).
- Hypoesthesia to pain and temperature on the opposite side of the body is due to a lesion of the spinothalamic tract.
- Falling or veering to the side of the lesion as well as ipsilateral limbs clumsiness and incoordination are due to involvement of the inferior cerebellar peduncle. Ataxia is the most common symptom at onset (Sacco et al.).
- Horner's syndrome is due to a lesion of the sympathetic system and tachycardia is due to involvement of the dorsal motor nucleus of the vagus.
- Hoarseness indicates involvement of the nucleus ambiguus.

Once localized to the neurological structures involved, it is important to determine if the event is vascular, neoplastic, or the result of an infectious or inflammatory process.

Wallenberg's syndrome is usually caused by vertebral artery or posterior inferior cerebellar artery occlusion.

In the vignette, there was clearly a previous transitory episode in the same vascular territory (dizziness, nausea, one episode of veering to the left), suggesting a thrombotic occlusive lesion. The patient also has risk factors for both large artery disease (smoking) and small-vessel disease (hypertension). She has a heart murmur, but no causes of cardiac embolism, such as atrial fibrillation, are indicated in the vignette. The vascular occlusive etiology remains the best explanation in the vignette. Other causes include hemorrhage due to a vascular malformation; abscess; metastatic tumor, and substance abuse (cocaine) (Brazis).

Therapy

See further discussion.

Vertebrobasilar (Top of the Basilar) Artery Syndrome

Vignette

A 45-year-old construction worker, after a bout of uncontrollable coughing, suddenly fell backward on the couch while watching TV. His wife was unable to rouse him. In the emergency room, he was arousable only to deep pain. His eyes were deviated laterally and the pupils were 6 mm and not reactive. A left Babinski sign was noted. Only his right leg withdrew to pain. He had a history of angina and had smoked a pack of cigarettes a day for many years before quitting the previous year. The wife recalled that for the past two weeks he had complained of brief episodes of vertigo and ringing in his ears.

Summary A 45-year-old male with sudden onset of reduced level of consciousness, bilateral third cranial nerve palsy, and left hemiparesis. Some previous transitory episodes of vertigo and tinnitus also were reported. He had a history of angina and cigarette smoking.

Localization

These symptoms localize the lesion to the rostral brainstem and right cerebral peduncle. It is important to differentiate a subtentorial lesion, such as an intrinsic lesion within the midbrain, that can be vascular, neoplastic or infectious from a supratentorial expanding mass compressing the midbrain, such as massive hemispheric infarct, intracerebral, epidural, or subdural hematoma, tumor, complicated by hemorrhage and pituitary apoplexy. The clinical findings identified in the vignette indicate a lesion involving the Edinger-Westphal nucleus in the midbrain, causing fixed, dilated pupils. Altered level of consciousness results from infarction of the rostral medial reticular formation. An acute brainstem infarction therefore localizing the lesion as subtentorial can be suspected when signs of midbrain or pontine damage accompany the onset of coma (Plum et al.).

The patient in the vignette is relatively young with a history of heart disease (angina) and risk factors for large artery occlusive disease (smoking). In consideration of a subtentorial intrinsic lesion, an embolic occlusion of the rostral portion of the basilar artery can explain the symptoms presented by this patient. The basilar artery progressively tapers as it extends more rostrally. An embolus small enough to traverse the vertebral artery would not block the basilar artery, except distally (Caplan 1980). A source of embolization—cardiac or intraarterial—should be aggressively considered in this patient. The patient had transient episodes of vertigo and ringing in his ears that might point toward a vertebral artery source, but he also had cardiac risk factors (angina) that need to be investigated.

Diagnosis and Treatment

Neuroimaging studies should exclude a supratentorial space-occupying lesion compressing the brainstem. The picture of bilateral thalamic infarcts sometimes associated with infarcts in the posterior cerebral artery territory may indicate embolism of the top of the basilar artery (Caplan 1996). Magnetic resonance angiography is very sensitive in showing the basilar artery. Transcranial Doppler can help in the possibility of high-grade stenosis of the vertebral or basilar artery. Angiography is the test of choice in demonstrating the severity and the area of the stenosis.

Clinical Features

Occlusion of the top of the basilar artery may cause the occurrence of infarction of midbrain and thalamus, associated with infarction of parts of the temporal and occipital lobes.

Occlusion of the rostral portion of the basilar artery is usually attributed to an embolic mechanism with sources originating from the heart or proximal vertebrobasilar artery. The infarction can cause extensive neurological damage but parameters such as size of the clot, duration of the obstruction, and presence of an adequate collateral flow play a critical role. Brainstem and/or hemispheres can be affected.

Clinical findings of rostral brainstem infarction include

- Pupillary dysfunction: The size of the pupils can be small or large, or they can be in midposition.
- Ocular movement abnormalities that can manifest with different clinical pictures, such as vertical gaze palsies particularly upgaze paralysis, convergence abnormalities (hyperconvergence, convergence-retraction nystagmus), skew deviation pseudosixth due to deficit on full abduction on lateral gaze in patients with upper brainstem lesions (Caplan 1996).
- Altered consciousness and behavior abnormalities with hypersomnolence, coma, hallucinations (peduncular-hallucinations which are vivid visual hallucinations) (Caplan 1996).
- Memory disturbances particularly occur with thalamic infarction.

Clinical signs and symptoms of infarction of the posterior cerebral artery include (Caplan 1980)

- Visual field defects: Hemianopia, awareness of the visual deficits, absence of neglect.
- Behavior abnormalities (acute delirium, agitation if bilateral).
- Somatosensory abnormalities: Sensory loss in the absence of motor weakness.
- Cortical function abnormalities.

Posterior cerebral artery infarction is discussed later in this chapter.

Proximal Basilar Artery Occlusion

Vignette

A 65-year-old retired postal worker was found by his daughter lying in bed unable to move his right arm and leg and slurring his words. He could follow commands and complained of severe occipital headache and buzzing in both ears. In the emergency room two hours later he was drowsy with incomprehensible speech. He had severe weakness on the right side, including the face, and mild weakness on the left. Some myoclonic jerks were noted in both shoulders. There was horizontal gaze paresis and the only horizontal eye movement was abduction with nystagmus on the left. Both plantar responses were extensor. For the past two months he had complained of double vision and occipital headache, and one time had momentary buckling of his legs. He had a history of hypertension and diet-controlled diabetes.

Summary and Localization

The differential diagnosis first needs to consider an acute vascular ischemic or hemorrhagic event. The sudden onset of right hemiparesis and dysarthria may initially suggest an anterior circulation vascular lesion, such as deep infarct of the left middle cerebral artery or subcortical small-vessel disease. But the the patient in the vignette developed bilateral neurological signs and had a prior history of transitory ischemic attacks of double vision and leg weakness. All these symptoms strongly suggest a vertebrobasilar localization. The bilateral corticospinal tract involvement and the gaze abnormality localize to the basis pontis with extension also to the left tegmentum with involvement of the left parapontine reticular formation and medial longitudinal fasciculus. This is called "one-and-a-half syndrome." Therefore, the patient could have basilar artery occlusion. The history of transitory ischemic attacks characterized by diplopia, vertigo, tinnitus, and hemiplegia that can alternate sides is an indication of ischemia in the vertebrobasilar territory. Dysarthria may be very severe and a right hemiplegia of pontine origin may reduce the patient's speech to an unintelligible "growl" (Fisher). Other signs of brainstem involvement include transient diplopia, horizontal nystagmus, bilateral extensor plantar response, and transient sensation of blockage of the ear canals (Fisher). Occipital headache can also be experienced by the patient.

In the differential diagnosis of the case presented we also need to consider other vascular events such as pontine hemorrhages or hemorrhages due to vertebrobasilar aneurysm rupture. Space-occupying lesions, such as posterior fossa tumor abscess and extradural or subdural hematoma, also need to be differentiated, as do basilar migraine and central pontine myelinolisis.

Clinical Features

The most common cause of basilar artery occlusion is atherosclerosis of the proximal basilar artery near the anterior inferior cerebellar artery branches. Thrombotic occlusion of the basilar artery is often preceded by transitory ischemic attacks and occipital headache. The transitory attacks that last a few minutes consist of vertigo, tinnitus, diplopia, alternating hemiparesis, tetraparesis, perioral numbness, and so on. Since the pons, particularly the basis pontis, is supplied by the basilar artery, an occlusion will often cause a bilateral involvement sometimes with extension into the median tegmentum.

Clinical signs and symptoms of basilar artery occlusion include

- Paralysis of all extremities and bulbar muscles due to lesion of the corticobulbar and corticospinal tract within the basis pontis. Bilaterality of both motor signs is an important point, but the weakness may be asymmetrical (Caplan 1996).
- Bulbar dysfunction characterized by dysphagia, severe dysarthria, dysphonia, and facial weakness. Mutism can also occur.
- Oculomotor abnormalities include a wide range of manifestations:
  —Diplopia.
  —Internuclear ophthalmoplegia due to lesion of the medial longitudinal fasciculus.
  —Paralysis of conjugate lateral or vertical gaze.
  —Horizontal, vertical dissociated nystagmus.
- Sixth nerve palsy.
- Skew deviation.
- Ocular bobbing: Vertical movement of the eyes.
- One-and-a-half syndrome.
- Altered level of consciousness and coma caused by bilateral pontine and midbrain tegmental lesions affecting the reticular activating system.
- Sensory symptoms as well as cerebellar abnormalities can be absent due to the fact that only the paramedian structures of the pontine base are affected.

Posterior Cerebral Artery Infarction

Vignette

A 62-year-old accountant suddenly became confused and agitated while at work. He was irritable, restless, and seemed not to know the names of his employees. In the emergency room he did not know what he had for breakfast, could not name simple objects, and recalled none of three items after five minutes. A right homonymous hemianopia was noted. He could not stand with his eyes closed. Pain, temperature, and position sense were markedly reduced on the right. Strength was full, DTR symmetrical, and plantar responses were flexor.

Summary A 62-year-old man with sudden change in mental status, difficulty naming persons and objects, memory impairment, right homonimous hemianopia, right sensory loss, and normal motor function.

Localization

Left occipital-temporal and deep structures concerned with memory are affected. In this patient manifesting sudden changes in mental status and focal findings, an acute vascular event should be considered first, particularly a left posterior cerebral artery (PCA) territory infarction. The combination of hemisensory loss with hemianopia without motor weakness is suggestive of infarction in the PCA territory (Caplan 1993). Other clinical findings described in the vignette can also be explained by such an event. Left PCA territory infarct can cause difficulty naming objects (anomic or transcortical sensory aphasia) and marked memory dysfunction. Visual field defect associated with awareness of the deficit and sensory abnormalities (subjective with paresthesias or objective with hypoesthesia to pain, touch, and position sense) are other characteristics. PCA territory infarction is usually due to an embolic mechanism.

Other etiological considerations for the case presented are space-occupying lesions causing sudden changes in mental status, such as tumor, abscess, or subdural hematoma, and also basilar artery occlusion, and so on.

Clinical Features of PCA Infarction

Visual field defects can be summarized as

- Hemianopia with awareness of the defect.
- Visual hallucinations in the blind part of the visual field.
- Visual perseverations.

Somatosensory dysfunction can be marked:

- Hypoesthesia or anesthesia to touch, position, and pain.
- Motor function can be preserved.

Behavioral and cortical abnormalities are represented by

- Anomia (amnestic aphasia) alexia without agraphia and visual agnosia (with left PCA infarct).

Bilateral lesions may be responsible for

- Changes in mental status with delirium and restlessness.
- Korsakoff's amnestic states.
- Cortical blindness with preservation of pupillary reactions and normal optic disc.
- Balint's syndrome characterized by optic ataxia, visual disorientation, and inability to voluntarily scan the visual field, in absence of any eye movement abnormality.

Weber's Syndrome

Vignette

A 60-year-old female elementary teacher with diet-controlled diabetes complained of diplopia and left-sided weakness two days after undergoing a hysterectomy for carcinoma of the uterus. On examination there was a partial right ptosis; paresis of right upward, downward, and medial gaze; and a large poorly responsive right pupil. On the left, muscle strength was 4/5. A left Babinski's sign was noted.

Summary A 60-year-old diabetic woman with onset of right third nerve palsy and left hemiparesis.

Localization

Lesions at different areas can cause a third nerve dysfunction:

- Nucleus.
- Fascicular portion within the midbrain.
- Subarachnoid space.
- Cavernous sinus.
- Orbit.

Localization in the vignette is a third nerve fascicular lesion. Deficits of the oculomotor fasciculus are characterized by the presence of associated brainstem signs, such as for instance involvement of the long motor tract in a crossed distribution. Third nerve dysfunction plus contralateral hemiparesis are typically due to involvement of the ipsilateral cerebral peduncle (Weber's syndrome). Causes responsible for this clinical picture include vascular occlusion, metastasis, and demyelination.

Carotid Artery Disease

Vignette

A 52-year-old male telephone operator complained of intermittent episodes of right hand shaking, sometimes with speech difficulty. During one episode there were 20 seconds of wavering movements with the right hand, which made it difficult for him to hold his fork while eating. One time he was thought to be drunk because he was using the wrong words. He had smoked two packs of cigarettes a day for 20 years and had borderline hypertension. His mother had multiple sclerosis. During the last six months his left eye had bothered him with sudden blurriness, especially under sunlight.

Summary A 52-year-old man with episodes of right hand shaking, speech difficulties, and left eye blurriness worsened by sunlight.

Localization

Before localizing, it is important to decide if these episodes of transitory neurological dysfunction represent a vascular event, partial seizure, or complicated migraine. The etiology also needs to be clarified. Are these events vascular in origin or is there an underlying infectious, inflammatory, demyelinating, or space-occupying process? The presence of several risk factors, such as smoking and hypertension, places a vascular mechanism at the base of these episodes a high possibility.

The constellation of symptoms localizes to the anterior circulation (carotid territory). Involuntary episodic abnormal movements are a rare but well-described symptom of occlusive disease of the carotid artery (Leira et al.). The movements are described as "shaking," "trembling," "twitching," "flapping," or "wavering." Attacks appear to cease following carotid endarterectomy (Tatemichi). The mechanism underlying shaking, transient ischemic attack (TIA), is presumed to be hemodynamic insufficiency (Tatemichi).

Speech difficulty with transitory aphasia is also an important sign of carotid disease. According to Barnett et al., the most common symptoms of carotid involvement are motor and sensory deficit of the contralateral limbs, followed by pure motor dysfunction, then pure sensory dysfunction, and, less commonly, isolated dysphasia. The duration of the transitory attack is brief, usually less than 10 minutes.

Finally, the blurriness of the left eye, especially under sunlight, experienced by the patient in the vignette indicates another possible characteristic of carotid dysfunction or amaurosis fugax. Transient episodes of visual loss have been characterized as brief monocular visual obscuration, "blur," "cloud," "fog," or "shade," which usually lasts less than 15 minutes (Barnett et al.). It has also been reported that exposure to bright light (often sunlight) precipitates transient unilateral visual loss (Barnett) in patients with high-grade stenosis.

Considering these vascular transitory events, the localization resides in the left anterior circulation (carotid artery) territory.

These episodes can be caused by an embolic mechanism with sources originating from the heart or from atherothrombotic carotid plaques. Also, severe hypoperfusion due to high-grade carotid stenosis is another mechanism. A cardiac source seems unlikely in the patient described because there are no known cardiac factors and the transitory attacks do not involve multiple vascular territories as seen with cardiac embolization.

Other important causes to be considered in the differential diagnosis are primary and secondary inflammatory vascular disorders. Primary inflammatory vascular disorders include systemic vasculitis, systemic lupus, antiphospholipid antibody syndrome, and others. Secondary inflammatory vascular disorders occur with infections, drugs, irradiation, and so on. Important factors that lead to the right diagnosis are systemic features, such as weight loss, anorexia, headache, malaise, low-grade fever, arthralgia, livedo reticularis, and so on. Arterial dissection is another possibility to be kept in mind as cause of TIA or stroke and is usually related to trauma.

As stated earlier, the differential diagnosis of transient focal neurological symptoms of acute onset includes the following:

- Migraine aura (with or without headache), usually manifests in younger patients with a family history of migraine. Visual symptoms are important and consist of light flashes, scintillations or fortification spectra, and so on. Sensory and motor disturbances may also be present and spread over a period of minutes in a marching fashion (like seen in cheiro-oral migraine).
- Partial seizures can cause sudden sensory or motor positive phenomena with rapid involvement of contiguous body parts. Postictal or Todd's paralysis may occur after a partial motor seizure or a generalized seizure with focal onset.
- Structural brain lesions such as neoplasms, AVMs, and intracranial aneurysms, can present with transient neurological deficits through various mechanisms, such as

partial seizures, spreading depression, vascular steal phenomenon, intracranial hypertension, and so on.
- Multiple sclerosis can rarely cause focal neurological symptoms that simulate TIA, but is usually easily distinguished by other clinical manifestations.

Carotid Artery Dissection

Vignette

A 25-year-old female ballet dancer started experiencing right arm numbness and weakness while eating lunch. For the last three days she had complained of throbbing headache, left retroorbital and facial pain, "sparkles" in front of her eyes, and a bad taste in her mouth. In the emergency room, the weakness and numbness resolved. On examination, her left pupil was 2 mm and her right 3 mm. There was mild left ptosis. Fundi were normal. Left hemilingual atrophy was noted. Past medical history was unremarkable. She had recently returned from a ski trip in Utah.

Summary A 25-year-old woman experiencing left side headache, facial pain, sparkles in front of her eyes, and dysgeusia, as well as transitory episodes of right weakness and numbness. Neurological examination shows left Horner's syndrome and left twelfth nerve involvement (hemilingual atrophy).

Localization

Before localizing the lesion, consideration needs to be given to the history reflecting one episode of possible TIA (right sided weakness and numbness that resolved) and neurological findings described as left Horner's syndrome, dysgeusia, and left hemilingual atrophy. The diagnosis of Horner's syndrome is related to associated findings. Horner's syndrome is clinically characterized by the presence of miosis resulting from paralysis of the dilator of the pupil, a partial or pseudoptosis due to paralysis of the upper tarsal muscle, and ipsilateral facial anhidrosis.

The lesions causing Horner's syndrome can be classified as central (first-order neuron), preganglionic (second-order neuron), or postganglionic (third-order neuron). The neurological signs and symptoms help localize the lesion. The pupillary findings remain the same in all localizations. Central causes of Horner's syndrome include Wallenberg's syndrome and other brainstem infarctions, cerebral and hypothalamic infarctions and tumors, AVM, syrinx and trauma involving the cervical cord, and demyelinating disease. Preganglionic lesions include tumors of the thoracic area and the neck and traumatic lesions. Pancoast's apical lung tumor, in particular, is included in this group but also breast metastasis, chest tube, neck dissection, and so on. Postganglionic causes are neck surgery or trauma, endarterectomy, migraine/cluster headaches, and cavernous sinus lesions.

In the differential diagnosis, internal carotid artery (ICA) dissection should rank high in the list of the possibilities. The causative trauma can be significant or even minor due to neck manipulation, sudden turning while skiing, prolonged head turning, and so on. The first symptom is usually head pain that can be throbbing and localized on the side of the dissection, often associated with face pain and neck pain. Facial pain is considered to be mediated through the trigeminal nerve from activation of pain receptors in the adventitia of the ICA.

Incomplete Horner's syndrome can be present due to involvement of sympathetic fibers of the internal carotid plexus extending along the distended vessel wall. Ipsilateral facial anhidrosis is not found in carotid dissection as in other postganglionic sympathetic pathology.

The ischemic manifestations are represented by TIAs, stroke, or both, involve the territory of the internal carotid artery and are due to an embolic mechanism.

Cranial nerves, particularly the vagus, spinal accessory, or hypoglossus, can be affected due to vascular compromise. Hemilingual atrophy has also been described.

Diagnosis

Stenosis of the artery can be demonstrated on angiography with various findings from irregular narrowing to the characteristic string sign if marked stenosis is observed.

Treatment

The treatment is based on the use of anticoagulants for three months in order to prevent embolization, followed by antiplatelet therapy for a similar length of time. In the case of dissection extending into the intracranial segment of the ICA, a more cautious approach is suggested when using anticoagulation due to the possibility of subarachnoid hemorrhage.

The indication for surgical intervention remains the presence of a residual dissecting aneurysm that may cause embolization or the occurrence of subarachnoid hemorrhage due to a leaking intracranial dissection or dissecting aneurysm.

Carotid Cavernous Fistula

Vignette

A 50-year-old man developed headache, left eye pain, redness, and double vision two days earlier.

On examination there was mild exophthalmus, decreased visual acuity, left VI and III nerve palsy, and decreased left corneal reflex. Motor and sensory examinations were intact. He had no previous history, except for being involved in a motor vehicle accident two-and-a-half days prior, with resultant mild head concussion.

Summary A 50-year-old man presenting with headache, diplopia, left eye pain, redness, exophthalmus, ophthalmoplegia (VI, III), and involvement of the fifth nerve (decreased corneal reflex). History is significant for a motor vehicle accident.

Localization

Several localizations are considered:

- Orbit.
- Cavernous sinus.
- Parasellar area.
- Posterior fossa.

The history of motor vehicle accident with mild concussion makes a carotid cavernous fistula rank high on the list. This condition is usually traumatic but can also be due to intracavernous aneurysm rupture or connective tissue disorders (e.g., Ehlers-Danlos). Symptoms include painful ophthalmoplegia affecting primarily the sixth nerve but also the third and fourth, visual loss, and exophthalmus. In the case described in the vignette, other conditions, such as cavernous sinus thrombosis, endocrine exophthalmus, retroorbital tumors, or orbital vascular malformations need to be excluded.

Temporal Arteritis

Vignette

An 82-year-old diabetic woman was taken to the emergency room by her daughter. The woman had called her daughter upon awakening that morning because she was unable to see out of her left eye. For the past three months she had complained of generalized aching of both shoulders and stiffness of the legs when climbing stairs. She had lost weight and at times complained of severe, generalized headache, mainly at night, as well as transitory diplopia. Her primary physician had given her medication for arthritis, which improved her symptoms. Upon examination the left pupil reacted only to consensual light. Left disc edema was noted. Strength was 5-/5 in the lower extremities. Knee jerks were trace and ankle jerks absent.

Summary An 82-year-old diabetic woman with sudden onset of left eye blindness and history of headache, diplopia, generalized aching, and weight loss.

Localization

The localization points to an optic nerve dysfunction in association with systemic symptoms.

Protracted visual loss in an elderly patient like the one presented in the vignette, often with an antecedent history of transitory visual loss (amaurosis fugax) as well as headache and systemic involvement, should immediately bring to your consideration giant cell arteritis (GCA). The prompt diagnosis and aggressive management of this condition will prevent further visual loss. Visual loss that can be sudden and painless and starting upon awakening is characteristic of ischemic optic neuropathy. Anterior ischemic optic neuropathy has been distinguished into nonarteritic and arteritic. Nonarteritic anterior ischemic optic neuropathy that has been found in association with hypertension, diabetes, atherosclerosis, and hypotension is not preceded by premonitory symptoms and the visual loss is maximum at the initial presentation.

Giant cell arteritis is a systemic disorder involving the medium and large arteries, in particular, the extracranial branches of the carotid arteries and can be responsible for the occurrence of severe visual loss in elderly patients. Headache, often described as a stabbing, deep, or annoying pain that can be constant or intermittent, is an important complaint in over half the patients and often an early symptom. Older patients complaining of recent onset of headache or new characteristics of a preexisting headache should be cautiously investigated for the possibility of temporal arteritis. Polymyalgia rheumatica and jaw claudication can also be part of the systemic involvement. Often the area of the temporal artery reveals tenderness to touch and nodularity but the appearance can be normal without excluding the diagnosis.

Visual dysfunction in GCA is associated commonly with anterior ischemic optic neuropathy and less frequently with posterior ischemic optic neuropathy and central retinal artery occlusion (Kay).

Transitory visual loss (amaurosis fugax) can precede the permanent visual loss but diplopia and ophthalmoplegia can also manifest. The pattern of permanent visual loss is usually of sudden onset with symptoms manifesting over hours to a day, or less frequently, over weeks. Jaw claudication presenting with difficulty on chewing due to pain and weakness occurs in over half the patients. Systemic manifestations characterized by generalized malaise, fatigue, low-grade fever, poor appetite, and weight loss, often in conjunction with stiffness and myalgia, can precede or be associated with the visual symptoms.

Diagnosis

The most common diagnostic studies for GCA are the blood erythrocyte sedimentation rate (ESR) and temporal artery biopsy. Almost all patients with GCA have an ESR markedly elevated in the range of 100. Temporal artery biopsy shows features of necrotizing arteritis with multinucleated giant cells. The biopsy should include a segment longer than 1 cm and preferably 2 cm in length, considering that GCA does not affect an artery continuously but tends to skip areas and should be taken from the superficial temporal artery on the side of the visual loss.

Treatment

If administered acutely, high doses of oral or intravenous corticosteroids (500 to 1000 mg methylprednisolone every 12 hours) may reverse acute visual loss (Kupersmith and Carlow). Visual recovery depends on various factors and complications, such as degree of ischemic involvement of the retina or optic nerve. If the patient does not have visual symptoms, an initial daily dose of 60 to 80 mg of prednisone with progressive tapering after one month has been recommended, if clinical improvement is obtained and the ESR is normalized. If symptoms tend to occur again, the prednisone is increased in increments of 10 mg a day until control is obtained. Corticosteroids represent the first line of treatment, but in addition dapsone and cytotoxic drugs have been considered.

Treatment of Acute Ischemic Stroke

Thrombolytic Therapy

Thrombolytic therapy has been used to recanalize the site of the occlusion and provide partial or total resolution of the neurological deficits in the treatment of acute stroke. Intravenous t-PA, whose mechanism of action is based upon the transformation of plasminogen to plasmin leading to a fibrinolytic action on the blood clots, has been approved in the treatment of acute stroke within three hours of onset. The recommended dose of t-PA based on several studies is 0.9 mg/kg with a maximum of 90 mg administered over one hour with 10 percent given as a bolus. Thrombolytic therapy carries a risk of intracranial hemorrhage, particularly during the first 36 hours and should be cautiously monitored in the intensive care unit, looking for changes in mental status or worsening of the symptoms. The blood pressure should be attentively monitored.

Stroke study: Inclusion and Exclusion Criteria for IV Thrombolysis

Inclusion criteria:

- Clearly determined time of onset of symptoms.

- Within 3 hours of onset of symptoms.
- A deficit measurable on NIHSS.
- Patient older than 18 years of age.

Exclusion criteria:

- Evidence of intracranial hemorrhage.
- Stroke or head trauma experienced in last three months.
- Major surgery within 14 days.
- Significant hypertension: systolic blood pressure greater than 185 mmHg and diastolic greater than 110.
- Rapidly improving or minor symptoms.
- Symptoms indicating subarachnoid hemorrhage, or history of intracranial hemorrhage, arteriovenous malformation, aneurysm, or cerebral neoplasm.
- Gastrointestinal or genitourinary hemorrhage within 21 days.
- Arterial puncture at a noncompressible site within last seven days.
- Seizure at the onset of the stroke or uncontrolled chronic seizure disorder.
- Patient taking oral anticoagulant with a PT greater than 15 seconds or heparin.
- Recent myocardial infarction.
- Platelet count less than 100,000/mm^3.
- Glucose less than 50 or greater than 400 mg/dl.
- Coma or severe lethargy.
- Caution is advised with NIHSS score more than 22.

Antithrombotic Therapy

The treatment of acute ischemic stroke is based on the use of anticoagulants and antiplatelet agents.

Anticoagulants

Heparin is indicated when there is a cardiac source increasing the risk of recurrent embolization, particularly in patients with atrial fibrillation complicated by hypertension or congestive heart failure or patients with mechanical heart valves or intracardiac thrombi. The use of short-term heparin therapy is suggested for patients with progressive ischemic stroke, particularly in the vertebrobasilar circulation (Sacco). Heparin inhibits thrombin, factor Xa and factor IXa, by binding to antithrombin III. Therefore, it interferes with fibrin formation and thrombus propagation. The effects of heparin therapy are assessed by monitoring the aPTT, which should reach the therapeutic range of 1.5 to 2.5 times the control aPTT value.

The use of heparin in the treatment of acute ischemic stroke is still debated, particularly regarding issues such as the indication and duration of treatment, the use of a loading dose, the preferable level of anticoagulation, and so on. Complications, particularly the occurrence of extracranial and intracranial hemorrhages, are dose re-

lated. Thrombocytopenia can also occur with the use of heparin.

Low-molecular-weight heparins, such as nadroparin and heparinoids, have been assessed for the prevention or treatment of deep venous thrombosis and as an alternative to the use of heparin in cases of complications. The nadroparin study showed treatment benefit at six months, with a significant dose-dependent reduction in the rate of poor outcome.

The trial of acute stroke treatment evaluated the effect of early treatment with the heparinoid danaparoid sodium in acute stroke. The treatment benefit at six months showed no benefit except in the subgroup of patients with large artery atherosclerotic disease. Also patients were more likely to have major bleeding than the placebo group.

Warfarin sodium, which inhibits coagulation factors by interfering with vitamin K metabolism, is effective in reducing the risk of stroke in atrial fibrillation. Particularly at risk of stroke are those patients with atrial fibrillation and additional complications such as hypertension, congestive heart failure, TIA, systemic embolism, prior CVA, or older age (over 70). An INR between 2 and 3 should be mantained unless there is a high risk of hemorrhage. Patients with mechanical prosthetic valves also need anticoagulation with an INR maintained between 3 and 4. Other situations at risk where anticoagulation is recommended are cardiomyopathy, heart failure, rheumatic heart disease, and patent foramen ovale (in selected cases). Lone atrial fibrillation that occurs in the absence of other complications in a younger age group (before 60) has a low risk of stroke and does not need warfarin but can be treated with aspirin if some prevention is sought.

Aspirin is also recommended if the risk of bleeding is an issue, such as in patients with liver dysfunction, coagulation disorders, older age, thrombocytopenia, and so on.

Antiplatelet Agents

Several antiplatelet agents, such as aspirin, ticlopidine, and clopidogrel, have been used for the prevention of stroke. Aspirin, which inhibits platelet function by inactivating cyclooxygenase, is available for secondary stroke prevention and has been administered in a dose that varies between 75 and 325 mg a day. The main adverse effects are gastrointestinal.

Ticlopidine hydrochloride is an inhibitor of platelet aggregation by acting on adenosine diphosphate (ADP). In the ticlopidine aspirin stroke study (TASS), ticlopidine (250 mg bid) was more effective than aspirin (650 mg twice daily), showing a 21 percent risk reduction of stroke compared with aspirin. Adverse effects of ticlopidine include neutropenia, particularly during the first 3 months, diarrhea, rash, and so on. A CBC with differential is usually obtained during the first 3 months with close monitoring of the neutrophils.

Clopidogrel (Plavix) is an antiplatelet drug that inhibits adenosine diphosphate.

The usual dose is 75 mg daily. Adverse effects include purpura, diarrhea, and rash. Contraindications include peptic ulcer, intracranial hemorrhage, or bleeding diathesis.

References

Sinus Thrombosis

Ameri, A. and Bousser M.G. Cerebral venous thrombosis. Neurol. Clin. 10:87–111, 1992.

Aminoff, M. Neurology and General Medicine. New York: Churchill-Livingstone. 487–503, 1989.

Biousse, V. and Bousser, M.G. Cerebral venous thrombosis. Neurologist, Nov. 1999.

Bousser, M.G. Cerebral venous thrombosis: Nothing, heparin or local thrombolisis. Stroke vol. 30:481–483, 1999.

Bousser, M.G. and Russell, R.R. Cerebral Venous Thrombosis. Philadelphia: W.B. Saunders, 1997.

Broderick, J.P. Cerebral venous thrombosis. Curr. Diagnosis Neurol. 74–79, 1994

Cantu, C. and Barinagarrementeria, F. Cerebral venous thrombosis associated with pregnancy and the puerperium: Review of 67 cases. Stroke 24:1880–1884, 1993.

Donaldson, J. Neurology of Pregnancy, ed 2. Philadelphia: W.B. Saunders, 1989.

Vinken P.J. and Bruyn, G.W. Handbook of Clinical Neurology, Vol. 12. Amsterdam: North Holland, 434–440, 1972.

Subarachnoid Hemorrhage

Adams, H.P. Jr. Clinical manifestations and diagnosis of subarachnoid hemorrhage. Semin. Neurol. 4:304–314, 1984.

Bendock, B.R. et al. Treatment of aneurysmal subarachnoid hemorrhage. Semin. Neurol. 18:521–531, 1998.

Caplan, L.R. Stroke: A Clinical Approach, ed. 2. Boston: Butterworth-Heinemann, 389–423, 1993.

Caplan, L.R. Vascular diseases, part A. Continuum, Jan. 1996.

Caplan, L.R. Should intracranial aneurysms be treated before they rupture? N. Engl. J. Med. 24:1774–1775, 1998.

Kassell, N.F. et al. Cerebral vasospasm following aneurysmal subarachnoid hemorrhage. Stroke 16:562–572, 1985.

Khajavi, K. and Chyatte, D. Subarachnoid Hemorrhage. Neurobase medLink, Arbor Publishing, 2000.

Weir, B. Subarachnoid Hemorrhage: Causes and Cures. Contemporary Neurology Series. New York: Oxford University Press, 1998.

Cerebellar Hemorrhage

Adams, R.D. and Victor M. Cerebrovascular diseases. In: Principles of Neurology, ed. 5. New York: McGraw-Hill, 718–723, 1993.

Amarenco, P. Cerebellar stroke syndromes. In: Stroke Syndromes. Cambridge: Cambridge University Press, 1995.

Bogousslavski, J. and Caplan, L. Cerebellar stroke syndromes. In: Stroke Syndromes. Cambridge: Cambridge University Press, 344–357, 1995.

Caplan, L.R. Intracerebral hemorrhage. In: Stroke: a clinical approach, ed. 2. Boston: Butterworth-Heinemann, 425–468, 1993.

Caplan, L. Posterior circulation disease: Clinical findings, diagnosis and management. New York: Blackwell, 608–614, 1996.

Case records of the Massachussets General Hospital. Case 35. N. Engl. J. Med. 423–428, 1967.

Ropper, A.H. and Kennedy, S.F. Management of nontraumatic brain hemorrhage in neurological and neurosurgical intensive care, ed. 2. Philadelphia PA: Williams & Wilkins, 209–217, 1988.

Stieg, P.E. and Kase, C.S. Intracranial hemorrhage: Diagnosis and emergency management. In: Neurol. Clin. North Am. 16:373–390, 1998.

Cerebral (Lobar) Hemorrhage

Greenberg, S.M. The clinical spectrum of cerebral amyloid angiopathy. Neurology 43:2073–2079, 1993.

Bassetti, C., Bogousslavski, J., and Regli, F. Sensory syndromes in parietal stroke. Neurology 43:1942–1949, 1993.

Barnett, H.J.M., Mohr, J.P., Stein, B.M., and Yatsu, F.M. Stroke Pathophysiology: Diagnosis and Management, ed 2. New York: Churchill Livingstone, 1994.

Case Records of the Massachusetts General Hospital. Case 22. N. Engl. J. Med. 335:189–195, 1996.

Feldmann, E. Intracerebral hemorrhage. Stroke vol. 22:684–691, 1991.

Kase, C.S. Intracerebral hemorrhage: Non-hypertensive causes. Stroke 17:590–594, 1986.

Sacco, R. Lobar intracerebral hemorrhage. N. Engl. J. Med. 342:276–279, 2000.

Warlow C.P. et al. Stroke: A practical guide to management. New York: Blackwell, 287–321, 1996.

Wallenberg's Syndrome

Brazis, P. Ocular motor abnormalities in Wallenberg's lateral medullary syndrome. Mayo Clinic Proc. 67:365–368, 1992.

Brazis, P. et al. Localization in Clinical Neurology, ed. 2. New York: Little Brown, 272–274, 1990.

Caplan, L.R. Stroke: A Clinical Approach, ed. 2. Boston: Butterworth-Heinemann, 237–271, 1993.

Caplan, L.R. Vascular disease. Continuum: Jan. 1996.

Caplan, L.R. and Gorelick, P. Salt and pepper on the face: Pain in acute brainstem ischemia. Ann. Neurol. 13:344, 1983.

Johnson, M.H. and Christman, C.W. Posterior circulation infarction anatomy, pathophysiology and clinical correlation. Semin. Ultrasound CT MRI 16:237–252, 1995.

Lie-Gan Chia and Wu-Chung Shen. Wallenberg's lateral medullary syndrome with loss of pain and temperature sensation on the contralateral face: Clinical, MRI and electrophysiological studies. J. Neurol. 240:462–467. 1993.

Lincoff, N.S. Neuroophthalmologic signs found in brainstem

stroke. Cerebrovascular disease. American Academy of Neurology, 49th Annual Meeting, Boston, April 12–19, 1997.

Sacco, R.L. et al. Wallenberg's lateral medullary syndrome: Clinical–magnetic resonance imaging correlations. Arch. Neurol. 50:609–614, 1993.

Posterior Circulation Syndromes

Barnett, H.J.M. et al., Vertebrobasilar Occlusive Disease in Stroke: Pathophysiology, Diagnosis and Management, ed. 2. New York: Churchill Livingstone, 443–515, 1992.

Berguer, R. and Bauer R.B. Vertebrobasilar Occlusive Disease: Medical and Surgical Management. New York: Raven, 1984.

Brazis, P.W. Localization of lesions of the oculomotor nerve: Recent concepts. Mayo Clinic Proc 66:1029–1035, 1991.

Caplan, L.R. Top of the basilar syndrome. Neurology 30:72–79, 1980.

Caplan, L. Basilar artery occlusive disease. In: Posterior Circulation Disease: Clinical Findings, Diagnosis and Management. New York: Blackwell, 324–380, 1996.

Ferbert, A. et al. Clinical features of proven basilar artery occlusion. Stroke 21:1135–1142, 1990.

Fisher, M. The herald hemiparesis of basilar artery occlusion. Arch. Neurol. 45:1301–1303, 1988.

Liu, J. et al. Premonitory symptoms of stroke in evolution to the locked-in state. Neurol. neurosurg. psych. 46:221–226, 1983.

Mehler, M.F. The neuro-ophthalmologic spectrum of the rostral basilar artery syndrome. Arch. Neurol. 45:966–971, 1988.

Patrick, B.K. et al. Temporal profile of vertebro-basilar territory infarction: Prognostic implications. Stroke 11:643–648, 1980.

Plum F. and Posner J.B. The diagnosis of stupor and coma. F.A. Davis PA 1980.

Carotid Artery Disease

Baquis, G.D. et al. Limb shaking: A carotid TIA. Stroke 16: 3:444–448, 1985.

Barnett, H.J.M. et al. Internal carotid artery disease. In: Stroke: Pathophysiology, Diagnosis and Management, ed. 2. New York: Churchill Livingstone, 1994.

Bogousslavski, J. and Caplan L. Stroke Syndromes. Cambridge: Cambridge University Press, 91–100, 1995.

Leira, E.C. et al. Limb shaking: Carotid transient ischemic attacks successfully treated with modification of the antihypertensive regimen. Arch. Neurol. 57:904–905, 1997.

Tatemichi T.K. et al. Perfusion insufficiency in limb shaking transient ischemic attacks. Stroke 21:341–347, 1990.

Warlow, C.P. et al. Stroke: A Practical Guide to Management. New York: Blackwell, 25–79, 1996.

Carotid Artery Dissection

Barnett, H.J.M. et al. Stroke: Pathophysiology, Diagnosis and Management. New York: Churchill Livingstone, 769–786, 1998.

Caplan, L.R. Stroke: A Clinical Approach, ed. 2. Boston: Butterworth-Heinemann, 299–306, 1993.

Glaser, J.S. Neuroophthalmology, ed. 2. Philadelphia: J.B. Lippincott, 475–479, 1990.

Mokri, B. Spontaneous dissections of internal carotid arteries. Neurologist 3:104–119, 1997.

Carotid Cavernous Fistula

Adams, R. and Victor, M. Principles of Neurology, ed. 5. New York: McGraw-Hill, 751–752, 1993.

Glaser, J.S. Neuroophthalmology. Philadelphia: J.B. Lippincott, 535–540, 1990.

Temporal Arteritis

Barnett, H.J.M. et al. Stroke: Pathophysiology, Diagnosis and Management, ed. 2. New York, Churchill Livingstone, 691–700, 1996.

Goodwin, J. Temporal arteritis. Neurobase MedLink. Arbor, 1993–2000.

Hunder, G.G. Giant cell arteritis. Rheum. Dis. Clin. North Am. 16:399–408, 1990.

Kay, M.C. Ischemic optic neuropathy. Neurol. Clin. 9:115–129, 1991.

Kupersmith, M.J. and Carlow T. Giant cell arteritis. American Academy of Neurology, 52nd Annual Meeting, San Diego, April 29–May 6, 2000.

Tang, R.A. Giant cell arteritis: Diagnosis and management. Semin. Ophthalmol. 3:244–248, 1998.

Stroke Therapy

Biller, J. Practical Neurology. Philadelphia: Lippincott, 379–391, 1997.

Biller, J. Stroke therapy in the new millennium. Semin. Neurol. Vol. 18, No. 4, 1998.

Cerebrovascular disease. American Academy of Neurology, 52nd Annual Meeting, San Diego, April 29–May 6, 2000.

8
Movement Disorders

Multiple System Atrophy

Vignette

A 56-year-old hospital clerk had complained for the past three years of stiffness and clumsiness, mainly affecting his right hand more than the left and later involving both hands. This progressed to the point that he became unable to write. At the same time, his balance became a problem, causing him to fall several times. His wife complained that she could barely understand his voice at times because he was mumbling. The last six months he had difficulty swallowing. He was no longer able to walk without the assistance of two persons, and felt severe dizziness after standing suddenly or after sitting for 30 minutes. He had a long history of impotence and constipation with difficulty initiating micturition. Neurological examination showed an expressionless, thin man with severe dysarthria, some upward gaze limitation, and pupillary anisocoria (left 3 mm, right 2.5 mm). There was rigidity in all four extremities, with very brisk deep tendon reflexes. A right plantar extensor response was noted. A fine action tremor predominantly on the right was noted.

Summary A 56-year-old man with progressive neurological deterioration evolving over a few years. The clinical characteristics are:

- Extrapyramidal features represented by rigidity, hypomimia, and dysarthria in combination with pyramidal signs (right Babinski, very brisk deep tendon reflexes).
- Dysphagia.
- Orthostatic hypotension, urinary retention, impotence, and other signs of autonomic dysfunction.
- Action tremor (cerebellar system).

Localization and Differential Diagnosis

There is symmetrical involvement suggesting a parkinsonian syndrome rather than idiopathic Parkinson's disease where asymmetry of findings is more common (Rodnitzky). The presence of prominent, relatively early, autonomic symptoms in combination with involvement of other systems such as pyramidal and cerebellar is not usually consistent with idiopathic Parkinson's disease. It is not possible to pinpoint to a single localization since different neurological systems seem to be involved, which most likely indicates a degenerative process. The main clinical features of the vignette are represented by parkinsonism with findings consistent of rigidity, decreased facial expression and dysarthria, associated with signs of marked autonomic dysfunction such as orthostatic hypotension, impotence, and urinary retention. This combination of symptoms suggests a diagnosis other than idiopathic Parkinson's disease.

Disorders characterized by parkinsonian symptoms in association with signs of neurological dysfunction due to degeneration of other systems are defined as multiple system atrophies or parkinsonism-plus syndromes. If a distinction from Parkinson's disease can present some initial difficulties, the full constellation of symptoms and signs clearly helps to assess the correct diagnosis. The involvement of at least two major neuronal systems, one of which is represented by the autonomic nervous system, in the absence of any other precisely defined etiology is consistent with the diagnosis of Shy-Drager syndrome (SDS) (Mathias and Williams). The incidence is unknown. Men are preferably affected, with the onset of symptoms usually after the fifth decade. Clinical manifestations of SDS are due to involvement of the extrapyramidal, cerebellar, and autonomic systems. Severe dysautonomia manifests with the following symptoms:

- Orthostatic hypotension, attributed to a cerebral ischemic mechanism and presenting with dizziness, weakness, lightheadedness, and syncope after changing posture such as from lying to sitting or standing.

- Anhidrosis: Decreased tears and saliva.
- Diarrhea, constipation, or fecal incontinence, and dysphagia due to gastrointestinal dysfunction.
- Urinary retention and incontinence; erectile dysfunction and impotence.
- Pupillary abnormalities (anisocoria, Horner's syndrome, and Adie's-like pupil).

Severe early autonomic dysfunction manifesting with orthostatic hypotension, impotence, constipation, urinary retention, and incontinence, is not typically observed in idiopathic Parkinson's disease (Rodnitzky). These symptoms commonly manifest in the later stages of idiopathic Parkinson's disease and can be worsened by the use of dopaminergic and anticholinergic drugs.

The extrapyramidal features of Shy-Drager syndrome are characterized by prominent rigidity and bradykinesia, bilateral involvement, absent or minimal tremor, and poor response to levodopa treatment.

With worsening of the disorder, prominent postural instability and orthostatic hypotension represent a difficult problem to manage. Other clinical manifestations are due to cerebellar and pyramidal system involvement.

Diagnosis

Magnetic resonance imaging may demonstrate hypointensity in the putamen on a T_2-weighted image due to deposition of iron and other paramagnetic substances. Atrophy of the cerebellum and brainstem can also be seen.

Autonomic tests (tilt-table tests, sweat tests, barium studies, urodynamic studies) may be important in demonstrating the autonomic failure.

Treatment

There is little or no response to dopaminergic agents. This is consistent with positron emission tomography (PET) studies that demonstrate diminished striatal D2 binding (Mathias and Williams). Anticholinergic drugs may worsen bladder dysfunction. Symptomatic and supportive therapy may be beneficial, particularly for managing postural hypotension, which can result in significant morbidity.

Progressive Supranuclear Palsy

Vignette

A 70-year-old Italian man was brought to your attention at the insistence of his family. His wife was very frantic over his progressive physical and mental decline over the past two years. She says he has become irritable, depressed, or apathetic; suddenly changing from a sad mood to a happy one, or having uncontrollable crying spells or outbursts of rage. He is totally neglectful of his real estate business. He is unsteady and seems to fall out of the blue all the time. He cannot ascend stairs, falling backward when he steps up with the right leg. His speech is slurred and he reports problems choking on his food. He has difficulty with eye focusing and is unable to read the newspaper, but also descending stairs has become an impossible task. He was told that his vision remained unchanged and that he did not need to change his glasses. His family doctor told his wife that he has Alzheimer's disease and should be placed in a nursing home.

Summary A 70-year-old man with chronic progressive palsy.

- Impaired gait with resultant frequent falls.
- Personality changes.
- Visual disturbances.

The core of the vignette consists of

- Postural instability.
- Pseudobulbar signs: dysphagia, dysarthria, emotional lability.
- Visual dysfunction described in the vignette as difficulty reading or descending stairs. The patient was told that he did not need to change glasses because his vision was unchanged. This suggests a dysfunction of vertical gaze.

Localization and Differential Diagnosis

Prominent gait imbalance occurring at a relatively early stage is a red flag for the diagnosis of progressive supranuclear palsy (PSP). In PSP, an important presenting sign is marked balance dysfunction resulting in frequent falls due to early loss of postural reflexes. Idiopathic Parkinson's disease instead may show marked imbalance gait and postural instability in more advanced stages (9 to 12 years after being diagnosed or longer according to Litvan).

It is not an easy task to distinguish PSP from Parkinson's disease during the first two years of symptom onset if postural instability or ophthalmoplegia manifest late in the course of PSP or when these patients may still benefit from levodopa (Litvan). Diffuse Lewy body disease characterized by spontaneous parkinsonism, dementia, and prominent psychiatric symptoms, particularly visual hallucinations, can be easily distinguished from PSP and ruled out. Rarely, diffuse Lewy body disease can be associated with oculomotor dysfunction and simulate PSP.

Cortical basal ganglionic degeneration (CBGD) is an important part of the differential diagnosis and can be misdiagnosed as PSP. In CBGD, visual disturbances, such as supranuclear downgaze paresis, as well as postural instability, frontal lobe signs, dysphagia, dysarthria, and lack of response to levodopa can occur as in PSP (Cardoso and Jankovic in Calne). However, certain distinctive features may help the differentiation in favor of cortical basal ganglionic degeneration. These include the presence of asymmetrical rigidity, dystonic posturing in the hand, athetosis, orolingual dyskinesia, postural and action tremors, ideomotor apraxia, stimulus-sensitive myoclonus, alien limb phenomena (one limb behaves in a way not recognized by the patient as belonging to him or her), and so on (Cardoso and Jankovic in Calne).

Other disorders rarely seen, such as Gerstmann-Straussler-Scheinker disease, which is related to prions, should be easily differentiated. This condition is usually familial with an autosomic dominant transmission and characterized by progressive dysarthria, marked cerebellar and pyramidal signs, dementia, and supranuclear vertical gaze palsy, predominantly upgaze.

Because of the frontal lobe symptoms also exhibited in the vignette, Pick's or Alzheimer's diseases need to be considered. However, there are no other signs of cortical dementia indicated in the vignette, and therefore PSP should rank very high in the differential diagnosis.

Clinical Features

PSP is the most common form of degenerative parkinsonism after Parkinson's disease (Litvan). Common manifestations include early gait dysfunction, abrupt falls with a tendency to fall backward due to loss of postural reflexes, and ocular disturbances. Falls are usually the presenting manifestation and according to Litvan more than one half of patients with PSP have repeated falls during the first year of symptom onset. Characteristic clinical signs include bradykinesia, axial rigidity, and nuchal dystonia. The rigidity particularly involves the axial musculature causing a posture characterized by hyperextension of the knees and cervical spine. The involvement is usually symmetrical. Resting tremor, which is a prominent feature of idiopathic Parkinson's disease, is not usually seen in PSP or, if present, shows slight amplitude (Collins et al.).

PSP patients manifest important ocular findings, such as supranuclear vertical gaze palsy, particularly downgaze that can be overcome by oculocephalic maneuvers. Limitation of upward gaze is frequently seen in elderly people. Supranuclear vertical gaze palsy is not specific for PSP but may also be observed in other disorders, such as corticobasal degeneration, dementia with Lewy bodies, Creutzfeld-Jacob disease, vascular parkinsonism, Whipple's disease, and so on (Litvan).

Signs of corticobulbar and corticospinal tract involvement can also be commonly present in PSP with dysarthria, dysphagia, emotional lability, Babinski's signs, and so on. The dysarthric speech has a combination of spastic, hypokinetic, and ataxic features (Litvan). Cognitive and behavioral dysfunction suggestive of a frontal lobe pathology can manifest with apathy, depression, changes in personality with emotional lability, disinhibition, perseveration, and so on.

The diagnosis of PSP is predominantly clinical. Tests such as CT, MRI, or PET scan, can be useful for exclusion of other disorders. CT scan of the brain and MRI may show atrophic changes in the midbrain and in the area of the third ventricle. PET study shows hypometabolism in the striatal and frontal regions (Litvan).

Treatment

The treatment is only symptomatic. The use of levodopa or dopamine agonists usually shows only minimal benefits. This is because PSP is characterized by significant loss of the postsynaptic D2 receptors due to the loss of the postsynaptic striatal neurons (Jankovic in Calne).

Wilson's Disease

Vignette

An 18-year-old high school student started complaining of hand tremor at the age of 16. His handwriting became irregular and coarse. He could not drink without spilling. Gradually, the tremor became more pronounced and his speech became slurred and poorly articulated. He was apathetic and irritable and his school performance deteriorated. He was treated with psychotherapy without success. A psychiatrist noted that the patient's speech was monotonous and hardly intelligible and that when the arms were outstretched, a wing-beating tremor occurred. The family history was significant for an alcoholic father who died of liver cirrhosis. One maternal great uncle had Alzheimer's disease.

Summary An 18-year-old male with progressive tremor, dysarthria and behavior changes. The vignette can also be titled: parkinsonism in young adults.

Differential Diagnosis

It is essential to consider Wilson's disease in young patients presenting with progressive neurological dysfunction, in particular when the extrapyramidal system is involved. Also, young patients with progressive psychiatric symptoms should be investigated for Wilson's disease, particularly if combined with neurological deterioration.

Wilson's disease, or hepatolenticular degeneration, is an autosomal recessive disorder due to abnormal copper metabolism that consists of decreased biliary excretion of copper and decreased rate at which copper is incorporated into ceruloplasmin. The urinary copper excretion increases in patients with Wilson's disease (to >100 mcg/day) but is unable to compensate for the reduced biliary excretion of copper. In Wilson's disease characteristic cyst formation and cavitation can be observed in the lenticular nuclei (putaminal and pallidal). These findings can also be present in the thalamus, subthalamic region, red nucleus, or dentate nucleus. In some cases, central pontine myelinolysis can be observed (Hoogenraad). Microscopic studies show loss of neurons with gliosis and marked hyperplasia of protoplasmic astrocytes (Alzheimer's, type II astrocytes).

Clinical Features

The excessive deposition of copper in several tissues is responsible for the multiplicity of symptoms. Hepatic involvement in Wilson's disease is manifested with the occurrence of jaundice, organomegaly (hepatomegaly and splenomegaly), and symptoms of anorexia, nausea, and vomiting. Liver dysfunction can present as acute hepatitis, chronic active hepatitis, cirrhosis, and fulminant liver failure (Hoogenraad). Other systems can be involved, particularly renal, musculoskeletal, and hematological, resulting in nephrosis, osteoporosis, and hemolytic anemia.

The neurological manifestations represent the initial presentation in about 40% of patients (Menkes). The most common initial neurological symptoms are dysarthria, dysphagia, and behavioral abnormalities (Fink). According to Hoogenraad, in the juvenile form that starts before age 20, hyperkinetic and dystonic symptoms predominate; in the early adult type (after age 20), tremor (intentional and postural) is more common (Hoogenraad). A distinction of the different neurological manifestations can also be made based on the most prominent symptoms into a parkinsonian syndrome where tremor, rigidity, and bradykinesia predominate, ataxic syndrome where tremor and ataxia predominate, and a dystonic syndrome (segmental and generalized). Often many symptoms coexist in the same patient. Tremor can be intentional or resembles the parkinsonian alternating type. A wing-beating tremor that occurs with extension of the arms can also be observed. Speech abnormality is a constant feature of patients with neurological involvement (Fink et al.). The dysarthria is often of the mixed type with ataxic, hypokinetic, and dysphonic features (Hoogenrad), and varies in severity. Cognitive and behavioral dysfunction are common.

Wilson's disease can manifest with a variety of psychiatric symptoms, such as depression, psychosis, emotional lability, personality changes, aggressive behavior, and so on.

The ophthalmological signs of Wilson's disease include the Kayser-Fleischer ring observed with slit-lamp examination that is invariably present in all patients with neurological manifestations and is caused by the accumulation of copper in Descemet's membrane at the limbs of the cornea.

Diagnosis

The following laboratory tests should be obtained:

- Plasma ceruloplasmin level which is absent or low, with values ranging from 0 to 10 mg/dl in the majority of patients.
- 24-hour urinary copper excretion in symptomatic patients exceeds 100 mcg per 24 hours.
- Liver biopsy to determine the hepatic copper content (the most reliable diagnostic test).
- Slit-lamp examination for evidence of the Kayser-Fleischer ring.
- MRI of the brain may show abnormal signal in the basal ganglia, atrophy, and ventricular dilatation.
- DNA analysis is also important in siblings of an affected patient. The Wilson's disease gene has been linked to chromosome 13q14.3.

Treatment

Penicillamine remains the primary drug used in the treatment of Wilson's disease. The initial dose is 250 mg a day that can be increased weekly by 250 mg until reaching the dose of 1 g a day divided in four doses. Adverse effects include fever, skin rash, thrombocytopenia, nephrotic syndrome, and acute arthritis. Other complications are lupus, nephropathy, and myasthenia gravis. Trientine has been used in patients who cannot tolerate penicillamine and requires doses up to 1 gm a day. Side effects include fever, skin rash, renal insufficiency, and bone marrow suppression. Ammonium tetratiolmolybdate is an important alternative to penicillamine and trientine. Zinc acetate given orally is effective for maintenance therapy. Liver transplantation is indicated for severe cases of hepatic failure and very advanced liver disease.

Parkinson's Disease

Vignette

A 30-year-old housewife has a six-month history of left hand tremor at rest, slowness, and a decrease in dexterity. She denies any difficulty with speech or balance. Family history is negative except for a maternal aunt with Alzheimer's disease.

Summary A 30-year-old woman with six-month history of left hand tremor at rest and slowness.

Localization: Extrapyramidal System

Asymmetrical tremor, bradykinesia, and loss of dexterity make Parkinson's disease (PD) rank high in the list of differential diagnosis. Resting tremor is an important sign of PD. The typical tremor of PD usually involves one side and is asymmetrical, even though it may spread and involve the other side. The differential diagnosis in this case needs to exclude other causes, including Wilson's disease (hepatocerebral degeneration). Toxic, metabolic, infectious, postinfectious, pharmacological, and other causes of parkinsonism will be discussed in the next vignette.

Treatment

Selegiline (monoamine oxidase type B inhibitor) can be the initial treatment for mild PD. Anticholinergics for tremor or amantadine can be used (see discussion on treatment).

Parkinson's Disease vs. Parkinsonism

Vignette

A 53-year-old farmer was brought to your attention because of left hand tremor, slowness, drooling, especially at night, and depression. On examination, he showed increased tone with resting tremor on the left, decreased arm swing, and a slow gait.

Summary A 53-year-old farmer with left hand tremor at rest, bradykinesia, and other features suggestive of extrapyramidal system dysfunction.

Localization

The asymmetry of symptoms at presentation (left side in the patient described), tremor at rest, bradykinesia, and a positive response to levodopa when treated favor a diagnosis of idiopathic Parkinson's disease rather than parkinsonism related to other causes. Parkinson's disease typically presents with an asymmetrical pattern but asymmetry can also be observed in other disorders, such as cortical basal ganglionic degeneration and hemiparkinsonism–hemiatrophy. It is important to distinguish Parkinson's disease from secondary parkinsonism.

Causes of Parkinsonism

Infectious and postinfectious processes

- Encephalitides (encephalitis lethargica, Japanese B).
- Syphilis.
- Creutzfeld-Jacob disease.
- AIDS.

Toxic causes

- Manganese.
- Carbon monoxide.
- Carbon disulfide.
- Organophosphate.
- MPTP.
- Methanol.
- Cyanide.

Drug-induced

- Neuroleptic agents (dopamine blockers).
- Reserpine, alpha-methyl-dopa.
- MAO-inhibitors.
- Lithium.
- Calcium channel blocking agents.
- Cytosine arabinoside.

Trauma/anoxia

- Subdural hematoma.
- Anoxic encephalopathy.
- Dementia pugilistica.

Vascular disorders

- Multiple cerebral infarctions.
- Binswanger's disease.

Metabolic causes

- Hypoparathyroidism and basal ganglia calcification.
- Chronic hepatocerebral degeneration.
- Wilson's disease.

Others

- Normal pressure hydrocephalus.
- Brain tumors.

Hereditary disorders

- Neuroachantocytosis.
- Rigid variant of Huntington's disease.
- Hallervorden-Spatz disease. (
- Ceroid lipofuscinosis.

Parkinsonism and dementia

- Alzheimer's disease.
- Diffuse Lewy body disease.

Parkinson's-plus syndrome

- Progressive supranuclear palsy.
- Corticobasal ganglionic degeneration.
- Multisystem atrophy: olivopontocerebellar atrophy (OPCA), striatonigral degeneration (SND), Shy-Drager syndrome.

Parkinsonism in the Young

Hereditary diseases

- Wilson's disease (described in this chapter).

- Huntington's disease.
  - Autosomal dominant.
  - In children and young adult-onset, a rigid form predominates.
  - Juvenile HD is characterized by cognitive and behavioral abnormalities and seizures.
  - Tremor may be present, mainly action related.
- Hallervorden-Spatz disease.
  - Onset in the first decade of life.
  - Clinically characterized by tremor, dysarthria, rigidity, dystonia, choreoathetosis.
  - Pathologically there is abnormal iron and pigment disposition in the basal ganglia.
- Juvenile Parkinson's disease.

Infectious and postinfectious causes

- Postencephalitis: subacute sclerosing panencephalitis. (SSPE)

Toxins

- Manganese.
- Carbon monoxide.
- Carbon disulfide.
- Cyanide.
- MPTP.

Drug-induced

- Neuroleptics.
- Reserpine.
- Tetrabenazine.
- Lithium.
- Meperidine.

Treatment of Parkinson's Disease

A brief description is presented. For more information, consult textbooks and articles.

The treatment of Parkinson's disease is based on the use of levodopa, which is given in combination with a decarboxylase-inhibiting drug in order to interfere with the systemic conversion of levodopa into dopamine. Formulations available are tablets of carbidopa-levodopa 10/100, 25/100, and 25/250 mg. Also, the extended-release tablets are 25/100 and 50/200 mg. A new preparation combining carbidopa-levodopa and entacapone (COMT inhibitor) is also available.

It is suggested to use the lowest dose of levodopa that will provide a good clinical response. Side effects of levodopa treatment include nausea, vomiting, and hypotension. Adverse effects caused by the chronic use of this drug include motor fluctuations, dyskinesias, and psychiatric disturbances with hallucinations.

Dopamine agonists, which act directly on striatal dopamine receptors, are used either as monotherapy or in addition to levodopa. Bromocriptine and pergolide are ergot-derived dopamine agonists. Bromocriptine (Parlo-

del) is a strong D2 receptor agonist and a weak D1 receptor antagonist. The starting dose is half of 2.5 mg a day with slow increase up to 40 mg a day. Adverse effects consist of nausea, vomiting, hypotension, hallucinations, dyskinesias, pulmonary and retroperitoneal fibrosis, and Raynaud's-like phenomena. Pergolide (Permax) is a strong D2 and a weak D1 receptor agonist. The initial dose is 0.05 mg a day with maximum of 3 mg per day. Side effects are similar to those of bromocriptine.

The new dopamine agonists pramipexole (Mirapex) and ropirinole (Requip) are non-ergot with high selectivity for the D2 receptor group. Pramipexole is given as an initial minimal dose of 0.125 mg tid and increased up to 1.5 mg a day over one month. The maximum dose is 4.5 mg a day. Pramipexole has demonstrated to markedly ameliorate motor function and decrease the duration and severity during on and off periods. Adverse effects include lethargy, syncope, hypotension, hallucinations, agitation, dyskinesias, and pedal edema. Ropirinole is started at a low dose and increased up to a maximum of 3 to 8 mg tid.

TABLE 8.1. Treatment of Parkinson's Disease

Indications	Agents	Notes
Early-stage PD: When signs are mild and do not interfere with daily activities	Neuroprotective treatment: selegiline	
	Symptomatic therapy for tremor and bradykinesia: anticholinergic medications, amantadine	
Early-stage PD: When signs and symptoms are progressively worse and troublesome to the patient	Dopamine agents (ergots): pergolide, bromocriptine	Dopamine agents help delay the complications that occur with levodopa treatment
	Dopamine agents (non-ergots): pramipexole, ropirinole	
	Carbidopa/levodopa	Carbidopa/levodopa useful in elderly patients (over age 70) and when psychosis and hallucinations related to dopaminergic agents become an issue
	COMT inhibitors	COMT inhibitors are important in increasing the amount of levodopa available to enter the brain
Moderate PD	Levodopa	

COMT inhibitors interfere with the action of COMT, one of the enzymes that metabolize dopamine. COMT inhibitors prevent the conversion of levodopa to 3–0 methyldopa, increasing the quantity of levodopa available to enter the brain. The COMT inhibitors entacapone (Comtan) and tolcapone (Tasmar) have been used as adjunctive therapy to levodopa in the treatment of PD. The dose of entacapone varies from 600 to 1600 mg/day. Tolcapone has a usual daily dose of 300 to 600 mg/day. Adverse effects include dopaminergic side effects, particularly dyskinesia, orthostatic hypotension, syncope, hallucinations, confusion, nausea, severe diarrhea, and elevation of liver enzymes. Tolcapone patients need monitoring of liver function.

Dementia with Lewy Bodies

Vignette

A 70-year-old retired history professor had shown progressive mental decline for the past two years. His daughter first noticed some problems with balance, with a tendency to fall, slowness of his movements, and poor dexterity. He began to have sleep difficulties, including irritability, agitation, and vivid dreams, and then visual hallucinations that seemed to be very distressful. He could never remember to take his blood pressure medications and often confused his nephew for his deceased son. His behavior and mental functions appeared to vary during the course of the day and week by week, alternating between confusion and reasonable lucidity. On examination, he was oriented to place only. He showed mild apraxia, bradykinesia, hypophonic monotonous speech, and mild bilateral rigidity. No other motor or sensory findings were noted.

Summary A 70-year-old man with progressive cognitive impairment, psychiatric disturbances (visual hallucinations), parkinsonian features (bradykinesia, rigidity, hypophonic speech), and fluctuation of the symptoms.

Localization and Differential Diagnosis

The relentless progression of the symptoms suggests a degenerative disorder involving the cortical and subcortical areas. When insidious and progressive mental decline is combined with signs of extrapyramidal dysfunction, dementia associated with parkinsonism is a preferred diagnosis rather than Alzheimer's disease. In the differential diagnosis, several degenerative and nondegenerative conditions need to be considered. Among the degenerative disorders with associated dementia and parkinsonism, dementia with Lewy bodies (DLB) ranks high on the list of diagnoses. It is a characteristic disorder that typically manifests with dementia, fluctuation of the symptoms, visual hallucinations, and parkinsonism. The visual hallucinations in DLB are described as vivid and occur in 40 to 75 percent of patients (Galasko) compared with the lower percentage (5 to 20 percent) of Alzheimer's disease patients experiencing hallucinations.

Other disorders characterized by the presence of dementia and Parkinsonism include progressive supranuclear palsy and corticobasal ganglionic degeneration. PSP has distinctive features, such as prominent axial rigidity, vertical ophthalmoparesis, postural instability, dysarthria, dysphagia, frontal lobe signs, and so on. Corticobasal degeneration is usually characterized by an asymmetrical presentation of the symptoms and clinical features such as alien limb phenomenon, limb dystonia, reflex myoclonus, postural and action tremor of the affected limbs, severe apraxia, cortical sensory loss, and so on. The dementias of CBD and PSP are usually less prominent than dementia with Lewy bodies. The motor abnormalities and clinical features usually create an easy distinction from dementia with Lewy bodies on clinical grounds.

Striatonigral degeneration and mesolimbocortical dementia can also present with dementia and extrapyramidal symptoms. In these rare disorders, signs of frontal lobe dysfunction predominate with marked behavior abnormalities such as irritability, and decreased judgment and insight associated with memory dysfunction and signs of parkinsonism.

Alzheimer's disease (AD) with extrapyramidal signs and Parkinson's disease dementia are the other important considerations in the differential diagnosis. In AD, the parkinsonian signs are usually distributed bilaterally and symmetrically with mild rigidity and bradykinesia and less commonly tremor, and are not an early finding but tend to occur in later stages of dementia. Delusions in AD are more common than the vivid visual hallucinations typically present in a majority of DLB patients. A distinction can also be made between Parkinson's disease and DLB. In Parkinson's disease the characteristic findings of rigidity, bradykinesia, and resting tremor usually assume an asymmetrical and unilateral distribution. Cognitive dysfunction is usually not a feature of early PD, and hallucinations are drug induced, for example, secondary to dopaminergic agents.

Among the nondegenerative conditions that enter in the differential diagnosis of DLB, consideration needs to be given to the following:

- Chronic infections: meningitis, encephalitis.
- Neoplastic and paraneoplastic disorders (limbic encephalitis).
- Prion disease: Creutzfeld-Jacob disease.

- Metabolic and toxic abnormalities.
- Nutritional and endocrine disorders; organ system failure.
- Subdural hematoma.
- Normal pressure hydrocephalus.

Clinical Features

Dementia with Lewy bodies, characterized by the presence of Lewy bodies in the cortical and subcortical areas, is now considered the second most common neuropathological cause of dementia after Alzheimer's disease. Dementia, defined as progressive decline of memory and other cognitive functions causing impairment in functional ability, is an essential feature for the diagnosis. The dementia can have cortical and subcortical characteristics.

Other features include fluctuation of symptoms, visual hallucination and spontaneous Parkinsonism. Fluctuation can be defined as a significant variation in a patient's cognitive or functional abilities, or periods of confusion or decreased responsiveness alternating with reasonable lucidity (Galasko). This is a distinctive characteristic and can vary in duration from minutes to days or weeks. Fluctuation can present as episodic confusion, inattention, decreased level of arousal, and even speech arrest.

Visual hallucinations are often a prominent feature and have been described in 40 to 75 percent of patients with DLB (Galasko). The hallucinations are represented by vivid images of animals, people, or children and can be very disturbing to the patient.

Parkinsonian features are also found in DLB, particularly rigidity and bradykinesia and less commonly resting tremor.

Other clinical findings include syncope, loss of muscle tone, transient loss of consciousness, delusions, and so on.

Treatment

The treatment is symptomatic with the use of anticholinesterase and antipsychotic and neuroprotective agents. The response to levodopa is variable among subjects.

Pick's Disease and Frontotemporal Dementia

Vignette

A 60-year-old woman has a five-year history of irritability, forgetfulness, apathy, decreased speech, and poor concentration. Lately she had became more restless, irritable, and agitated, at times having a compulsive desire to micturate or to disrobe in public. On examination she is alert and echoes some of the examiner's questions. She simulates hand gestures, but does not follow verbal commands. She can name none of the common items that are shown to her. Cranial nerve functions are normal. There is no rigidity or gait abnormality.

Summary A 60-year-old woman with progressive behavior and speech abnormalities over the course of five years.

Localization, Diagnosis, and Differential Diagnosis

The patient presented in the vignette has symptoms indicative of marked behavior and speech abnormalities with progressive aphasia.

The behavior abnormalities characterized by apathy, disinhibition, compulsiveness, poor social skills, and inappropriate conduct, suggest a frontal lobe dysfunction. The speech disorder consists of severe expressive and receptive aphasia. There is also mention of memory deficits. The vignette seems to indicate a localized cortical process with predominant involvement of the frontal and temporal regions. Different categories of disorders need to be considered.

In this patient the relentless progression without remission during five years suggests a degenerative disorder. Alzheimer's disease is the most common degenerative disorder affecting the cerebral cortex and is usually characterized by progressive memory decline in the early stages and only occasionally by marked signs of frontal lobe dysfunction at onset. With progression of the disorder, vocabulary becomes restricted and progressive aphasia manifests. Inappropriate behavior due to lack of judgment and social function appears as AD progresses.

Other degenerative disorders that need to be considered are diseases presenting with prominent frontal lobe symptoms or progressive aphasia, such as Pick's disease and frontal lobe dementia (dementias with nonspecific cortical pathology). In Pick's disease, usually there are marked behavior abnormalities with loss of social skills, judgment, and insight at the early stages compared with Alzheimer's disease where gradual development of forgetfullness is the major initial symptom.

Lewy body dementia also enters the differential diagnosis but, with its characteristic features of marked fluctuation of cognitive or functional abilities, visual hallucinations that occur without a provoking factor, and parkinsonism, can be easily clinically excluded from the vignette.

Corticobasal degeneration, which presents with clinical features of apraxia, alien limb phenomenon, visuoconstructive problems, myoclonus, tremor, and parkinsonism, only in few selected cases has shown marked frontal involvement that can simulate FTD. PSP patients can present with frontal lobe dysfunction, but postural instability with frequent falls, bradykinesia, rigidity, and vertical ophthalmoplegia are the hallmarks of this syndrome.

Other disorders, such as infectious, inflammatory, toxic, neoplastic, and traumatic disorders, can cause cognitive impairment but are unlikely with lack of systemic manifestation and in view of the long duration (5 years) and relentless progression. These disorders are mentioned for didactive purposes and include:

- Neoplasm, primary and metastatic.
- Chronic traumatic lesions: subdural hematoma.
- Prion diseases: Creutzfeld-Jacob disease, Gerstmann-Straussler-Scheinker disease.
- Metabolic: nutritional, endocrine, organ system dysfunction.

Clinical Features

Pick's disease is included in the broad class of disorders termed frontotemporal degeneration. Personality and behavioral dysfunctions represent major clinical features with characteristics described as impulsiveness and compulsiveness, loss of social propriety, inappropriate behavior that does not show restraint, hyperorality, disinhibition, lack of judgment and insight, and decreased executive functions.

The clinical manifestations depend upon the underlying neurochemical deficits and the predominant location of pathology, which can be bilateral and symmetrical or asymmetrically left-sided or right-sided (Miller). If the pathology is predominantly localized to the frontotemporal lobes of the left hemisphere, language dysfunction with progressive aphasia may appear. The Lund and Manchester dementia research group has established diagnostic criteria for the frontotemporal dementias defined as progressive disorder of insidious onset characterized by marked cognitive impairment and behavior dysfunction with loss of judgment, disinhibition, impulsivity, social misconduct, social withdrawal, and out of proportion to anterograde amnesia (Peterson et al.). The linkage of FTD to chromosome 17q21–22 in several extended families with phenotypic variation has been described. Tau protein mutations have been associated with FTD.

Treatment

No treatment is available except for symptomatic therapy. Some behavioral symptoms may respond to selective serotonine reuptake inhibitors.

Huntington's Disease

Vignette

A 44-year-old lawyer started having problems coping with new work responsibilities for the past two years. According to his wife, he has been irritable, anxious, and slightly paranoid with frequent outbursts of rage. He did not respond to psychiatric treatment, but became more forgetful, clumsy, and fidgety, especially with his hands. There was no history of alcohol or drug abuse. The patient's paternal grandmother had Parkinson's disease and died in a psychiatric hospital. He was orphaned at a young age. On examination, he had difficulty with memory, orientation, writing, and following three-step commands. There was involuntary grunting during speech. His saccadic eye movements were slow and he had difficulty fixating on command. When sitting, he moved his arms back and forth from the arms of the chair to his lap, and he could not keep his arms still when extended. Gait was wide-based with excessive lateral swing, variable cadence, and irregular, rapid flowing movements.

Summary A 44-year-old man with progressive dementia and psychiatric symptoms, associated with involuntary movements and gait disorder. The involuntary movements (involuntary grunting during speech; irregular, rapid flowing movements) and the gait dysfunction describe a choreic type of disorder. There is no clear family history except for a paternal grandmother with Parkinson's disease, who died in a psychiatric hospital. (This family history may underlie the possibility of a movement disorder with dementia in a relative.)

Localization and Differential Diagnosis

Chorea, characterized by involuntary arrhythmic, purposeless movements that flow from one body part to another, seems to be associated particularly with loss of medium spiny striatal neurons projecting to the lateral pallidum. Among the differential diagnoses, first hereditary and degenerative disorders need to be described. Huntington's disease is the first to be considered and should rank high on the list of possible diagnoses of a patient presenting with choreic movements and progressive behavior and cognitive decline. It is an autosomal dominant disorder characterized by involuntary choreiform movements, behavioral abnormalities, and progressive mental deterioration.

Neuroacanthocytosis may manifest clinically with generalized chorea, cognitive decline, and personality changes. Other typical features not mentioned in the vignette include seizures, orolingual dystonia, lip and tongue biting often causing self-mutilation, motor neuropathy with muscle wasting, and hyporeflexia, and should create a distinction from HD. The diagnosis may be confirmed by the presence of acanthocytes (thorny or spiky appearance of erythrocytes).

Wilson's disease can present with cognitive dysfunction, behavioral abnormalities, and involuntary movements. The most common neurological features include dysarthria, tremor, dystonia, rigidity, and behavioral disturbances. Rarely choreoathetosis is a prominent feature, but subtle chorea of the fingers and wrists can sometimes be observed.

Dentatorubropallidoluysian atrophy (DRPLA), which is a hereditary disorder transmitted with an autosomal dominant trait and caused by CAG repeat expansion in an abnormal gene located on chromosome 12, may also be included in the differential diagnosis because it can be characterized by chorea and cognitive impairment, but other features such as ataxia and oculomotor abnormalities represent significant characteristics.

Other hereditary degenerative disorders can present with chorea and mental status changes, such as Pelitzeus-Merzbacher disease (PMD) or Hallervoden-Spatz disease (HSD), but the accompanying neurological signs and symptoms should help pinpoint the correct diagnosis. PMD is characterized by symptoms such as prominent nystagmus, choreoathetosis, corticospinal tract dysfunction, dysarthria, cerebellar ataxia, and mental decline. HSD has extrapyramidal signs, such as rigidity and bradykinesia, associated with corticospinal signs and cognitive impairment.

Among the nonhereditary or degenerative disorders to be considered are other causes of chorea and mental status changes. In the vignette, the long course and lack of systemic symptoms easily rule out most of these disorders. Following are nonhereditary choreas associated with mental status changes:

- Infectious causes such as bacterial: poststreptococcal, Lyme disease, neurosyphilis, or viral: encephalitis, Creutzfeld-Jacob disease, subacute sclerosing panencephalitis, herpes encephalitis, AIDS.
- Inflammatory/autoimmune disorders: systemic lupus erythematosus, Behcet's disease, periarteritis nodosa.
- Metabolic disorders: hypo/hypernatremia, hypocalcemia, hepatic encephalopathy, uremic encephalopathy.
- Endocrine abnormalities: hyperthyroidism, hypoparathyroidism, psueudohypoparathyroidism, hyperparathyroidism, Addison's disease.
- Intoxications: alcohol, carbon monoxide, mercury, manganese, thallium.
- Drug related: neuroleptics, levodopa, anticonvulsants, bromocriptine, noradrenergic stimulants, lithium, oral contraceptives, steroids.
- Cerebrovascular disorders: basal ganglia infarction, hemorrhage, subdural hematoma, Moya Moya disease.
- Trauma, kernicterus, senile chorea.
- Migraine.
- Multiple sclerosis.
- Neoplastic: primary and metastatic brain tumors, CNS lymphoma, paraneoplastic syndromes.

Clinical Features

Huntington's disease is a hereditary disorder transmitted with an autosomal dominant pattern characterized by movement disorder, typically chorea, and behavioral abnormalities that manifest between the ages of 35 and 50. Chorea is characterized by purposeless, involuntary, flowing movements that occur randomly and vary in severity. Dystonia and parkinsonian features, such as bradykinesia, rigidity, and postural instability, can occur. Depression is an early symptom. Mental status changes are due to a subcortical type of dementia with characteristic bradyphrenia. Personality changes include anxiety, irritability, apathy, and antisocial personality disorder.

Diagnosis

CT and MRI demonstrate striatal atrophy. Progressive caudate atrophy correlates with the degree of mental deterioration, therefore the measurement of the bicaudate diameter has been used to assess the progression of the cognitive decline. Elevated levels of lactate in cortex and basal ganglia have been shown in patients with HD. The HD gene is localized near the tip of the short arm of chromosome 4. The abnormal gene contains extra expansion of the repeats of the trinucleotide CAG (cytidine-adenine-guanidine).

Treatment

The treatment is symptomatic with medication that helps reduce the chorea, such as dopamine blockers (Haloperidol) or benzodiazepines, particularly clonazepam. Psychiatric symptoms are treated with antidepressant and antipsychotic medications.

References

Multiple System Atrophy

Case Records of the Massachusetts General Hospital. Case 23. N. Engl. J. Med. 1406–1414, 1983.

Mathias, C.J. and Williams, A.C. Shy-Drager syndrome and multiple system atrophy. In: Neurodegenerative Diseases. Philadelphia: W.B. Saunders, 743–767, 1994.

Parkinson's Disease. Continuum, Part A. August 1995.

Rodnitzky, R. The Parkinsonisms: Identifying what is not Parkinson's disease. Neurologist 5:300–312, 1999.

Wenning, G.K. et al. Clinicopathological study of 35 cases of multiple system atrophy. J. Neurol. Neurosurg. Psychiatry 58:160–166, 1995.

Progressive Supranuclear Palsy

Calne, D.B. Progressive Supranuclear Palsy. In: Neurodegenerative Disease. Philadelphia: W.B. Saunders, 769–786, 1994.

Case Records of the Massachusetts General Hospital. Case 46.
N. Engl. J. Med. 1560–1566, 1993.

Collins, S.J. et al. Progressive supranuclear palsy: Neuropath-
ologically based diagnostic clinical criteria. J. Neurol. Neurosurg. Psychiatry 58:167–173, 1995.

Fahn, S. et al. Movement Disorders. Continuum, Part A. 1994.

Goetz, C.G. Parkinson's disease. Continuum, Part A. August
1995.

Johnson, R.T. and Griffin, J.W. Movement disorders. In: Current Therapy in Neurologic Disease, ed. 5. St. Louis: Mosby,
279–282, 1997.

Litvan, I. Progressive supranuclear palsy revisited. ACTA Neurol. Scand. 98:73–84, 1998.

Rodnitzky, R.L. The Parkinsonisms: Identifying what is not Parkinson's disease. Neurologist 5:300–312. 1999.

Wilson's Disease

Berg, B.O. Principles of Child Neurology. New York: McGraw-
Hill, 1167–1170, 1996.

Calne, D.B. Wilson's disease (progressive hepatolenticular degeneration). In: Neurodegenerative Disease. Philadelphia:
W.B. Saunders, 667–683, 1994.

Feldmann E. Current Diagnosis in Neurology. St. Louis: Mosby,
217–221, 1994.

Fink, J.K. et al. Hepatolenticular degeneration (Wilson's disease). Neurologist 5:171–185, 1999.

Hellenberg J.H. et al. Etiology of Parkinson's Disease. New
York: Marcel Dekker, 1–49, 1995.

Hoogenraad, T. Wilson's Disease. Major Problems in Neurology.
Philadelphia: W.B. Saunders, 1996.

Jankovic, J. and Tolosa, E. Wilson's disease. In: Parkinson's
Disease and Movement Disorders, ed. 2. Baltimore: Williams
& Wilkins, 217–33 1993.

Johnson, R.T. and Griffin, J.W. Current Therapy in Neurologic
Disease, ed. 5. St. Louis: Mosby, 352–355, 1997.

Menkes J.H. Textbook of Child Neurology, Ed. 4. Philadelphia:
Lea and Febiger, 114–121, 1990.

Panteliadis, C. and Darras, B.T. Movement disorders. In: Pediatric Neurology: Theory and Praxis. Thessaloniki, 457–
468, 1995.

Parkinson's Disease

Djaldetti, R. and Melamed, E. Management of response fluctuations: Practical guidelines. Neurology 51(Suppl. 2):S36–
S40, 1998.

Fahn, S. Medical treatment of Parkinson's disease. J. Neurol.
245(Suppl. 3):15–34, 1998.

Hubble, J.P. Drug therapy in Parkinson's disease. American
Academy of Neurology, 52nd Annual Meeting, San Diego,
2000.

Lang, A.E. and Lozano A.M. Parkinson's disease, parts I and
II. N. Engl. J. Med. Oct., 1130–1142, 1144–1154, 1998.

Quinn, N.P. Classification of fluctuations in patients with Parkinson's disease. Neurology 51(Suppl. 2):S25–29, 1998.

Dementia with Lewy Bodies

Galasko, D. A clinical approach to dementia with Lewy bodies.
Neurologist 5:247–257, 1999.

Galasko, D. Dementia with Lewy bodies: A clinical syndrome.
American Academy of Neurology, 52nd Annual Meeting,
San Diego, 2000.

Hohl, U. Diagnostic accuracy of dementia with Lewy bodies.
Arch. Neurol. 57:347–351, 2000.

Kaufer, D.I. Dementia with Lewy bodies. Mediguide Geriatr.
Neurol. 1:1–8, 1997.

Pick's Disease

Case Records of the Massachusetts General Hospital. Case 6.
N. Engl. J. Med. 326:397–404, 1992.

Case Records of the Massachusetts General Hospital. Case 16.
N. Engl. J. Med. 314:1101–1111, 1986.

Case Records of the Massachusetts General Hospital. Case 11.
N. Engl. J. Med. 342:1110–1117, 2000.

Mathuranath, P.S. et al. Corticobasal ganglionic degeneration
and/or frontotemporal dementia: A report of two overt AD
cases and review of literature. J. Neurol. Neurosurg. Psychiatry 68:304–312, 2000.

Miller, B.L. Pick's disease and frontotemporal dementias:
Emerging clinical and molecular concepts. Neurologist 5:
205–212, 1999.

Neary, D. Frontotemporal degeneration, Pick disease and corticobasal degeneration. Arch. Neurol. 54:1425–1429, 1997.

Peterson, R.C. et al. Case studies in Alzheimer's disease non-
Alzheimer dementia. American Academy of Neurology, 52nd
Annual Meeting, San Diego, 2000.

Huntington's Disease

Adams, R. and Victor, M. Principles of Neurology, ed 5. New
York: McGraw-Hill, 969–973, 1993.

Calne, D.B. Neurodegenerative Diseases. Philadelphia, W.B.
Saunders, 685–704, 1994.

Case Records of the Massachusetts General Hospital. Case 2.
N. Engl. J. Med. 326:117–125, 1992.

Fahn, S. Movement Disorders. Continuum, Part A. 1994.

Harper, P.S. Huntington's disease. Philadelphia: W.B. Saunders,
1991.

Martin, J.B. and Gusella, J.F. Huntington's disease: Pathogenesis and management. N. Engl. J. Med. 315:1267–1276,
1986.

Watts, R. and Koller, W.C. Movement Disorders: Neurologic
Principles and Practice. New York: McGraw-Hill, 477–518,
528–539, 1997.

9
Tumors

Pineal Tumors

Vignette

A 25-year-old legal secretary has been having problems concentrating for the last four weeks, often forgetting important appointments. She attributed her problems to some morning headache. The day of the examination she had vomited twice and felt that her vision was blurry. In the emergency room, the examining resident noticed that visual acuity and visual fields were normal. The left pupil was 4 mm, the right pupil was 3.5 mm, and both were sluggish. When asked to look at her wristwatch, her eyes remained immobile. She had sustained gaze-evoked upbeat nystagmus and reduced upward saccades. Optic disc margins were blurry. Gait was unsteady particularly during tandem or quick turns.

Summary A 25-year-old woman with difficulty concentrating, headache, vomiting, and blurry vision. The examination shows pupillary anisocoria, paralysis of accommodation, upward gaze paralysis and nystagmus, papilledema, and unsteady gait.

Localization and Differential Diagnosis

The vignette includes nonlocalizing signs due to increased intracranial pressure represented by headache, papilledema, and vomiting, and neuroophthalmological signs localizing to the midbrain. In particular, the midbrain center for convergence and vertical gaze lies in the roof of the midbrain. These ocular findings include

- Anisocoria with poorly reactive pupils (the left pupil is 4 mm and the right is 3.5 mm and both are sluggish).

- Paralysis of vertical gaze particularly upward gaze paralysis rather than downward gaze, with sustained gaze-evoked upbeat nystagmus.
- Paralysis of convergence (the eyes remain immobile when the patient is asked to look at the wristwatch).

In a patient presenting with signs of increased intracranial pressure and ophthalmologic signs localizing to the roof of the midbrain (pineal region) the differential diagnosis first needs to include the likely possibility of tumors. Pineal tumors usually manifest with headache and signs of increased intracranial pressure due to obstruction of the aqueduct. Other pathological processes that are part of the differential diagnosis include arteriovenous malformations, trauma, vascular occlusions, encephalitis, posterior fossa aneurysm, demyelinating lesions, and Wernicke's encephalopathy.

Tumors of the pineal region include the following:

- Germ cell tumors (germinoma, teratoma).
- Pineal parenchymal cell tumors
    Pineocytes (pineocytoma, pineoblastoma).
    Glia (astrocytoma, ependynoma).
- Others
    Meningioma.
    Hemangiopericytoma.
    Arachnoid cysts.

Neurological manifestations characteristic of pineal region involvement include the following (Packer et al.):

- Hydrocephalus.
- Parinaud's syndrome.
- Decreased level of alertness.
- Signs of pyramidal tract involvement with spastic weakness.
- Ataxia.

There are characteristic visual signs and symptoms related to involvement of the superior colliculus and pretegmental area. These consist of

- Paralysis of vertical gaze, particularly upward gaze paralysis, an important feature of Parinaud's syndrome. Doll's head maneuver or Bell's phenomenon causes upward elevation of the eyes, therefore confirming the supranuclear type of paralysis.
- Convergent-retraction nystagmus when attempts at upward saccades.
- Light-near dissociation: The pupils are mid-dilated and fixed to the light, but react to near effort.
- Paralysis of convergence when the eyes try to move to a near target.
- Papilledema.

The compression of the cerebral aqueduct is responsible for hydrocephalus and intracranial hypertension. This could also be due to obstruction of the third ventricle. Increased intracranial pressure manifests with headache, decreased level of alertness, vomiting, and changes in mental status. Headache and papilledema represent the most important signs of pineal tumors.

Diagnosis

Computed tomography and magnetic resonance imaging are important in order to detect the characteristics of the tumor such as size, position, possible cystic or hemorrhagic components, and presence of hydrocephalus. Germinomas may cause an increased level of serum human chorionic gonadotropin and serum alpha-fetoprotein.

Treatment

The treatment is based on shunt insertion for the management of hydrocephalus, radiotherapy, or surgical intervention such as stereotactic biopsy or operative exploration.

Acoustic Neuroma

Vignette

A 58-year-old housewife started complaining of dizziness attributed by her primary physician to her long-standing hypertension. Her right ear was bothering her and sometimes she had difficulty listening to her daughter on the phone and had to switch the receiver to her other ear. When probed for more history of her symptoms, she said that she felt irritation and dryness of her right eye and some numbness of her face. She denied any headache or visual disturbances. On examination, there was right lateral gaze nystagmus. She had difficulty closing her right eye and did not blink when the right cornea was stimulated. When a vibrating tuning fork was applied to the forehead, she only felt the vibration to the left.

Summary A 58-year-old woman with progressive right hearing loss. Midforehead tuning fork test (Weber) localizes to normal ear in sensory-neural hearing loss. (The patient described in the vignette felt the vibration to the left when a vibrating tuning fork was applied to her forehead.) The irritation and dryness of the eye and facial numbness represent early signs of trigeminal nerve dysfunction. Depression or absence of the corneal reflex is the most consistent early clinical sign (Rengachari). The incomplete closure of the eyelid is an early sign of facial nerve involvement.

Localization

The localization is extrinsic to the brainstem at the level of the cerebellopontine angle. Lesions localized on the surface of the brainstem are characterized by involvement of nearby cranial nerves, and by late and only modest, if any, involvement of the long sensory and motor tracts (Adams and Victor). The triad of unilateral hearing loss, ipsilateral corneal anesthesia, and incomplete facial nerve paresis is virtually pathognomonic of a cerebellopontine angle mass, usually acoustic neuroma (Rengachari). Following are the most common tumors of the CPA angle in adults:

- Acoustic schwannoma.
- Meningioma.
- Epidermoid cyst.
- Glomus jugular tumor.
- Choroid plexus papilloma.

Clinical Features

The incidence of diagnosed acoustic tumors is about 1 per 100,000 population per year (Avezaat and Pauw). The presentation is usually unilateral but bilateral manifestations typically can be found in neurofibromatosis type 2. Clinical signs include progressive hearing loss, which is the initial symptom in the majority of patients. It can be accompanied by tinnitus and vertigo.

The size of the tumor influences the multitude of symptoms, which are due to compression of adjacent cranial nerves, particularly the fifth and the seventh and less often the ninth and tenth. Further expansion of the tumor causes compression of the pons and lateral medulla and obstruction of the cerebrospinal circulation. The involvement of the trigeminal nerve manifests with facial pain, numbness and paresthesias as well as decreased or absent corneal reflex. Seventh nerve dysfunction causes paralysis of the hemiface, hemifacial spasm, or twitching of the orbicularis oculi.

Compression of the cerebellum is responsible for ataxia of gait.

Signs of involvement of lower cranial nerves and long tract dysfunction with hyperreflexia and extensor plantar responses are usually a late manifestation.

Diagnosis

The diagnosis is based on audiological evaluation that reveals a sensory-neural type of hearing loss typically in the high frequency range. MRI is the imaging of choice, particularly for detection of small intracanalicular tumors. The findings may demonstrate isointensity to mild hyperintensity on T_1, slight hyperintensity on T_2, moderate gadolinium-DTPA enhancement, and in some cases widening of the ipsilateral cerebellopontine angle.

Treatment

The treatment is based on the surgical removal of the tumor. Operative complications depend on the size of the tumor and mainly involve damage to the seventh nerve with various degrees of facial paralysis.

Pituitary Adenoma

Vignette

A male, 45-year-old mailcarrier had experienced headache and occasional visual obscuration during the past six months. He had a tendency to bump into objects while walking and noticed difficulty seeing cars passing by while driving. He had experienced a 15-pound weight gain and impotence. Visual acuity was 20/200 on the right and 20/60 on the left. Right optic atrophy was also noted. A temporal visual field defect was noted more dense on the right.

Summary A 45-year-old man presenting with progressive headache, visual obscuration, peripheral vision dysfunction, weight gain, and impotence. The neurological examination reveals decreased visual acuity on the right and right optic atrophy associated with bitemporal hemanopia more dense on the right.

Localization and Differential Diagnosis

The clinical signs and symptoms localize to the optic chiasm and right optic nerve. Involvement of the chiasm in the majority of patients is caused by extrinsic tumors such as pituitary adenomas, suprasellar meningiomas, and craniopharyngiomas or by aneurysms. Other disorders include gliomas, chordomas, melanomas, and metastases.

Infectious and inflammatory processes involving the pituitary gland, such as abscess, cysticercosis, sarcoidosis, tuberculosis, and lymphocytic hypophisitis, can also be responsible for a chiasmal syndrome (Van Der Lely).

Clinical Features

Pituitary adenomas usually cause visual and endocrine abnormalities and can frequently present with signs and symptoms of chiasmal dysfunction, in particular complete or partial bitemporal hemianopia. They are called microadenoma if the diameter is less than 10 mm and can be particularly active, especially in secreting prolactin. Adenoma associated with the secretion of prolactin are the most common microadenoma and cause the constellation of symptoms such as amenorrhea and galactorrhea.

Adenomas wih size larger than 10 mm cause expansion of the sella turcica and, with increasing growth, induce compression of adjacent structures. In particular, a lateral extension may cause dysfunction of the cavernous sinus, a superior extension is associated with compression of the optic chiasm and infundibulum, and an inferior extension may produce erosion of the sella turcica and invasion of the sphenoid sinus.

Hemorrhage and necrosis can occur in the setting of a pituitary tumor. A severe complication is pituitary apoplexy, which is characterized by acute onset of excruciating headache that simulates SAH, extraocular nerve palsies, rapidly progressive visual loss, and diminished sensorium. It is due to hemorrhage into a preexisting adenoma and is a surgical emergency.

Diagnosis

MRI is more sensitive than CT in the visualization of small microadenoma and can clearly visualize macroadenoma, especially in case of enlargement of the sella turcica and expansion beyond its confines. Angiographic studies may rule out the possibility of an aneurysm.

Treatment

Different forms of treatment are available, including drug therapy (bromocriptine), operative intervention, and radiotherapy.

Pseudotumor Cerebri

Vignette

A 29-year-old laboratory technician has been complaining of severe throbbing pain localized in the forehead and behind her eyes for the past six months. She is now becoming more concerned be-

cause for the past two weeks, she has noticed some episodes of blurry vision and one of complete visual obscuration lasting less than one minute. Her blurry vision seems somehow exacerbated by straining or coughing. The examination shows bilateral limitation in eye abduction and blurriness of the fundi.

Summary A 29-year-old woman with headache, transient binocular visual loss, bilateral abducens palsy, and papilledema.

Localization

The vignette indicates signs of increased intracranial pressure, such as

- Headache.
- Papilledema.
- Bilateral sixth nerve palsy.

(Increased intracranial pressure often causes a false localizing sixth nerve palsy [pseudosixth] that can be bilateral and also asymmetrical caused by stretching of the nerve in its course along the clivus.)

Differential Diagnosis

The differential diagnosis of transient binocular visual loss includes the following possibilities:

- Papilledema due to increased intracranial pressure.
- Pseudotumor cerebri.
- Venous thrombosis.
- Complicated migraine such as basilar migraine.
- Vertebrobasilar TIA in the territory of the top of the basilar artery or posterior cerebral artery.
- Demyelinating disorder: multiple sclerosis.
- Occipital seizures.
- Head trauma (especially in children).
- Hypertensive encephalopathy.
- Preeclampsia.
- Cerebral vasculitis.
- Hematological abnormalities: anemia/thrombocythemia/polycythemia and coagulopathies
- Drug toxicity (cyclosporine, methotrexate).
- Hydrocephalus.
- Space-occupying lesions
    Tumors: primary and metastatic.
    Cerebral hemorrhage.
- Infectious/inflammatory disorders
    Bacterial: syphilis.
    Viral: meningitis/encephalitis.
    Parasitic.
    Sarcoidosis, systemic lupus erythematosus.

Considering the patient described in the vignette, all the clinical possibilites need to be assessed before making the preferred diagnosis, in this case, pseudotumor cerebri, which is mainly a diagnosis of exclusion. Therefore, it is important to properly address all the possible etiologies in the differential diagnosis.

Clinical Features

Pseudotumor cerebri or benign intracranial hypertension manifests with signs and symptoms of increased intracranial pressure in the absence of localizing neurological findings and in a patient who has an alert sensorium. Except for the elevated opening CSF pressure all other diagnostic studies, particularly neuroimaging studies, should be normal and conditions such as brain tumors and sinus thrombosis need to be cautiously ruled out. The incidence is 0.9 per 100,000 in the general population per year, or 19.3 per 100,000 in obese women ages 20 to 44 (Friedman and Jacobson).

The main clinical manifestations are represented by headache and visual dysfunction. The headache is often chronic and manifests on a daily basis but has also been described as throbbing, resembling migraine headache. The pain can be localized in the retroorbital area and may be exacerbated by eye movements. In some cases, it can be associated with nausea, vomiting, photophobia, and neck and low back pain. Visual disturbances can manifest with a constellation of symptoms such as brief episodes of transient visual obscuration lasting several seconds, horizontal diplopia, blurred vision, sparkles (photopsia), and so on. Intracranial noises such as a pulsatile tinnitus has also being described in over half of patients. The ophthalmoscopic examination shows evidence of papilledema. In severe cases of PTC, the visual acuity may decline rapidly.

Diagnosis

The visual function can be assessed by perimetry that can discover visual field dysfunctions such as enlargement of the blind spot, generalized field constriction, and nasal defects (Friedman and Jacobson). Neuroimaging studies are obtained before a lumbar puncture is performed. An empty sella can be demonstrated in over 50% of patients with pseudotumor cerebri. The cerebrospinal fluid examination in a patient with pseudotumor cerebri shows an opening pressure above 200 mm of water in the non-obese and above 250 mm of water in the obese. Cell count and protein studies are normal.

Treatment

The medical treatment of PTC is based on the management of increased intracranial pressure, weight loss, and the use of diuretics such as acetazolamide and furosemide (lasix) and, infrequently, corticosteroids. A series of lumbar punctures have also been performed but are traumatic for the patient.

The indication for surgical intervention is progressive visual deterioration that requires optic nerve sheath fenestration. Lumbar peritoneal shunt can be used for intractable headache or failed nerve sheath surgery (Wall). Optic nerve sheath fenestration can effectively reverse visual loss in most cases but carries several complications, such as hemorrhagic complications, transitory diplopia, retrobulbar hemorrhage, central and retinal branch occlusion, and so on.

Limbic Encephalitis

Vignette

An 80-year-old retired stockbroker started becoming forgetful, agitated, and confused over the past three months. He was awake and combative at night and drowsy by day. Several treatments were prescribed, including neuroleptics and benzodiazepines. During the last few weeks he was more agitated, unable to recognize his relatives, and disoriented to time and place. He recently lost 10 pounds. He was hospitalized after the occurrence of a generalized tonic-clonic seizure. His past medical history was unremarkable. He denied ever using alcohol but had smoked about one pack of cigarettes a day for 30 years. On examination, he was thin and withdrawn, but cooperative. Recent memory was severely impaired, while memory for remote events was preserved. Reading, comprehension, writing, and repetition were intact. No focal signs were observed except for some mild wide gait instability.

Summary An 80-year-old man with progressive changes in mental status and one generalized seizure. The most significant aspect of the vignette is the patient's mental status and behavior abnormalities represented by confusion, agitation, disorientation, memory loss of subacute onset, with preservation of the higher cortical functions. An important part of the vignette is the history of heavy smoking that can bring into consideration the possibility of malignancy with all the related complications.

Localization and Differential Diagnosis

Memory disorders can be attributed to abnormality of the medial temporal lobe and its connection to the mammillary body and upper brainstem. Dysfunction of the limbic system can be responsible for behavior abnormalities characterized by anxiety, depression, confusion, agitation, hallucinations, and severe abnormality of recent memory.

The differential diagnosis includes several possibilities. First, metabolic, toxic, and nutritional disorders need to be considered. Metabolic disorders can often cause delirium and changes in mental status and can be due to electrolyte dysfunction, such as hypokalemia and hypercalcemia; endocrine abnormalities, such as thyroid and parathyroid disease and Cushing's disease; or organ failure, such as hepatic and uremic encephalopathy.

Among the toxic disorders are alcohol intoxication and withdrawl, arsenic and heavy metal poisoning, and toxic effects of medications. Nutritional disorders include vitamin B12 deficiency and Wernicke's encephalopathy, which should be particularly considered. Wernicke's encephalopathy is characterized by a global confusional state with prominent short-term memory dysfunction in combination with ocular abnormalities and ataxia. The diagnosis of Wernicke's disease is particularly based on the ocular signs but in isolated cases any one component of the triad (ocular signs, ataxia, confusional state) may be the sole manifestation of the disease (Adams and Victor). The patient in the vignette does not have a history of alcoholism, liver disease, or malnutrition.

Consideration needs to be given to infectious, inflammatory, traumatic, neoplastic, and paraneoplastic disorders. Among the infectious disorders, herpes simplex encephalitis needs special attention because of the predilection for limbic structures, but is usually characterized by an acute course with fever, headache, seizures, confusion, and personality changes. Chronic meningeal disorders, such as cryptococcal, tuberculosis, carcinomatous, neurosyphilis, and so on, can cause mental status changes with confusion, but are also characterized by chronic headache, meningeal signs, cranial nerve involvement, focal deficits and seizures.

Inflammatory disorders, such as vasculitis (SLE, polyarteritis nodosa, Wegener's granulomatosis) can cause encephalopathies, but are associated with systemic symptoms.

Primary and metastatic tumors as well as subdural hematoma, are other considerations and enter the differential diagnosis of mental status changes. There is no prior history of trauma or any etiologic factor that may suggest chronic subdural hematoma. The history of heavy smoking may bring into consideration a possible diagnosis related to effect of a malignancy.

Among the paraneoplastic disorders, limbic encephalitis could well represent the clinical symptoms of the vignette. Paraneoplastic limbic encephalitis is associated with lung tumors, especially small cell cancer in at least 70 percent of cases (Aminoff). The limbic encephalitis often manifests before the tumor is diagnosed. Clinical manifestations are characterized by confusion, agitation, anxiety, depression and marked recent memory dysfunction with normal cognitive functions (Aminoff). Additional symptoms consist of seizures that can be partial or generalized and hallucinations.

Laboratory Tests

The CSF usually shows a pleocytosis and increased protein level.

Treatment

Treatment of the underlying malignancy may cause temporary improvement of the symptoms. Plasmapheresis has been used in selective cases.

Meningeal Carcinomatosis

Vignette

A 70-year-old retired handyman was in his usual state of health until six months ago when he started experiencing headache, on and off confusion, and twitching of his left face, with difficulty closing his eyelid. He was diagnosed with Bell's palsy and put on a short course of prednisone. He then complained of diplopia, right facial numbness, and hearing loss. For the past two weeks he had also experienced low back pain, difficulty climbing stairs, and burning pain across the left knee. On neurological examination, there was pupillary anisocoria, left ptosis, and limitation on left lateral gaze with abduction. There was bilateral facial weakness, right greater than left. Corneal reflexes were absent. Hearing was diminished on both sides. There was mild weakness of the left hip flexion, knee extension, and foot inversion. Left knee jerk was absent. He had a history of atrial fibrillation, depression, and heavy cigarette smoking, which stopped three years earlier following a lung resection.

Summary A 70-year-old man presenting with headache, on/off confusion, and progressive multiple cranial nerve dysfunction (third, fifth, seventh, eighth), associated with low back pain, and left leg weakness.

Localization

The vignette presented has multifocal signs and symptoms involving cerebral hemispheres (with signs of headache and confusion) multiple cranial nerves (third, fifth,

seventh, and eighth), and lumbar roots (L1–L3, L2–L4, and L4–L5). Considering first multiple cranial neuropathies, the cause can be a lesion, intrinsic or extrinsic, to the brainstem. Lesions extrinsic to the brainstem manifest with involvement of nearby cranial nerves and with late and only modest (if any) involvement of the long sensory and motor tracts and segmental structures lying within the brainstem (Adams and Victor). Intrinsic lesions of the brainstem often cause early involvement of long tracts producing a crossed sensory or motor syndrome.

Neuromuscular disorders such as myasthenia gravis that can commonly involve multiple cranial nerves and have fatigable weakness that improves with rest can be easily ruled out by the hearing loss and sensory loss on the face.

Assuming that the localization is extrinsic to the brainstem, several categories need to be considered:

- Infectious disorders.
- Inflammatory disorders.
- Neoplastic disorders.

Infectious disorders responsible for multiple cranial neuropathies include bacterial, viral, and fungal diseases, such as tuberculosis, Lyme disease, neurosyphilis, and herpes zoster.

Inflammatory disorders comprise granulomatous and vascular disorders, such as sarcoidosis, Wegener's granulomatosis, polyarteritis nodosa, temporal arteritis and so on. These disorders need great consideration but their diagnosis is not supported in the vignette by the presence of systemic symptoms or multisystem disease.

Neoplastic disorders include primary or metastatic tumors.

Diffuse or multifocal infiltration of the leptomeninges by a tumor (meningeal carcinomatosis) can manifest with a constellation of symptoms, such as headache, cognitive changes, multiple cranial nerve dysfunction, signs of meningeal irritation, and spinal cord or root lesions. The man's history of cigarette smoking and lung resection suggest the possibility that complications due to a malignancy may have occurred, placing meningeal carcinomatosis high on the list of differential diagnosis. The signs and symptoms of meningeal carcinomatosis can initially be confined to one anatomical area, but multiple levels of the neuraxis become involved as the symptoms progress (Wasserstrom). These areas generally include the cerebral hemispheres, cranial nerves, spinal cord, and nerve roots.

Cerebral signs are characterized by headache, often associated with nausea and vomiting, drowsiness, cognitive impairment with confusion, memory dysfunction, and occasionally seizures or focal findings. Cranial nerve abnormalities particularly tend to affect the oculomotor nerves with varying degree of paralysis (third, fourth, and sixth) followed by facial weakness, hearing loss, and involvement of the optic, trigeminal, and hypoglossal nerves (Schiff and Batchelor). Involvement of nerve roots particularly in the lumbosacral region is responsible for asymmetrical weakness, paresthesias, reflex loss, and radicular pain.

Diagnosis

CSF analysis is important in establishing the diagnosis and may demonstrate evidence of malignant cells, particularly after repeated samples are obtained. Other findings include an elevated opening pressure, increased protein content, hypoglycorrhachia, and mononuclear pleiocytosis. Neuroimaging studies may show meningeal enhancement.

Treatment

The treatment is based on a combination of radiation therapy and chemotherapy.

Paraneoplastic Cerebellar Degeneration

Vignette

A 69-year-old registered nurse for the past three months has experienced headache, dizziness, unsteady gait, and double vision. She had described the dizziness as "feeling of spinning or movements of her body." There was no history of alcohol and the medical history was unremarkable except for a recent weight loss of 10 pounds. On examination there was mild dysarthria and a coarse downbeat nystagmus in the primary position. There was diplopia when looking upward (vertical) with a tendency for the left eye to assume a higher position. Gait was wide based and unsteady particularly during quick turns.

Summary A 69-year-old woman with subacute onset of vertigo, dysarthria, ataxia, and visual difficulties. Neurological examination shows dysarthria, ataxia, and specific visual signs:

- Downbeat nystagmus.
- Vertical diplopia.
- Skew deviation.

Localization and Differential Diagnosis

The vertigo and accompanying neurological signs and symptoms are indicative of a central lesion rather than peripheral vertigo and may localize to the cerebellum and its connection. Vertigo can be due to central or peripheral causes. The vertigo and also nystagmus are more protracted with central lesions. Nausea and vomiting, which can be prominent with peripheral causes, are variable in central lesions. Nystagmus associated with central pathology may be multidirectional and is worsened by visual fixation.

Downbeating nystagmus has the fast phase beating in a downward direction. It may localize to a lesion at the level of the craniocervical junction, or may be found in patients with diffuse cerebellar dysfunction. Downbeat nystagmus can be observed with the following disorders:

- Malformations of the craniocervical junction, such as Arnold-Chiari malformation, basilar invagination, and platybasia.
- Wernicke's encephalopathy and cerebellar dysfunction due to alcohol or drugs, such as phenytoin or lithium.
- Neurodegenerative disorders, such as spinocerebellar degeneration and familial cerebellar degeneration.
- Multiple sclerosis, encephalitis, or vascular and neoplastic disorders involving the brainstem and cerebellum.
- Paraneoplastic cerebellar degeneration.

The vertical diplopia with the tendency of one eye to assume a higher position can be due to third nerve palsy or skew deviation. Skew deviation indicates brainstem or cerebellar involvement.

The differential diagnosis of the patient in the vignette should include all the disorders causing progressive cerebellar and brainstem dysfunction (mainly vestibulocerebellum and its connections). These include:

- Demyelinating disorders such as multiple sclerosis.
- Vascular disorders localized in the vertebrobasilar territory.
- Infectious: chronic meningitis, PML, Creutzfeldt-Jacob disease.
- Congenital malformations: Dandy-Walker malformation, Chiari malformation.
- Primary or metastatic tumors, lymphoma.
- Paraneoplastic disorders: paraneoplastic cerebellar degeneration due to remote effect of carcinoma.
- Toxic and metabolic disorders: alcohol and drugs, such as phenytoin, hypothyroidism.
- Hyperpirexia.
- Hereditary cerebellar degeneration, olivopontocerebellar atrophy.

Paraneoplastic cerebellar degeneration (PCD) is an important consideration. According to Bolla and Palmer, acute or subacute cerebellar degeneration presenting in older patients after the fifth decade of life is paraneoplastic in half of the cases. It can manifest months to years before a malignancy is discovered. This disorder has been described in association with carcinoma of the breast, ovary, and female genital tract, as well as small cell cancer of the lung and Hodgkin's lymphoma.

The clinical manifestation can present acutely or subacutely with signs of cerebellar involvement, such as truncal and limb ataxia, dysarthria, nystagmus, oscillopsia, and so on. Other symptoms include nausea and vomiting, and in some cases, changes in mental status with decreased sensorium, cognitive impairment, and limb weakness.

Therefore paraneoplastic cerebellar degeneration should be considered in a patient with progressive cerebellar dysfunction, particularly in middle-aged women presenting with severe ataxia, dysarthria and downbeat nystagmus.

Laboratory Tests

The discovery of circulating antineuronal autoantibodies in some PCD patients has supported the theory of an autoimmune etiology (Dropcho). Anti–Purkinje cell antibodies (APCA, also called anti-Yo) found in some cases may indicate the possibility of an underlying malignancy, in particular breast, ovarian, or female genital tract cancer.

Foster Kennedy Syndrome Due to Olfactory Groove Meningioma

Vignette

A 56-year-old accountant complained of incessant frontal headache of one year's duration. His family noted that he lost interest in his work, began acting inappropriately, and showed very little emotion to his wife's sudden death 4 months earlier. Neurological examination indicates a forgetful man with right anosmia, optic atrophy, and concentric narrowing of the visual field. A left disc edema is noted.

Summary 56-year-old man with headache, personality changes, memory loss, and focal findings:

• Right anosmia and optic atrophy.
• Left papilledema.

Localization

Frontal lobe: Subfrontal area with involvement of olfactory bulb or tract and ipsilateral optic nerve.

Diagnosis and Differential Diagnosis

Loss of smell can be an early and important symptom of intracranial neoplasm, particularly when considering meningiomas of the sphenoidal ridge and olfactory groove, gliomas of the frontal lobe, and parasellar masses causing compression of the olfactory bulbs or tracts (Brazis et al.).

The vignette typically describes the so-called Foster Kennedy syndrome, which can be found occasionally with olfactory groove or sphenoid ridge masses (especially meningiomas), or space-occupying lesions of the frontal lobe. The syndrome consists of three clinical signs:

• Ipsilateral anosmia caused by compression of the olfactory bulb or tract.
• Ipsilateral optic atrophy due to optic nerve dysfunction on the side of the lesion.
• Contralateral papilledema due to increased intracranial pressure caused by the space-occupying process.

References

Pineal Tumors

Glaser, J.S. Neuroophthalmology, ed. 2. Philadelphia: J.B. Lippincott, 408–410, 1990.
Packer, R.J. and Cohen, B.H. Germ cell tumors and pineal tumors. In: Handbook of Clinical Neurology. Vol. 24: Neuro-oncology, Part III. New York: Elsevier, 229–256, 1997.
Rengachari, S. and Wilkins, R.H. Principles of Neurosurgery. St. Louis: Mosby 29-2–29-16, 1994.
Schmidek, H.H. Pineal Tumors. New York: Masson, 21–55, 1977.
Van Der Lely, A.J. et al. Pituitary tumors. In: Handbook of Clinical Neurology. Vol. 24: Neuro-oncology, Part III. New York: Elsevier, 343–364, 1997.

Acoustic Neuroma

Adams, R.D. and Victor, M. Priciples of Neurology, ed. 5. New York: McGraw-Hill, 580–583, 1993.
Avezaat, C.J.J and Pauw, B.K.H. Vestibular schwannomas. In: Handbook of Clinical Neurology. Vol. 24: Neuro-oncology, Part II. New York: Elsevier, 421–464, 1997.
Rengachari, S.S. Principles of Neurosurgery. 30.2–30.7, 1994.

Pituitary Adenoma

Adams, R.D. and Victor, M. Principles of Neurology, ed. 5. New York: McGraw-Hill, 583–586, 1993.
Van Der Lely, A.J. et al. Pituitary Tumors. In: Handbook of Clinical Neurology. Vol. 24: Neuro-oncology, Part II. New York: Elsevier, 343–364, 1997.

Pseudotumor Cerebri

Boeri, R. The pseudotumor cerebri. Curr. Opin. Neurol. 7:69–73, 1994.
Friedman, D.I. and Jacobson, D.M. Pseudotumor cerebri. American Academy of Neurology, 52nd Annual Meeting, San Diego, 2000.

Johnston, J. et al. The pseudotumor syndrome. Arch. Neurol. 48:740–747, 1991.

Wall, M. Idiopathic intracranial hypertension: Mechanisms of visual loss and disease management. Semin. Neurol. 20:89–95, 2000.

Wall, M and George, D. Idiophatic intracranial hypertension: A prospective study of 50 patients. Brain 114:155–180, 1991.

Limbic Encephalitis

Adams, R. and Victor, M. Principles of Neurology, ed. 5. New York: McGraw-Hill, 593–594, 1993.

Aminoff, M.J. Neurology and General Medicine. New York: Churchill Livingstone, 1989.

Bakheit, A.M.O. et al. Paraneoplastic limbic encephalitis: Clinico-pathologic correlations. J. Neurol. Neurosurg. Psychiatry, 53:1084–1088. 1990.

Paraneoplastic limbic encephalitis N. Engl. J. Med. 319:849–860, 1988.

Posner J.B. Paraneoplastic syndromes involving the nervous system. In: Aminoff, M.J. Neurology and General Medicine. New York: Churchill Livingstone, 341–364, 1989.

Meningeal Carcinomatosis

Case Records of the Massachusetts General Hospital. Case 32. N. Engl. J. Med. 366–375, 1987.

Case Records of the Massachusetts General Hospital. Case 33. N. Engl. J. Med. 426–436, 1988.

Mollman, J.E. et al. Neurooncology. Continuum, Part A 1:63–77, 1994.

Schiff, D., Batchelor, T. Neurologic emergencies in cancer patients. Neurol. Clin. North Am. 16:449–483, 1998.

Van Oostenbrugge, R.J. et al. Presenting features and value of diagnostic procedures in leptomeningeal metastases. Neurology, 53:382–385, 1999.

Wasserstrom, W.R. Leptomeningealogy metastases. In: Wiley, R.G. Neurological Complications of Cancer. New York: Marcel Dekker, 45–71, 1995.

Paraneoplastic Cerebellar Degeneration

Anderson, N.E. et al. Paraneoplastic cerebellar degeneration: Clinical immunological correlations. Ann. Neurol. 24:559–567, 1988.

Bolla, L. and Palmer, R.M. Paraneoplastic cerebellar degeneration. Arch. Intern. Med. 157:1258–1262, 1997.

Case Records of the Massachusetts General Hospital. Case 34. N. Engl. J. Med. 321:524–534, 1989.

Dropcho, E.J. Paraneoplastic disorders: antineuronal antibodies and therapeutic options. Semin. Neurol. 14:179–187, 1994.

Olfactory Groove Meningioma

Adams, R.D. and Victor, M. Principles of Neurology, ed. 5. New York: McGraw-Hill, 586–587, 1993.

Brazis, P. et al. Localization. In: Clinical Neurology, ed. 2. Boston: Little Brown, 93–98, 1990.

10
Infections

Herpes Simplex Encephalitis

Vignette

A 62-year-old man was taken to a local hospital by his family because he seemed agitated and combative. He vomited once and was complaining of a smell of rotten eggs. In the emergency room he had a generalized tonic-clonic seizure. Twenty days before he had experienced some flu-like symptoms and a dry cough which lasted several days and was complaining of pain at both temples and the lower back. During examination he was confused, uncooperative, and mildly febrile. He perseverated in saluting when asked to say goodbye. His speech was paraphasic and he could not understand complex commands. Right toe was extensor.

Summary A 62-year-old man presenting with acute confusional state and focal neurological findings consisting of aphasia and right Babinski's sign. Also described are a generalized tonic-clonic seizure and olfactory hallucination (smell of rotten eggs).

Localization

The history and neurological examination provide a clue for the localization. Headache and back pain may be signs of meningeal irritation. Confusion, seizures, aphasia, and olfactory hallucinations point to a cortical involvement. Olfactory hallucinations may occur with pathology involving the inferior and medial parts of the temporal lobe particularly the region of the hippocampal convolution of the uncus (Adams and Victor). The aphasic syndrome characterized by fluent speech with paraphasic errors and trouble understanding complex commands also help to localize to the dominant temporal lobe.

Differential Diagnosis

A patient presenting with fever, meningeal signs, focal neurological deficits, and an abnormal mental status should raise highly the suspicion of an underlying central nervous system infectious process. Viral encephalitis is an important primary consideration. Herpes simplex encephalitis (HSE) is the most common cause of sporadic encephalitis in the United States, with an estimated frequency of 1 in 250,000 to 500,000 persons per year (Rubeiz and Roos). HSE should rank high in the list of the diagnostic possibilities when a patient presents with fever, headache, changes in mental status, focal or generalized seizures, or any acute focal sign that points to a lesion involving the frontal or temporal lobes. It is important to promptly identify the cases of possible HSE because of the high mortality rate in the absence of specific treatment (according to Tyler the mortality exceeds 70 percent if the infection is not appropriately treated).

Other herpes viruses include varicella-zoster virus, Epstein-Barr virus, and cytomegalovirus (CMV). Herpes zoster-varicella virus is not commonly responsible for severe encephalitis unless other factors coexist, such as older patients, immunosuppression, and disseminated cutaneous zoster (Rubeiz and Roos). Epstein-Barr virus usually causes a milder form (infectious mononucleosis) which only rarely involves the CNS. Encephalitis related to Epstein-Barr virus can manifest with changes in mental status, seizures, hallucinations, ataxia, and so on. CMV encephalitis usually develops in immunodepressed patients and, if symptomatic, can present with changes in mental status, fever, and signs of meningeal irritation (Rubeiz and Roos).

According to Rubeiz and Roos, the arboviruses cause 10 percent of all encephalitis cases reported annually as compared with the 2 percent of cases due to the enteroviruses.

In the differential diagnosis, consideration also needs to be given to other infections and space-occupying lesions. A brain abscess can present with headache, fever, changes in mental status, drowsiness, focal and generalized seizures, and focal motor or sensory neurological deficits. In the vignette there is no mention of any source of infection, such as the middle ear, sinuses, or heart, and there are no signs of increased intracranial pressure. Septic embolism also enters the differential diagnosis and is usually responsible for a mutifocal symptomatology in patients with endocarditis (not described in the vignette).

Other infections considered in the differential diagnosis include tuberculosis, cryptococcal infections, toxoplasmosis, and so on. Tuberculous meningitis presents with headache, fever, confusion, meningeal signs, and often cranial nerve involvement. Cryptococcal infections can manifest with headache, fever, and signs of increased intracranial pressure, particularly in patients immunosuppressed due to AIDS, lymphoma, leukemia, and so on. Toxoplasmosis can result in meningoencephalitis, particularly in immunocompromised patients, with confusion, mental status changes, seizures, and signs of meningeal irritation. The vignette does not indicate that the patient was immunodepressed.

Finally, space-occupying lesions, such as tumor and subdural hematoma, need to be ruled out. Tumors usually present with headache, signs of increased intracranial pressure, seizure, or localizing focal cerebral signs but the evolution is not as acute as the case presented unless a hemorrhage has occurred in the tumor. In acute subdural hematoma, the relation with traumatic etiology is clear. Chronic subdural hematoma where the history of previous trauma can be less obvious is characterized by a progressive evolution with headache, mental status changes, and, less often, focal lateralizing signs.

Therefore the best tentative diagnosis is herpes encephalitis.

Clinical Features

HSE is the most common cause of sporadic encephalitis in the United States, with an incidence of 1 in 250,000 to 500,000 individuals per year (Rubeiz). Herpes simplex virus (HSV) type 1 is responsible for herpes encephalitis. Type 2 infection can cause acute encephalitis in the neonatal period or aseptic meningitis in adults. The infection with HSV type 1 takes place through contaminated saliva or respiratory secretions. Latent HSV is discovered in the trigeminal ganglia of 75 percent of HSV-1 seropositive individuals (Tyler). The infection can be primary, occurring in cases where there is no prior exposure, or can be the result of reactivation of endogenous latent virus from the trigeminal ganglia.

The clinical symptoms of HSE usually manifest with abrupt onset of fever, headache localized in the frontal and retroorbital area, altered consciousness with lethargy, confusion, delirium, and coma. Also there can be audi-

tory, olfactory, and visual hallucinations, as well as seizures, focal or generalized. Focal neurological findings include hemiparesis, ataxia, cortical blindness, visual field defects, and so on.

Diagnosis

CSF examination reveals lymphocytic pleocytosis but the fluid can be xanthochromic. The pressure is frequently elevated and protein content mildly increased with a normal glucose level. The virus is cultured in the CSF in a minority of cases but in most patients HSV-specific DNA can be demonstrated by PCR.

MRI is more sensitive than CT of the brain and may show abnormalities in the orbitofrontal and temporal area, with variable degrees of parenchymal necrosis, mass effect, and edema. EEG can reveal generalized slowing, predominantly in the frontotemporal area, focal arrhythmic delta activity, and pseudoperiodic complexes.

Biopsy is rarely suggested and only in selected cases.

Treatment

The acute treatment includes respiratory care and treatment of seizures. Acyclovir is the drug of choice and is recommmended in a dosage of 10 mg/kg every 8 hours intravenously for a minimum of 14 days (Tyler). Side effects include elevation of BUN, liver function test abnormality, and trombocytopenia. Neurological symptoms of toxicity include changes in mental status, tremors, ataxia, and seizures (Tyler).

Herpes Zoster Vasculitis

Vignette

A 36-year-old legal secretary started experiencing speech difficulty and right-side weakness. She had a history of mild arthritis in the past that did not require treatment but denied hypertension, heart disease, diabetes, or smoking. Six weeks ago she had noted a painful maculopapular rash around the left forehead and periorbital area, which had resolved. In the emergency room she was slightly lethargic. She had diminished speech output. She uttered a few short words and perseverated these. She had no movements of the flaccid right limbs except a triple flexion of the right leg to pinch. Pinprick was decreased on the right. A right Babinski's sign was present.

Summary A 36-year-old woman with abrupt onset of aphasia and right hemiplegia with sensory loss.

Localization

The localization is cortical and points to a lesion in the left middle cerebral artery distribution.

This is a difficult vignette. A clue in the diagnosis is the maculopapular rash that occurred six weeks before the acute neurological symptoms. When an acute event, possibly vascular, occurs in a young patient who has no known risk factors for stroke, consideration needs to be given to other etiological factors that can be responsible for the brain ischemia.

The prior history of a rash may lead to consideration of infectious processes that can cause arteritis. Bacterial, spirochetal, fungal, and viral infections can be responsible for many cases of vasculitis. Herpes varicella-zoster (HVZ) virus is a well-known and documented etiological agent among the viral arteritides (Caplan).

The painful maculopapular rash described on the left forehead and periorbital area should bring the suspicion of herpes ophthalmicus. A distinctive central nervous system syndrome associated with HVZ is that of herpes zoster ophthalmicus (HZO) followed by ipsilateral cerebral angiitis and consequent contralateral hemiparesis (Hilt et al.). Transitory ischemic attacks may precede the onset of the stroke in some cases. Generally the stroke follows weeks to months after the HZO and affects the cerebral hemisphere ipsilateral to the zoster infection (Bourdette).

Other causes of arteritis include bacterial, spirochetal, and fungal infections. Bacterial meningitis can be complicated by the occurrence of strokes but the usual initial presentation includes fever, headache, meningeal signs, and altered sensorium. Meningo-vascular syphilis can cause strokes in young adults characterized by acute onset of motor and sensory weakness, aphasia, and visual loss, but this complication follows several years after the original infection. Other focal or multifocal lesions, such as brain abscess (bacterial or fungal), toxoplasmosis and other parasitic infections, Lyme disease, and autoimmune vasculitides, should also be considered in the differential diagnosis.

Clinical Features

Varicella zoster virus is responsible for the occurrence of varicella (chicken pox) and herpes zoster. Herpes zoster tends to preferentially involve the thoracic dermatometers and the ophthalmic division of the trigeminal nerve. The involvement of the ophthalmic division of the fifth nerve causes the occurrence of ocular complications, including possible corneal anesthesia and scarring. Uveitis, scleritis, and episcleritis can also occur.

A characteristic syndrome called Ramsay Hunt syndrome or herpes zoster oticus presents with ipsilateral facial weakness, loss of taste in the anterior two thirds of the tongue, and a painful vescicular rash in the external auditory meatus, and is due to the presence of an herpetic infection in the geniculate ganglion.

Varicella zoster virus infections are more common in elderly patients as well as in patients immunocompromised due to cancer, lymphoma, leukemia, and AIDS. The cutaneous lesions appear as eryhematous macules or papules that may progress into pustular or hemorrhagic lesions with superficial necrosis and then develop into crusts. The dermatological lesions occur in successive groups (crops) over several days (Hirschmann). Neurological complications of herpes zoster include postherpetic neuralgia, stroke, encephalitis, arteritis, myelitis, motor neuropathy, and so on. Postherpetic neuralgia is defined as protracted or paroxysmal pain of more than one month's duration in the area affected by the herpetic lesions and described as a throbbing, burning, aching, stabbing, itching sensation.

Motor neuropathies tend to affect cranial nerves, particularly the VII nerve and the ophthalmic branch of the V. Ramsey Hunt syndrome characterized by facial paralysis, loss of taste of the anterior two thirds of the tongue, earache, and dermatologic lesion in the external auditory canal as described above is a typical example of motor neuropathy. When there is involvement of the ophthalmic branch of the trigeminal nerve, there can be involvement of the extraocular muscles due to lesion of cranial nerves particularly third, fourth, and sixth.

Vasculitic complications may cause delayed brain infarction and hemiplegia contralateral to herpes zoster ophthalmicus. Symptoms of acute weakness, sensory loss, or aphasia can occur weeks to months after the herpetic infection. According to Hilt and colleagues the mortality is approximately 25% and the prognosis is guarded.

Encephalitis (zoster encephalitis) usually tends to affect patients immunosuppressed due to AIDS or other causes and presents with symptoms of headache, mental status abnormalities, nuchal rigidity, ataxia, cranial nerve palsies, and seizures.

Zoster myelitis is a rare complication that can manifest before or after the occurrence of the rash with weakness initially on one side and then bilaterally. Sensory and sphincteric dysfunction are also present.

Varicella zoster virus infection has also been associated with acute inflammatory demyelinating polyradiculoneuropathy and Reye's syndrome in rare cases (Lefond and Jubelt).

Diagnosis

The diagnosis of HZ is based on the characteristics of the painful rash. The vasculitic complication of herpes ophthalmicus should be kept in mind as a diagnostic consideration in a patient presenting with acute neurological signs (weakness, hemisensory loss, and aphasia) weeks or months following a herpetic facial lesion, usually involving the eye. The delayed hemiplegia is contralateral to the herpetic lesion.

Neuroimaging studies (CT scan and MRI of the brain) may show ischemic infarcts in the distribution of the middle cerebral artery and its branches. Cerebral angiography may demonstrate segmental narrowing of the proximal middle and anterior cerebral arteries.

Treatment

The treatment of varicella zoster virus is based on the use of oral or intravenous acyclovir. Famciclovir, used in the acute phase is presently the drug of choice for herpes zoster and has been shown to reduce the duration of postherpetic neuralgia in patients over age 50 (Lefond and Jubelt). The vasculitic complications of HZO-associated hemiparesis have been treated with corticosteroids or anticoagulants with varying results.

Progressive Multifocal Leukoencephalopathy

Vignette

A 52-year-old carpenter seemed uninterested in his usual activities for the last six weeks, often acting inappropriately and forgetful at work. Three days prior to this visit he did not return home and was found confused and disheveled at the train station. He was also noticed bumping into objects while walking. In the emergency room he was confabulating, but did not talk spontaneously, at times lying motionless and silent. His short-term memory was very impaired. No optokinetic nystagmus (OKN) was noted, in either direction. He did not respond to visual threats on the left and a left homonymous hemianopia was noted. He urinated once on the floor. He had a five-year history of chronic lymphocytic leukemia and mild hypertension. His brother had Parkinson's disease and his father died at 78 with Alzheimer's disease.

Summary A 52-year-old man with progressive cognitive, speech, and visual impairment. Past medical history is significant for chronic lymphocytic leukemia.

Localization and Differential Diagnosis

The vignette describes a patient with subacute behavior and mental status changes and focal neurological localizing findings. Abulia, apathy, confabulation, memory dysfunction, sphincter abnormalities, and inappropriate social conduct (urinating on the floor) point to a frontal lobe pathology. The absence of OKN suggests a localization to a lesion involving the inferior parietal lobule. The left homonymous hemianopia indicates a retrochiasmatic pathology.

Since the patient in the vignette has a history significant for chronic lymphocytic leukemia, consideration must be given first to the neoplastic and paraneoplastic causes of encephalopathy. Encephalopathies associated with malignancy and also immunosuppression can be due to metabolic or nonmetabolic causes. Metabolic abnormalities associated with malignancy usually cause symmetrical signs and symptoms and lack focal or lateralizing deficits. Nonmetabolic complications associated with malignancy and immunosuppression include

- Metastatic disease.
- Embolism.
- Tumors, such as lymphoma.
- Paraneoplastic disorders, such as limbic encephalitis.
- Infections, such as progressive multifocal leukoencephalopathy (PML).

Metastatic disease involving the nervous system can present as meningeal metastasis, intracranial metastasis, skull, dural, and brain metastasis. Involvement of the CNS in leukemia is often due to infiltration with leukemic cells and is called meningeal leukemia (Aminoff). Meningeal leukemia is characterized by headache, mental status changes such as lethargy and coma, seizures, papilledema, nausea, vomiting, and signs of meningeal irritation. Cranial nerve or spinal nerve root dysfunction can occur due to a mechanism of compression or infiltration by the leukemic deposits. There is a preferential involvement of the seventh, sixth, third, and fifth cranial nerves (Reich). This clinical picture does not seem to relate to the vignette presented. Localized leukemic foci may be responsible for focal neurological deficits influenced by the localization and can present with cranial nerve palsies, seizures, motor weakness, visual field defects, aphasia, and so on (Aminoff). These complications are rare when effective systemic therapy of leukemia is instituted.

Multiple cerebral emboli (marantic endocarditis or nonbacterial thrombotic endocarditis) associated with disseminated cancer can manifest with a wide variety of neurological symptoms and signs characterized by acute onset of focal or multifocal deficits in the territory of the carotid or vertebrobasilar artery, but preferentially occur with solid tumors, such as adenocarcinoma of the lung or pancreas or cardiac neoplasm. Stroke or encephalopathy is often the first clinical manifestation (Aminoff).

Primary central nervous system lymphoma, which is more common in immunocompromised patients, can present with a unifocal or multifocal bilateral cerebral involvement. Clinical manifestations include headache, behavioral dysfunction, seizures, changes in mental status, signs of intracranial hypertension, and lateralizing signs that suggest the underlying pathology. It is always a consideration in immunosuppressed patients.

Paraneoplastic diseases, particularly limbic encephalitis, must be considered in a patient with a history of cancer and immunosuppression. Clinically it is characterized by agitation, confusion, severe recent memory impairment, depression, seizures, and memory loss. Limbic encephalitis is usually associated with lung cancer, especially small cell cancer, in at least 70 percent of cases (Aminoff).

Progressive multifocal leukoencephalopathy is a demyelinating disorder due to JC virus and associated with immunosuppression, particularly due to AIDS, but also to lymphoproliferative and mycloproliferative disorders, such as chronic lymphocytic leukemia, Hodgkin's disease, and other lymphomas, as well organ transplantation, sarcoidosis, tuberculosis, or chronic use of steroid or antineoplastic agents. The symptoms start insidiously with cognitive abnormalities, mental status changes, visual abnormalities, particularly visual field defects rather than ophthalmoparesis, speech difficulties, motor weakness, and seizures. The course of the disease is subacute but the prognosis remains poor.

Diagnosis

In PML, the lesions involve the cerebral hemispheres in an asymmetrical and multifocal pattern that tends to affect preferentially the frontal and parietooccipital areas (Berger and Major). Neuroimaging studies, particularly MRI, reveals hyperintense lesions on T_2-weighted images in the affected regions. CSF study is helpful in excluding other disorders and may show a mild protein content elevation. Brain biopsy is the gold standard for diagnosis but is not always available. Berger describes the histopathology of PML as a triad of multifocal demyelination, hyperchromatic enlarged oligodendroglial nuclei, and bizarre astrocytes with lobulated hyperchromatic nuclei. The JCV can be detected in the oligodendroglial cells by electron microscopy.

Treatment

There is no effective treatment for PML. Cytosine arabinoside has been used and may have beneficial effects.

Creutzfeldt-Jacob Disease

Vignette

A 52-year-old cemetery worker, previously healthy, started experiencing unsteady gait, blurry vision, difficulty concentrating, and memory loss. Two months later his gait had worsened with frequent falls and he complained of diplopia on lateral gaze. While watching TV, he would scream that the images were enlarged and moving toward him. During the last four months he had become depressed, forgetful, and apathetic and had experienced inappropriate behavior, such as urinating or disrobing in public. His wife stated that he had episodes of uncontrollable agitation and body tremors diagnosed as possible seizures. On neurological examination a striking startle response to loud sounds was noted. He responded only to his name and was echolalic. He had slow eye movement, limited upward gaze, and marked ataxia and rigidity. Bilateral Babinski's signs were noted.

Summary A 52-year-old man with progressive dementia, gait and visual disturbances, and possible seizures.

Localization

An exaggerated startle response suggests a form of myoclonus. The neurological symptoms are indicative of multiple localization, such as cerebellar, upper motor neuron, extrapyramidal, and cortical. The patient described has signs suggestive of progressive dementia associated with multifocal neurological findings and myoclonus.

Differential Diagnosis

The differential diagnosis of progressive dementia is extensive and includes various causes:

- Degenerative disorders, such as Alzheimer's disease, dementia with Lewy bodies, and the other dementias.
- Vascular disorders, such as multiinfarct dementia or amyloid angiopathy.
- Paraneoplastic processes, such as limbic encephalitis.
- Infectious/parainfectious/inflammatory disorders.
- Metabolic/endocrine/toxic abnormalities.
- Trauma.
- Others, such as normal pressure hydrocephalus.

Alzheimer's disease is considered the most common degenerative disease causing dementia. The clinical features usually include insidious and progressive cognitive decline without focal deficits or significant extrapyramidal signs. Other neurodegenerative diseases are also unlikely in this case. Frontal lobe dementias are characterized by significant behavioral abnormalities and abnormal judgment or social conduct out of proportion to the degree of anterograde amnesia. Dementia with Lewy bodies has characteristic clinical features dominated by spontaneous parkinsonism, marked fluctuation in alertness or cognitive abilities, and vivid visual hallucinations.

Metabolic disturbances, such as nutritional, endocrine, and organ system dysfunctions, can all cause cognitive impairment of subacute or chronic onset, but are not the first consideration in a previously healthy man, with no other systemic involvement.

There is also no indication in the vignette to suggest a vascular etiology for the dementia. This is usually attributed to multiple ischemic or hemorrhagic events in the cerebral hemispheres affecting patients with a typical history of dementia associated with strokes that show improvement following acute event and abrupt onset.

Paraneoplastic limbic encephalitis, which is also a cause of rapidly progressive dementia, is characterized by marked behavior abnormalities, such as confusion, agitation, hallucinations, and prominent recent memory impairment. Limbic encephalitis is associated with lung tumor, particularly small cell cancer, in the majority of patients but in some cases the primary tumor cannot be found.

Chronic subdural hematoma and normal pressure hydrocephalus can cause a progressive dementia but there is clearly no relation to these two diagnoses in the patient described in the above vignette.

Infectious processes, such as chronic meningitis can cause a subacute progressive dementia but other important symptoms are headache, fever, and meningeal signs.

Another diagnostic possibility in this case is prion disease, particularly Creutzfeld-Jacob disease (CJD). The vignette clearly describes its characteristic findings of progressive dementia associated with ataxia, myoclonus, and visual, cerebellar, pyramidal, and extrapyramidal signs.

Clinical Features

CJD, characterized by progressive dementia with myoclonus, has an incubation period that varies from 8 to 14 years (Ravilochan and Tyler). The usual duration of symptoms is less than 12 months and both sexes are affected equally, particularly in the sixth decade of life. Sporadic, iatrogenic, and familial forms are described. CJD can present with a prodrome characterized by fatigue, anxiety, asthenia, and depression followed by forgetfulness, behavior dysfunction, confusion, and severe intellectual deterioration. Hallucinations can also occur, particularly visual but in some cases also auditory, olfactory, or gustatory.

Focal neurological findings tend to involve different systems. According to Ravilochan and Tyler signs of pyramidal tract dysfunction are present in 40 to 80 percent of patients affected and consist of increased reflexes and tone and Babinski's signs. Cerebellar involvement manifests with incoordination, tremor, nystagmus, ataxia, and dysarthria and can be severe.

Visual disturbances can also be a prominent feature and occur in 40 to 60 percent of cases (Ravilochan and Tyler). They include visual field abnormalities, impairment of visual acuity, cortical blindness, visual hallucinations, visual illusions such as distortion of shape and form of images, and so on. Extrapyramidal symptoms with rigidity, bradykinesia, and in some cases dystonia are also features of this disorder.

The involvement of the lower motor neuron has been described in a minority of patients (10 percent according to Ravilochan and Tyler). Seizures can be present but are not a prominent sign.

The progression of the disorder is rapid and inexorable with severe cognitive impairment, stupor, and profound dementia. The most characteristic and constant sign is myoclonus, which is often stimulus-sensitive (Johnson). Myoclonus is characterized by irregular, involuntary contractions of various muscle groups that persist during sleep and first appear on one side but then became generalized. It is stimulus sensitive but can also occur spontaneously. In the end, the majority of patients are unresponsive, rigid, and akinetic.

Iatrogenic cases of CJD have been described after medical procedures such as corneal transplant, placement of human cadaveric dura mater grafts, contaminated neurosurgical instrumentation, and recipients of human growth hormone. The familial forms of CJD have an autosomal dominant transmission, tend to manifest earlier, and have a more prolonged course than the sporadic form.

CJD is distributed worldwide with an incidence of 0.5 to 2 cases per million population per year (Ravilochan and Tyler).

Diagnosis

The diagnosis "definite CJD" is based on pathological examination of brain tissue and staining for prion protein. The EEG can be useful. During the early phase of CJD the EEG can be normal or show nonspecific diffuse slowing. In advanced cases, repetitive, high voltage triphasic and polyphasic sharp discharges and burst suppression pattern are observed. The examination of the cerebrospinal fluid does not show evidence of inflammatory reaction but only a mild increase in the protein content. Neuroimaging studies show nonspecific findings such as atrophy, ventricular enlargement, or diffuse high signal abnormalities in the basal ganglia.

Treatment

Treatment is not available. Antiviral agents have shown no efficacy.

Lyme Disease

Vignette

A 35-year-old businessman started complaining of headache and fatigue while vacationing for the

summer in Connecticut. He then developed numb-
ness of the left fourth and fifth digits. This was fol-
lowed by right wrist drop and left foot drop asso-
ciated with painful paresthesias. His wife noticed
that his speech was slurred and his face looked
asymmetrical. On examination his speech was
hoarse and mildly dysarthric. He was unable to
close his eyes or wrinkle his forehead on the right,
where hyperacusis was noted. There was marked
weakness of right wrist extension and left foot dor-
siflexion and patchy sensory loss over the extremi-
ties, more so on the left fifth digit. DTR were absent
throughout. There was marked right ankle swelling.

Summary A 35-year-old man with history of headache
and fatigue who then developed right facial weakness,
left hand numbness, right wrist drop, left foot drop, and
patchy sensory loss and parasthesias, while vacationing
in Connecticut.

Localization and Differential Diagnosis

There is no question that there is involvement of the peripheral nervous system. Considering the facial weakness,
the examination indicates that there was associated hyperacusis. Hyperacusis, which consists of an abnormal
loudness to sounds on the side affected is due to paralysis
of the stapedius muscle. This finding localizes the lesion
in the geniculate region of the facial canal. The distribution of weakness and sensory loss, involving multiple
peripheral nerves—left ulnar, right radial, and left peroneal, is typical of mononeuritis multiplex (see also vignette on mononeuritis multiplex in Chapter 6). Mononeuritis multiplex is characterized by the asymmetrical,
stepwise progression of individual cranial or peripheral
neuropathies (Preston and Shapiro). The pattern of mononeuritis multiplex can typically be observed in several
categories of disorders.

Mononeuritis multiplex can be associated with vasculitis, including polyarteritis nodosa, Churg-Strauss syndrome, cryoglobulinemia, systemic lupus, and so on. Vasculitic neuropathies can manifest with a focal or
multifocal involvement. Onset of the deficit is usually
acute and associated with the symptoms of weakness,
numbness, and pain, particularly burning, dysesthetic
pain. The neuropathy can occur first but in many cases
systemic symptoms accompany the clinical picture and
help in pinpointing the correct diagnosis.

Diabetes can also be complicated by peripheral neuropathy in the form of mononeuritis multiplex. It is excluded in the vignette by the lack of any previous evidence of this metabolic disorder.

Neoplastic and granulomatous disorders such as sarcoidosis, lymphoma, leukemia, and so on, can also create
a picture of mononeuritis multiplex. In the clinical case
presented, there is no evidence of systemic signs or symptoms that may indicate this possibility.

Infections, particularly Lyme disease, HIV, and leprosy, can be responsible for the developing of mononeuritis multiplex. Lyme disease stands high on the list of
possibilities for the patient in the vignette who is a 35-
year-old, previously healthy man, vacationing in Connecticut, with a history significant for subacute cranial
neuropathies, and mononeuropathies, associated with fatigue, headache, and ankle swelling.

Clinical Features

Lyme disease can present with a multitude of clinical
manifestations that vary from the cutaneous lesion, typically the erythema migrans rash, to cardiac, ophthalmological, neurological, and rheumatological manifestations. The nervous system is affected in approximately
15 percent of cases (Halperin).

Frequently, the patients complain of headache, fatigue,
irritability, myalgia, and generalized malaise. Cranial
neuropathies have a predilection for the facial nerve that
can also be involved bilaterally. According to Logigian,
facial palsy occurs in about 50 to 75 percent of patients
with early neuroborreliosis. Other cranial nerves can be
affected, such as the optic nerve, resulting in optic neuritis, perineuritis, and optic disk edema, and the oculomotor nerves. The involvement of nerve roots and peripheral nerves is responsible for symptoms of
radiculoneuritis where the pain is often severe and the
weakness and hypoesthesia follow an asymmetrical distribution. Involvement of the spinal cord with symptoms
of paraparesis or tetraparesis has been described but is
rare. Meningitis may be the presenting symptom of Lyme
disease (Belman) and is characterized by headache, neck
stiffness, and lymphocytic pleocytosis.

Chronic Lyme disease may be associated with chronic
neuropathy, radiculopathy, and encephalopathy.

Diagnosis

Laboratory tests may demonstrate antibodies to *Borrelia
burgdorferi* in the blood or cerebrospinal fluid. The antibody assay ELISA is the method used by most diagnostic laboratories.

Treatment

Patients presenting with neurological complications
should be treated with parenteral antibiotics such as third
generation cephalosporins or penicillin.

Neurocysticercosis

Vignette

A 22-year-old woman, recently immigrated from Mexico, was taken to a local emergency room after experiencing two generalized tonic-clonic seizures. She had a six-month history of intermittent headache with nausea and vomiting and blurry vision and a 10-pound weight loss. During this time she had several episodes of abnormal behavior, confusion, and agitation lasting several hours. The examination showed that she was alert and cooperative with normal vital signs and supple neck. There was decreased venous pulsation on both optic fundi and a questionable right extensor plantar response. Her past medical history was unremarkable.

Summary A 22-year-old Mexican immigrant with new onset of generalized seizure, two episodes of abnormal behavior and confusion, headache, decreased venous pulsation noted on funduscopic examination, and possible right Babinski's sign.

Localization

The patient's history of generalized as well as partial seizures (episodes of abnormal behavior, confusion, and agitation) associated with a neurological examination indicating signs of increased intracranial pressure (headache, early papilledema) suggest a cortical localization.

Differential Diagnosis

The differential diagnosis includes several disorders:

- Neoplastic processes (primary or metastatic).
- Infectious and inflammatory disorders (abscess, vaculitis).
- Vascular disorders (arteriovenous malformations, multiple emboli).

Brain tumors account for 3.5 to 5 percent of all cases of epilepsy; however, seizures complicate brain tumors in up to 30 to 50 percent of cases (Ettinger). In adult patients experiencing new onset of focal or generalized epilepsy, the possibility of an underlying brain tumor should be highly considered.

A variety of symptoms are associated with brain tumors, depending upon the site of origin, the tumor type and aggressiveness, and the occurrence of increased intracranial pressure with signs of headache, vomiting, papilledema, ocular palsies, altered level of consciousness, and so on. Seizures associated with brain tumors may be focal or generalized and can represent the first presenting symptom. Focal neurological deficits may consist of motor weakness, sensory loss, aphasia, visual field defects, and so on. Cerebral metastases are an important cause of new onset of seizures. Secondary brain involvement is preferentially due to tumor of the lung, breast, kidney, and melanoma.

In this patient, brain tumors are an important consideration and cannot be clinically excluded based on the information provided by the vignette.

Infectious processes include bacterial, viral, fungal, and parasitic infections and can be complicated by epilepsy when there is cerebral involvement. Neurocysticercosis is the main cause of adult onset epilepsy in developing countries in which the disease is endemic (Barry and Kaldjian). In the patient described, who is a 22-year-old female recently immigrated from Mexico where cysticercosis is endemic, this diagnosis should be highly considered. Other areas at risk are South America, India, China, Indonesia, and so on. Parenchymal neurocysticercosis may manifest with epilepsy, focal neurological findings such as motor and sensory deficits, ataxia, visual loss, mental status changes, intellectual deterioration and signs of increased intracranial pressure. Encephalitis has also been described.

Another parasitic infection to be considered that can be responsible for new onset of seizures and increased intracranial pressure is cerebral toxoplasmosis but involvement of the CNS typically occur in cases of immunodeficiency or during congenital infection. In the vignette there is no mention to any immunodeficient state clinically and by history.

Another infection that may occur particularly in developing countries is due to *Echinococcus granulosus* that is responsible for hepatic and cerebral involvement. Echinococcal cysts involve the CNS in only a small percentage of cases and if this occurs, may cause signs of increased intracranial pressure such as headache, vomiting and papilledema as well as seizures.

Schistosomiasis can rarely be responsible for the occurrence of headache and seizures if the CNS is involved, usually with *S. japonicum* infection.

Amebiasis can manifest with acute and chronic encephalitis and cerebral abscesses in rare but fatal cases dominated by rapid neurological deterioration. Hepatic abscesses are usually present.

In summary, neurocysticercosis is the best option among the parasitic infections. Consideration needs to be given to bacterial infections that can present with focal neurological symptoms and signs of space-occupying lesions or seizures. In particular, tuberculomas in developing countries can cause new onset of focal or generalized seizures as well as other symptoms of space-occupying lesions, such as headache, papilledema, and focal deficits.

Considering other aspects of the differential diagnosis

in this young woman with new onset of seizures, headache, focal findings, and increased intracranial pressure, cerebral vascular malformations need to be ruled out. Also cerebral vasculitis and multiple emboli enter the differential diagnosis.

Inflammatory disorders, such as systemic lupus erythematosus and Behçet disease, and congenital disorders, such as tuberous sclerosis and neurofibromatosis, can be mentioned for completion, but are easily excluded by the vignette due to the lack of systemic and other characteristic accompanying findings.

Clinical Features

Neurocysticercosis is considered an important cause of epilepsy, particularly in endemic areas such as Mexico, Central and South America, China, India, and so on. It occurs when larvae of the pork tapeworm *Taenia solium* infect the CNS. Humans are the intermediate host in the lifecycle of the tapeworm and become infected by ingesting eggs from contaminated water or food. *Cysticerci* may invade almost every tissue of the host, but clinically significant disease is due to involvement of the nervous system.

There are four principal forms of neurocysticercosis:

- Parenchymal.
- Ventricular.
- Subarachnoid.
- Racemose.

Clinical symptoms include focal or generalized seizures, which are the most frequent manifestation, headache, neck stiffness, signs of increased intracranial pressure, ataxia, sensory deficits, intellectual deterioration, and so on. Rarely, encephalitis occurs due to a severe inflammatory response.

Diagnosis

Neuroimaging studies, particularly MRI, can detect active ventricular or subarachnoid cysts. CT scan is helpful in visualizing parenchymal calcifications. CSF studies may show lymphocytic pleocytosis, increased protein level, and decreased glucose in half the patients. Immunological tests have been developed to detect anticysticercal antibodies in serum and CSF.

Treatment

The treatment is based on the use of cysticidal drugs, such as albendazole and praziquantel. The combined use of steroids may decrease the inflammatory reaction. Albendazole may have side effects such as gastrointestinal symptoms, leukopenia, and elevated liver enzymes. Praziquantel may cause headache, fever, and gastrointestinal upset. Epilepsy, which is a main manifestation of neuro-

cysticercosis, needs anticonvulsant treatment. Hydrocephalus that can be communicating or obstructive has been treated with shunting.

Cytomegalovirus Polyradiculopathy

Vignette

A 35-year-old man with a history of intravenous drug abuse and AIDS started complaining of low back pain, leg paresthesias, difficulty urinating, and two episodes of fecal incontinence in the last two weeks. On examination there was symmetrical weakness of flexion and extension of the toes and ankles. Right knee jerk was reduced and ankle jerks were absent.

Summary A 35-year-old man with history of drug abuse and AIDS complaining of low back pain, paresthesia, distal weakness and areflexia, and sphincteric disturbances.

Localization and Differential Diagnosis

There is no doubt that the localization is in the peripheral nervous system (PNS) with involvement of multiple roots (cauda equina). Another important point of the vignette is the indication that the patient had a history of AIDS. In the differential diagnosis, peripheral nervous system manifestations of HIV infections, particularly progressive polyradiculopathy, must be considered.

A well-recognized complication of late HIV disease is cytomegalovirus (CMV) associated polyradiculopathy that clinically manifests with a picture of subacute or rapid asymmetrical lower extremities weakness, loss of reflexes, sphincteric disturbances, and radicular pain. The neurological dysfunction follows an ascending pattern usually with a rapid progression and only rarely involving the upper extremities or cranial nerves. Sensory symptoms are usually represented by paresthesias of the lower extremities and perineum with some hypoanesthesias over the saddle and genital area. CSF examination is characterized by polymorphonuclear pleocytosis, increased protein content and mild hypoglycorrhachia. PCR for CMV is always detected in viral CSF cultures (Clifford). Magnetic resonance imaging may demonstrate root and leptomeningeal enhancement along the conus medullaris to the cauda equina after gadolinium administration. Electromyography and nerve conduction studies show low amplitude motor response and widespread denervation in lower extremity and lumbar paraspinal muscles, all indicative of severe axonal dysfunction.

Other opportunistic infections in HIV patients need to be differentiated from CMV polyradiculitis. Varicella zoster virus in AIDS patients can cause radiculomyelitis in association with the typical cutaneous dermatomal lesions. Herpes simplex virus type 2 can present with a picture of radiculomyelopathy associated with myelitis and autonomic disturbances. Neurosyphilis, which is not uncommon in HIV patients, can be responsible for cases of polyradiculopathy or myelopathy with a positive VDRL in the serum and CSF. Other organisms, such as *Toxoplasma gondii,* can present with a conus medullaris syndrome and myelitis with progressive weakness, sphincteric dysfunction, and back pain. HTLV-1 and HTLV-2 infections can also coexist in HIV patients but usually cause an insidious and progressive myelopathy.

Alternative diagnoses not related to the HIV in the patient presented in the vignette are primary and metastatic spinal tumors and lumbosacral disc herniations.

Treatment

The treatment of CMV polyradiculitis is based on the prompt use of ganciclovir or foscarnet that can stabilize or improve the neurological symptoms.

Parasitic Infection: Toxoplasmosis

Vignette

A 32-year-old actor noted the gradual onset of headache, generalized malaise, and fatigue over the past two to three weeks. He then started experiencing sudden, violent, flinging movements of the proximal right arm and leg that interfered with his balance and were worsened by attempts to move. His past medical history was significant for AIDS. He had been on several antiviral agents but could not tolerate them and had stopped all the medications six months ago. No other history was elicited.

Summary A 32-year-old man with history of AIDS, experiencing progressive headache, fatigue, malaise, and involuntary movements, described as violent and flinging, involving the proximal right arm and leg.

Localization

The involuntary movements resemble the characteristics of hemiballism rather than those of a partial motor seizure. The history and clinical findings are indicative of a lesion involving the left subthalamic nucleus.

Differential Diagnosis

In the differential diagnosis several possibilities should be considered:

- Vascular lesions: Infarction or hemorrhage in the deep gray matter.
- Space-occupying lesions:
  —Neoplastic processes (tumor): Primary or metastatic.
  —Infectious processes (abscess): Tuberculous mass lesion, toxoplasmosis.
- Inflammatory disorders: Systemic lupus, Behçet's disease.

In a patient with history of AIDS, great consideration needs to be given to opportunistic infections that may be responsible for cerebral abscesses.

Toxoplasmosis is considered the most common opportunistic infection of the CNS in acquired immunodeficiency syndrome with frequency that fluctuates between 5 and 15 percent (Concha and Rabinstein). The clinical manifestations usually assume a subacute course over days or weeks and are characterized by fever, headache, generalized malaise, seizures, and focal neurological findings. Movement disorders particularly choreoathetosis and ballism have also been described as a manifestation of CNS toxoplasmosis in patients who had abscesses in the contralateral subthalamic nucleus, putamen, or multiple sites within the basal ganglia (Cohen).

The differential diagnosis of toxoplasmic encephalitis needs to exclude in particular primary CNS lymphoma, tuberculoma, and PML. Primary central nervous system lymphoma, which typically occurs in severely immunocompromised patients, may manifest with symptoms that can resemble toxoplasmosis, characterized by changes in mental status, drowsiness, confusion, memory loss, seizures and focal neurological deficits. Therefore, a distinction between toxoplasma encephalitis and lymphoma is not always possible based on clinical findings and often also on neuroimaging studies.

Tuberculomas also enter the differential diagnosis and can be difficult to distinguish from CNS toxoplasmosis or lymphoma. They can manifest with changes in mental status, signs of increased intracranial pressure, headache, focal deficits, and new onset of seizures.

Other less common processes that must be considered in this patient include progressive multifocal leukoencephalopathy; fungal, pyogenic, candidal or herpetic abscesses; infarction with hemorrhage; and metastatic Kaposi's sarcoma.

In addition the possibility of some non–HIV-related CNS pathology, such as metastatic or primary malignant brain tumor, arteriovenous malformations, multiple sclerosis, etc., must be considered.

Clinical Features

Toxoplasmosis is the most common cause of infectious mass lesions in the brain of HIV-infected persons (Cohen). Most cases of cerebral toxoplasmosis are due to reactivation of a previously acquired latent infection. This usually occurs in advanced HIV infection when the CD4 cell count is less than 100/mm^3. The clinical manifestations present over several weeks with headache, fever, changes in mental status, drowsiness, confusion, and focal neurological deficits, particularly hemiparesis, ataxia, visual field abnormalities, and aphasia, but also movement disorders, such as hemichorea and hemiballism.

Diagnosis

Serum antitoxoplasma antibodies can be obtained as well as PCR detection of *Toxoplasma gondii* in CSF which is specific but not sensitive for the diagnosis of toxoplasma encephalitis. MRI with gadolinium may show multiple ring enhancing lesions that tend to be localized in the corticomedullary junction or basal ganglia. SPECT scanning shows no uptake with toxoplasmosis (a positive result favors lymphoma). Brain biopsy is a consideration in selected cases when neuroimaging studies evidence a single lesion, or if the patient shows no improvement with the appropriate therapy and serology is negative.

Treatment

The treatment is based on a combination of pyrimethamine and sulfadiazine for six weeks. Side effects include myelosuppression, liver dysfunction, fever, rash, and diarrhea.

HTLV-1 Myelopathy

Vignette

A 45-year-old female immigrant from Santo Domingo started experiencing low back pain and left leg numbness two years ago. The numbness then spread to the other leg, together with stiffness and unsteady gait, and some urinary urgency. No significant family history was noted. On examination there was a 3/5 strength in both lower extremities. A bilateral Babinski was noted. Sensory examination showed impaired vibration and joint position sense, left greater than right, on both lower extremities. MRIs of cervical and thoracic spine were reported as normal.

Summary A 45-year-old woman with progressive spastic paraparesis and sensory loss.

Localization

Localization is the spinal cord.

Differential Diagnosis

The differential diagnosis is of progressive myelopathy. Different categories of disorders need to be considered:

- Infectious processes: Lyme disease, treponemal infection, HIV, HTLV-1, HTLV-2, herpes, cytomegalovirus, polio, abscess of the epidural and paraspinal area.
- Inflammatory disorders: systemic lupus, sarcoidosis, and so on.
- Demyelinating disorders: multiple sclerosis.
- Primary lateral sclerosis, ALS variant with pure upper motor neuron signs.
- Structural compressive disorders and spinal malformations: Spondylosis, abscess, foramen magnum tumors, extramedullary and intramedullary tumors, disk herniation, syringomyelia. A-V malformations of the spinal cord.
- Vascular disorders: Spinal myelopathy, ischemic and hemorrhagic.
- Nutritional deficiencies: vitamin B$_{12}$ and folate.
- Hereditary disorders: progressive spastic paraplegia.

Several infectious processes are responsible for the development of progressive myelopathy. A well-recognized disorder is HTLV-1 and HTLV-2 associated myelopathy/tropical spastic paraparesis, characterized by progressive weakness and sphincteric dysfunction, particularly bladder, associated with antibodies to HTLV Type 1 or Type 2 in serum and CSF. HIV may cause a noninflammatory vacuolar melopathy with paraparesis and sensory ataxia. CMV, herpes zoster, and herpes simplex can also be responsible for a myelopathy, particularly in immunodepressed patients.

Inflammatory disorders, particularly systemic lupus erythematosus, may be complicated by a myelopathy that can be acute, remitting, relapsing, or chronic progressive. Sarcoidosis usually causes multiple cranial nerve involvement and only rarely a myelopathy.

Progressive multiple sclerosis can present with a myelopathy but it is also important to rule out first structural and compressive lesions. Spinal cord tumors in particular are associated with radicular pain, paresthesias, sensory loss, Lhermitte sign, a partial or complete Brown-Séquard syndrome, weakness and wasting, The involvement of the thoracic area may cause a persistent thoracic pain. Signs of cord compression are characterized by progressive asymmetrical weakness, sensory loss, and sphincteric dysfunction.

Syringomyelia can manifest with segmental weakness and atrophy of the hands, hyporeflexia, dissociated sensory loss with hypoesthesia to pain and temperature and preservation of touch, spastic paraparesis, and ataxia.

Tumors of the foramen magnum are characterized by suboccipital pain and may include lower cranial nerve involvement. Spinal arteriovenous malformations can cause acute weakness associated with severe neck and back pain if a subarachnoid hemorrhage has occurred or may be responsible for insidious and progressive paraparesis and sphincteric abnormalities.

Primary lateral sclerosis, which is a variant form of ALS with only upper motor neuron signs, is diagnosed after other causes have been excluded.

Hereditary spastic paraplegias include several disorders with different modes of inheritance that manifest with progressive paraplegia often with other neurological signs such as optic atrophy, mental retardation, extrapyramidal and cerebellar involvement, and so on.

Nutritional deficiencies, in particular vitamin B_{12} deficiency may be responsible for the development of subacute, combined degeneration of the spinal cord. Symptoms usually include signs of involvement of the posterior and lateral columns with loss of vibration and position sense, weakness, and hyporeflexia associated with cognitive and behavior abnormalities. Pernicious anemia is the main hematological abnormality.

In conclusion, in the patient described in the vignette—a 45-year-old woman from the Caribbean with signs of progressive spastic paraparesis and a normal cervical and thoracic MRI—tropical spastic paraparesis should rank high in the list of diagnosis.

Clinical Features

The human T-cell lymphotropic virus type 1 that has different ways of transmission, such as sexual, parenteral, and perinatal, is endemic in the Caribbean Islands, Central and South America, southern Japan, and sub-Saharan Africa. A variety of clinical manifestations can be associated. Among them, the two most common are adult T-cell leukemia/lymphoma and HTLV-1 myelopathy/tropical spastic paraparesis (Araujo).

A diagnosis of probable and definite HAM has been established based on certain parameters. The definite diagnosis requires the occurrence of progressive symmetrical myelopathy due to corticospinal tract dysfunction and laboratory studies showing antibodies in both serum and CSF.

Clinical features include a disorder of gait with paraparesis, stiffness, and increased reflexes, with pathological signs, such as Babinski's and Hoffmann's signs, clonus, and sensory symptoms, more often subjective. Pain can occur, particularly in the lumbar area, and can be severe in some cases. Sphincteric dysfunction may include bladder disturbance, constipation, and impotence. Less frequently, cerebellar signs, optic atrophy, cranial nerve deficits, nystagmus, and absent or reduced ankle jerk may be observed. Signs of peripheral neuropathy and inflammatory myopathy are also described in association with HAM. The diagnosis is based on the demonstration of HTLV-I/antibody or antigen in both serum and CSF. MRI of the spine can have normal findings or show some degree of cord atrophy.

Treatment

The treatment is based on the use of steroids administered at high doses, such as methylprednisolone (1 gm/day) followed by oral prednisone (80 mg/day) with slow tapering after three to six weeks. Other treatments include intravenous immunoglobulins or interferon-alpha.

References

Herpes Simplex

Adams, R.D and Victor, M. Principles of Neurology, ed. 5. New York: McGraw-Hill, 1993.

Blume, G.M. and Tyler, K.L. Infectious diseases. In: Feldmann, E. Current Diagnosis in Neurology. St. Louis: Mosby, 88–92, 1994.

Case Records of the Massachusetts General Hospital. Case 44. N. Engl. J. Med. 301:987–994, 1979.

Irani, D.N. Viral infections. In: Johnson R.T. and Griffin, J. Current Therapy in Neurologic Disease, ed. 5. St. Louis: Mosby, 1997.

Rubeiz, H. and Roos, R.P. Viral meningitis and encephalitis. Semin. Neurol. 12:165–76, 1992.

Tyler, K. Herpes simplex infections of the nervous system. American Academy of Neurology, 51st Annual Meeting, Toronto, 1999.

Whitley, R.J. et al. Diseases that mimic herpes simplex encephalitis: Diagnosis, presentation and outcome. JAMA 262:234–239, 1989.

Herpes Zoster Vasculitis

Bourdette, D.N. Herpes zoster ophthalmicus and delayed ipsilateral cerebral infarction. Neurology, 33:1428–1432, 1983.

Caplan, L. Stroke: A clinical approach, ed. 2. Boston: Butterworth-Heinemann 299–348, 1993.

Hilt, D. et al. Herpes zoster ophthalmicus and delayed contralateral hemiparesis caused by cerebral angiitis: Diagnosis and management approaches. Ann. Neurol. 14:543–553, 1983.

Hirschmann, J.V. Herpes zoster. Semin. Neurol. 12:322–328, 1992.

Johnson, R.T. Viral Infections of the Nervous System, ed. 2. Philadelphia: Lippincott Raven, 151–160, 1998.

Lefond, C.A. and Jubelt, B. Varicella-zoster virus infections of the nervous system. In: Neurobase MedLink, Arbor, 2000.

Liesegang, T. Varicella zoster viral disease. Mayo Clinic Proc. 74:983–998, 1999.

Progressive Multifocal Leukoencephalopathy

Aminoff, M.J. Neurology and General Medicine. New York: Churchill Livingstone, 191–195, 1989.

Berger, J.R. and Major, E.O. Progressive multifocal leukoencephalopathy. Semin. Neurol. 19:193–200, 1999.

Case Records of the Massachusetts General Hospital. Case 1. N. Engl. J. Med. 316:35–42, 1987.

Case Records of the Massachusetts General Hospital. Case 20. N. Engl. J. Med. 332:1773–1780, 1995.

Fovner, D.M. and Weiner, L.P. Chronic viral disease of myelin. Semin. Neurol. 5:168–178, 1985.

Reich, H.H. Neurological complications of leukemia. In: Handbook of Clinical Neurology, Vol. 25, Part III. New York: Elsevier, 233–260, 1997.

Creutzfeld-Jacob Disease

Buttner, U. and Fuhry, L. Eye movements. Curr. Opin. Neurol. 8:77–82, 1995.

Case Records of the Massachusetts General Hospital. Case 17. N. Engl. J. Med. 328:1259–1266, 1993.

Case Records of the Massachusetts General Hospital. Case 28. N. Engl. J. Med. 341:901–908, 1999.

Johnson, R.T. Viral Infections of the Nervous System, ed. 2. Philadelphia: Lippincott Raven, 356–364, 1998.

Korczyn, A.D. Prion diseases. Curr. Opin. Neurol. 10:273–281, 1997.

Kretzschmar, H.A. et al. Diagnostic criteria for sporadic Creutzfeld-Jacob disease. Arch. Neurol. 53:913–920, 1996.

Ravilochan, K. and Tyler, K.L. Human transmissible neurodegenerative diseases (prion diseases). Semin. Neurol. 12:178–192, 1992.

Scheld, W.M. et al. (eds.). Infections of the Central Nervous System, ed. 2. Philadelphia: Lippincott Raven, 199–221, 1997.

Schlossber, D. (ed.). Infections of the Nervous System. New York: Springer-Verlag, 153–168, 1990.

Shimizu, S. et al. Creutzfeldt-Jacob disease with florid type plaques after cadaveric dura mater grafting. Arch. Neurol. 56:357–362, 1999.

Lyme Disease

Belman, A.L. Lyme disease. American Academy of Neurology, 51st Annual Meeting, Toronto, 1999.

Case records of the Massachusetts General Hospital. Case 51. N. Engl. J. Med. Vol. 319, No. 25, 1988.

Finchel, M.F. The progressive paralytic disorder associated with Lyme disease. Semin. Neurol. 13:299–304, 1993.

Halperin J. Lyme disease. Neurobase MedLink. Arbor, 1993–2000.

Logigian, E.L. Peripheral nervous system Lyme borreliosis (abstract). Semin. Neurol. 17:25–28, 1997.

Preston D.C. and Shapiro B. Electromyography and Neuromuscular Disorders. Boston: Butterworth-Heinemann, 358–359, 1998.

Neurocysticercosis

Adams, R.D. and Victor, M. Principles of Neurology, ed. 5. New York: Mc-Graw Hill, 618, 1993.

Barry, M. and Kaldjian L.C. Neurocysticercosis. Semin. Neurol. 13:131–143, 1993.

Case records of the Massachussetts General Hospital. Case 20. N. Engl. J. Med. 1446–1457, 1990.

Davis, L.E. Neurocysticercosis: Pathophysiology, diagnosis and management. Neurologist 2:356–364, 1996.

Davis, L.E. Neurocysticercrosis. Neurobase MedLink, Arbor, 1993–2000.

Del Brutto, O. Neurocysticercosis. Current Opin. Neurol. 10:268–272, 1997.

Del Brutto, O. Cysticercosis. In: Feldmann E. Current Diagnosis in Neurology. St. Louis: Mosby, 125–129, 1999.

Ettinger, A.B. Structural causes of epilepsy. In: Neurology Clin. Epilepsy II (special issue). 12:41–56, 1994.

Cytomegalovirus Polyradiculopathy

Clifford, D.B. Neurologic complications of human immunodeficiency virus infection. Neurologist 4:54–65, 1998.

Cohen, B.A. Neurologic prognosis of cytomegalovirus polyradiculopathy in AIDS. Neurology 43:493–499, 1993.

Eidelberg, D. et al. Progressive polyradiculopathy in acquired immune deficiency syndrome. Neurology 36:912–916, 1986.

McArthur, J.C. Neuropathies associated with cytomegalovirus infection. Neurobase MedLink, Arbor, 1993–2000.

Parry, G. J. Neuropathies related to HIV infection and its treatment. In: Handbook of Clinical Neurology, Vol. 27. Amsterdam: Elsevier, 353–365, 1998.

Simpson, D.M. and Tagliati M. Neurologic manifestations of HIV infection. Ann. Intern. Med. 121:769–785, 1994.

Tucker, T. Central nervous system manifestations of human immunodeficiency virus infection. In: Bradley, W.G. Neurology in Clinical Practice. Boston: Butterworth-Heinemann, 1098–1111, 1991.

Wulff, E.A. and Simpson, D.M. Neuromuscular complications of the human immunodeficiency virus type 1 infection. Semin. neurol. 19:157–164, 1999.

Parasitic Infections

Bradley, W. G. Neurology in clinical practice. Boston: Butterworth-Heineman, 1098–1106, 1991.

Clifford, D.B. Neurologic complications of human immunodeficiency virus infection. Neurologist 4:54–65, 1998.

Cohen, B.A. Neurologic manifestations of toxoplasmosis in AIDS. Semin. Neurol. 19:201–211, 1999.

Concha, M. and Rabinstein, A. Central nervous system opportunistic infections in HIV-1 infection. CNS Spectrum 5:43–60, 2000.

Marra, C.M. Opportunistic infections in AIDS. American Academy of Neurology, 52nd Annual Meeting, San Diego, 2000.

Simpson, D.M. and Tagliati M. Neurologic manifestations of HIV infection. Ann. Intern. Med. 121:769–785, 1994.

HTLV-1 Myelopathy

Araujo, A.Q.C. HTLV-1 myelopathy. American Academy of Neurology, 52nd Annual Meeting, San Diego, 2000.

Feldmann, E. Current Diagnosis in Neurology. St. Louis: Mosby, 96–101, 1994.

Johnson, R.T. and Griffin, J. Current Therapy in Neurologic Disease, ed. 5. St. Louis: Mosby, 167–169, 1997.

Younger, D.S. differential diagnosis of progressive spastic paraparesis. Semin. Neurol. 13:319–320, 1993.

11
Headache and Facial Pain

Painful Ophthalmoplegia

Vignette

A 32-year-old pediatric nurse was brought to your attention because of right eye pain. Apparently 4 weeks previously she started complaining of throbbing pain involving the right eye, accompanied by severe frontal and periorbital headache. She then developed double vision and drooping of her right eyelid, which persisted without fluctuations. The neurological examination showed a large, nonreactive pupil on the right, right ptosis, and loss of right eye movement in all directions. Motor and sensory examinations were intact.

Summary A 32-year-old woman with right eye pain and ophthalmoplegia. Clinical findings include right eye pain, ptosis, dilated pupil, and complete ophthalmoplegia, indicating a lesion of the third, fourth, and sixth cranial nerves.

Localization

The first consideration is to decide whether the lesion involves the peripheral nerve or if it is due to dysfunction of the muscle or the neuromuscular junction. Following are common localizations for multiple infranuclear nerve involvement:

- Cavernous sinus/parasellar area/superior orbital fissure region.
- Subarachnoid space.
- Brainstem/posterior fossa.
- Orbital area.

In a patient presenting with multiple ocular nerve paralysis, a lesion involving the cavernous sinus should be highly suspected particularly because of the anatomical composition of the sinus. The carotid siphon, oculosympathetic complex, and cranial nerves III, IV, V_1, V_2 and VI are important structures located within the cavernous sinus. Therefore disorders affecting the cavernous sinus may cause multiple cranial nerve involvement. Another important feature is the occurrence of pain which is attributed to trigeminal nerve dysfunction. Different disorders of the cavernous sinus can cause painful ophthalmoplegia, such as infectious, inflammatory vascular disorders, and primary and metastatic tumors (see later discussion on cavernous sinus syndrome).

Infectious and neoplastic infiltration of the subarachnoid space can also manifest with multiple cranial nerve paresis, including the ocular motor nerves. Leptomeningeal metastasis can affect the sixth, third, and fourth oculomotor nerves and cause diplopia. Facial paralysis and visual and hearing loss can also occur in combination with headache and altered level of consciousness. Leptomeningeal metastasis represents a late manifestation of systemic cancer.

An intrinsic parenchymal brainstem process can cause dysfunction of ocular cranial nerves and their nuclei, but signs of involvement of the long motor and sensory tract are also present. Lesions extrinsic to the brainstem, such as ruptured aneurysms of the posterior communicating artery, can present with painful ophthalmoplegia particularly affecting the oculomotor nerve, usually with pupillary involvement. Basilar artery aneurysms can be responsible for progressive cranial nerve palsies and hydrocephalus.

Pathological processes involving the orbital area are due to inflammatory pseudotumor infections, such as mucormycosis, particularly in patients with diabetes, inflammation of the contiguous sinuses, and so on (Glaser). Painful ophthalmoplegia can be associated with proptosis and, in the case of mucormycosis, can cause fatal complications.

Disorders of the muscles include acute orbital myositis, which is an inflammatory process localized to the extra-

carotid sinus { vascular → Anevsm, fistula, thrombosis
Neoplasm → primary { pituity Adenoma → acute-pituty Apoplex
meningiomas.
metastatic →
Inflamation —

112   11. Headache and Facial Pain

ocular muscles and responsible for the occurrence of orbital pain and limitation of eye movements, that usually resolves over a few weeks. Ocular myopathies (e.g., thyroid myopathy and progressive external ophthalmoplegia) can also be differentiated. In dysthyroid myopathy, pain is not common. Bilateral involvement, pupillary sparing, proptosis, and restrictive ophthalmoplegia are other features.

Disorders of the neuromuscular junction, such as myasthenia gravis and botulism, also can be easily excluded. Myasthenia gravis is characterized by fatigable weakness that improves with rest, and asymmetrical painless ophthalmoplegia with ptosis and without pupillary involvement. Botulism is responsible for acute onset of dysphagia, ophthalmoplegia with dilated pupils, and rapidly progressing limb weakness and respiratory distress.

Cavernous Sinus and Its Disorders

The cavernous sinus is a venous structure localized on either side of the sella turcica that expands from the superior orbital fissure to the petrous portion of the temporal lobe and is connected with the opposite sinus via the intercavernous space. Disorders affecting the cavernous sinus can be vascular, neoplastic, infectious, and inflammatory.

Vascular disorders include intracavernous aneurysms, cavernous sinus fistulas, and thrombosis of the cavernous sinus. Aneurysms of the internal carotid artery present with progressive diplopia, varying degrees of ocular paresis, Horner's syndrome, exophthalmus, and periorbital pain that can be severe. Aneurysmal rupture may cause subarachnoid, intraventricular, or parenchymal hemorrhage with fatal complications.

Carotid-cavernous sinus fistulas that can be spontaneous or may follow a trauma are characterized by an abnormal communication between the ICA or its branches and the cavernous sinus. Clinical manifestations are characterized by chemosis, pulsating exophthalmus, ophthalmoplegia that more commonly affects the sixth nerve, and visual loss.

Cavernous sinus thrombosis is caused by spreading of infections of the ethmoid, sphenoid, or maxillary sinuses, or the skin around the eyes and nose. Symptoms are unilateral but may became bilateral if the opposite sinus becomes involved. They include exophtalmus, edema of the eyelids, ophthalmoplegia preferentially involving the sixth nerve, retinal hemorrhages, papilledema, and severe orbital pain.

Neoplastic disorders involving the cavernous sinus can be primary or metastatic. Pituitary adenomas may invade the cavernous sinus by lateral extension resulting in progressive ophthalmoparesis preferentially involving the third nerve. A dramatic picture of severe headache ophthalmoplegia and rapid neurological deterioration is caused by pituitary apoplexy due to spontanous hemorrhage into a pituitary adenoma.

Other tumors such as intracavernous meningiomas can cause slowly progressive cranial nerve palsies and ophthalmoparesis.

Metastatic tumors can involve the cavernous sinus by direct extension, such as nasopharyngeal carcinoma, via perineural routes, such as squamous cell carcinoma of the face or neck or through the hematic and lymphatic systems in patients with cancer of the lung, breast, or prostate, or malignant lymphoma.

Inflammation within the cavernous sinus may result from infectious causes or may be idiopathic. Infectious processes may be due to bacterial, viral, or fungal organisms, such as those responsible for bacterial sinusitis or herpes zoster and fungal mucormycosis. Granulomatous inflammatory disorders are typically represented by the Tolosa-Hunt syndrome and sarcoidosis

Tolosa-Hunt Syndrome

The Tolosa-Hunt syndrome is an idiopathic inflammatory disorder of the cavernous sinus that clinically manifests with orbital and periorbital pain and varying degrees of ophthalmoplegia due to dysfunction of the third, fourth, and sixth cranial nerves in various combinations. Pupils can be spared or involved and be dilated or small. Horner's syndrome can occur if the sympathetic fibers are affected. The course can be acute or subacute and the treatment is based on the use of steroids.

Pituitary Apoplexy

Pituitary apoplexy, which is due to hemorrhagic infarction of the pituitary gland, is an acute event characterized by abrupt onset of excruciating headache, epistaxis, or cerebral fluid rhinorrhea, visual loss, nausea, vomiting, and ophthalmoplegia. The headache is frontal or retroorbital and is often the initial manifestation. A superior expansion of the blood may cause compression of the optic chiasm and bitemporal hemianopia, visual loss, or junctional scotomas. A lateral expansion may be responsible for a cavernous sinus syndrome. Sphenoid sinus involvement causes epistaxis or cerebrospinal fluid rhinorrhea. Signs of hypopituitarism can be present. The course is usually acute but a subacute evolution is also described with symptoms occurring over days or weeks.

Pituitary apoplexy has been described in patients who have large adenomas and factors such as pregnancy, bleeding disorders, hypertension, trauma, radiation therapy, adrenalectomy may increase the risk. Neuroimaging studies may show evidence of hemorrhage. Lumbar puncture may increase the risk of herniation and should not be performed. The treatment is based on corticosteroid and supportive therapy as well as decompression through the sphenoid sinus.

Subdural Hematoma

Vignette

A 42-year-old successful editor started complaining of throbbing generalized headache. At work she seemed more irritable and at times forgetful and apathetic, making a few mistakes. She woke up a couple of times at night with headache and vomiting. There was no history of alcohol consumption or drug abuse and previous medical history was unremarkable. She seemed to notice that the headache began after returning from a ski trip in Switzerland with friends six weeks before. During the examination she had trouble with memory and calculation and was uncooperative. Absence of venous pulsation on fundoscopic examination and a left pronator drift were noted.

Summary A 42-year-old previously healthy woman with chief complaints of headache associated with vomiting and cognitive impairment. The neurological examination shows signs of increased intracranial pressure (early papilledema) and a left pronator drift. The headache started after returning from a ski trip with friends (underlying the possibility of a trauma).

Localization and Differential Diagnosis

The differential diagnosis in a patient with headache, cognitive impairment, and focal neurological signs is extensive. Space-occupying lesions should be ruled out first. Intracranial tumors may manifest with intermittent headache exacerbated by positional changes, coughing, or straining, and associated with mental status abnormalities, such as irritability, apathy, forgetfulness, and signs of increased intracranial pressure or focal neurological findings.

Inflammatory disorders such as central nervous system vasculitis are also a consideration in the differential diagnosis. Isolated angiitis of the CNS, for example, is characterized by the occurrence of headache, changes in mental status, focal neurological findings, and seizures, in the absence of signs of systemic involvement. Subarachnoid hemorrhage, cranial nerve involvement and myelopathy can also occur. The diagnosis is mainly based on angiographic findings of diffuse segmental narrowing of the cerebral vessels and on the results of brain biopsy.

Infectious and parainfectious processes include bacterial, fungal, parasitic, and viral causes.

Chronic meningeal processes can manifest with headache, confusion, stiff neck, fever, seizures, and focal lateralizing signs. CSF findings include mononuclear pleocytosis, hypoglycorrhachia, and decreased protein level. The responsible organisms include *Mycobacterium tuberculosis* and *Cryptococcus neoformans*. Tuberculous meningitis is more common in immunosuppressed individuals, such as AIDS patients, organ transplant recipients, or patients who undergo chronic corticosteroid treatment. High-risk groups also include immigrants from areas where tuberculosis is highly endemic. Clinically it is manifested with intermittent headache, confusion, low-grade fever, multiple cranial nerve involvement, and progressive deterioration, often in absence of meningeal signs. CSF shows lymphocytic pleocytosis, increased protein level, and hypoglycorrhachia. Cryptococcal meningitis can present with subacute onset of headache, mental status and behavioral changes, increasing intracranial pressure, and in some cases meningeal signs and seizures.

Toxic, metabolic, or endocrine disorders can be associated with encephalopathies, but without focal or lateralizing signs.

Chronic subdural hematomas frequently manifest with moderate to severe headache, mental status changes, and focal deficits. Headache occurs in 30 to 90 percent of patients (Stein et al.). The diagnosis of chronic subdural hematoma can present some difficulties when the patient is confused or cannot recall a minor head trauma.

Clinical Features

Subdural hematomas can be traumatic when due to the effects of penetrating or nonpenetrating trauma to the head, or spontaneous when not related to trauma but due to aneurysmal rupture, bleeding disorder, use of anticoagulants, infections, low intracranial pressure due to removal of CSF, and so on.

Traumatic subdural hematomas can be acute, subacute, and chronic based upon the time of clinical presentation that varies between a maximum of 72 hours to over 20 days after the trauma.

In acute subdural hematoma, presenting signs are related to the area where it is located and the size of the hematoma, and include changes in mental status, such as confusion, lethargy, stupor, and coma; pupillary abnormalities with dilatation of the pupil ipsilateral to the hematoma; and focal signs, such as hemiparesis. Cranial nerve paralysis may preferentially affect the third and sixth cranial nerves. Other findings include hypertension, bradycardia, papilledema, decerebrate posture, and so on (Stein et al.).

In chronic subdural hematoma, the history of trauma is less recognizable and can be represented by a minor injury often forgotten, particularly in elderly confused patients. Stein et al. describe the most frequent presenting symptoms as headache, changes in mentation, and hemiparesis. The headache can be intermittent, mild or severe and may be associated with nausea or vomiting. It can be precipitated by straining, coughing, or physical activity. Mental status and behavioral changes vary and manifest with drowsiness, confusion, forgetfulness, personality changes, and apathy, and can typically fluctuate. Focal signs are never a prominent feature and are mainly represented by hemiparesis. Transient neurological deficits and seizures also occur in some cases.

Diagnosis

The diagnosis of traumatic subdural hematoma is based on neuroimaging studies. Subdural hematomas are due to tearing of bridging veins, causing signs of brain compression. Venous bleeding is usually arrested by the rising intracranial pressure. Acute subdural hematoma can be clearly diagnosed by CT scan of the brain, which will demonstrate a hyperdense lesion with concave inner margins. The hyperdense lesion gradually becames isodense over two weeks and can still be easily diagnosed if signs of mass effect or brain compression are recognized, such as obliteration of the sulci or compression of the ventricles. Chronic subdural hematomas result in a hypodense collection on CT scan.

On MRI, acute subdural hematomas present with decreased signal on T_2 due to the presence of deoxyhemoglobin. As deoxyhemoglobin converts to methemoglobin, high signal appears on T_1 around the periphery of the collection, later filling in completely. Chronic hematomas show isointensity on T_1 and hyperintensity on T_2.

Treatment

The treatment of subdural hematoma can be medical and surgical. Medical therapy is based on controlling intracranial hypertension and prevention of seizures as well as electrolyte imbalance. The surgical intervention is based on the evacuation of the hematoma, particularly in order to prevent cerebral compression and temporal lobe tentorial herniation.

Migraine Headache

Vignette

A 20-year-old waitress had a six-month history of several episodes that she described as "pins and needles" in the right fingers that advanced to involve the whole hand, right mouth, lips, and tongue.

Occasionally she felt clumsiness of her right arm for 30 minutes, or mumbled or jumbled correct words. By this time a slight right-sided headache had developed, which increased in intensity over a few minutes to become throbbing and severe. Her past history included a heart murmur since childhood and cigarette smoking (one pack per day) for five years.

Summary A 20-year-old female experiencing episodes of paresthesias and clumsiness of the right arm spreading from the fingers to the right mouth, lips, and tongue, associated with occasional speech difficulties and followed by headache.

Localization

The vignette points to a cortical localization particularly the frontoparietal area.

Differential Diagnosis of These Transitory Episodes

The differential diagnosis includes

- Migraine with aura: cheirooral migraine.
- Epileptogenic event.
- Transitory vascular event.

Migraine with aura can manifest with sensory phenomena such as paresthesias that may involve the fingers of one hand and then advance to involve the forearm up to the elbow and the tongue (cheirooral migraine). This usually occurs in a slowly progressive march evolving over several minutes rather than in a simultaneous manner. Speech difficulties or dysphasia may also occur in a left-dominant patient. Motor weakness can also be present and if prolonged may be consistent with hemiplegic migraine.

Somatosensory seizures may originate in the postcentral or precentral area and are characterized by localized paresthesias or numbness that may progress in a Jacksonian march within seconds as opposed to the slow march of migraine. Postictal numbness can occur corresponding to a sensory Todd's phenomenon (Engel).

The spread of paresthesias as seen in the case presented is rarely seen in cerebrovascular attacks, where the advance of the paresthesias is much quicker than in migraine (Campbell and Fumihiko). Sensory phenomena in migraine usually consist of a pins and needle sensation that gradually spreads over different areas. TIAs are more often described as numbness and heaviness rather than a positive phenomenon of paresthesias. Also, true paresis is rare in migraine with aura according to some authors who rather describe the weakness as sensory ataxia. Pure hemiplegic migraine is a rare syndrome reported in 0.3

percent of migraine patients (Varelas). Headache can also develop in cerebrovascular disorders, sometimes preceding the stroke or being associated with transitory attacks. According to Marks and Rapoport, ischemia in the territory of the posterior cerebral arterial system is more likely to cause headache than anterior circulation cerebral ischemia.

Secondary disorders that may cause migraine-like episodes, seizures, or TIAs include

- Vascular disorders, such as venous thrombosis, subarachnoid hemorrhage, Moya-Moya, vascular malformations, cardiac embolism, carotid dissection, and so on.
- Blood abnormalities, such as protein C, S, and antithrombin deficiency, antiphospholipidic antibodies, sickle cell disease, and so on.
- Infectious and inflammatory disorders responsible for arteritis and arteriopathies, such as syphilis, tuberculosis, herpes zoster, collagen vascular disorders, and so on.
- Space-occupying lesions, such as tumors, abscess, cyst, and so on.
- Familial disorders such as MELAS (mitochondrial encephalopathy, lactic acidosis, and stroke), familial hemiplegic migraine, and so on.
- Drug-induced/toxic disorders due to cocaine, heroin, estrogens, or associated with particular situations such as pregnancy or puerperium.

Clinical Differential Diagnosis of Migraine Headache

There are important clinical clues that help support the diagnosis of migraine headache in this patient such as age of presentation usually during youth, typically between ages 6 and 25 (Marks and Rapoport), slow development of symptoms, recurrent similar attacks, focal neurological deficits that do not follow a vascular distribution, temporal association of the aura that can precede or manifest simultaneously with the headache, family history of migraine, and normal neurovascular examination.

Diagnosis

The diagnosis of migraine headache is based on a comprehensive medical and family history and neurological examination. The characteristic of the headache should be emphasized, such as age of onset, quality, location, frequency, duration, triggering or exacerbating factors, premonitory symptoms, aura if present, and associated symptoms, such as nausea, vomiting, diarrhea, photophobia or phonophobia, lightheadedness, vertigo, and so on.

Neuroimaging studies are indicated if the pain is severe and different from previous attacks in terms of frequency

and persistence and also if it is the first and worst episode of migraine mimicking the headache of SAH. The occurrence of seizures or neurological deficits on examination are also an indication for further investigations, such as MRI of the brain and EEG. MRA and cerebral angiography are not routinely performed unless there is a high index of suspicion for certain pathology, such as arteriovenous malformations, cerebral aneurysm, or vasculitis.

CSF examination is obtained only in selected cases when SAH is suspected but neuroimaging studies are normal, or if an infectious process needs to be ruled out. Cardiac studies are useful in selected cases to exclude the possibility of cerebral embolism as a cause of the headache or neurological deficits. Laboratory investigations are particularly important in all elderly patients where an elevated ESR can be an indication of temporal arteritis or to exclude anemia, electrolyte imbalance, systemic infections, and so on.

Clinical Features

Migraine Headache

Migraine headache is defined as an episodic disorder characterized by gradual onset of pain that is described as throbbing, pulsating, or pounding of different intensity and duration. According to the International Headache Society, diagnostic criteria for migraine without aura include the occurrence of five or more episodes of moderate to severe unilateral headache described as pulsating and exacerbated by physical activity and with a duration that varies from 4 to 72 hours (untreated or unsuccessfully treated). The headache is accompanied by at least one of the following:

- Nausea and/or vomiting.
- Photophobia and phonophobia.

Also there should be no indication based on history and general and neurological examination of organic pathology or, if there is suggestion of this possibility, it should be ruled out by appropriate studies. If there is an underlying organic pathology, the migraine attacks do not manifest for the first time in close temporal relation to the disorder.

Migraine with Aura

The auras are characterized by transient focal neurological symptoms that may precede or occur during the headache but can also represent the only symptom. The visual type of aura is very common and consists of positive phenomena, such as visual hallucinations that consist of a flashing light, stars, or lines moving across the visual field, or negative phenomena (scotoma) with different visual field defects. Sensory and motor phenomena can also occur as well as distortion of perception with alterations of size, contour, and shape of objects.

The International Headache Society has established criteria to differentiate migraine with aura. They include the occurrence of two or more episodes characterized by at least three of the following:

- One or more aura symptoms that resolve completely and suggest focal cerebral cortical or brainstem dysfunction, or both.
- At least one aura symptom that occurs gradually over more than four minutes, or two or more symptoms that develop in succession.
- The symptoms related to the aura should not last more than one hour unless there is more than one aura symptom.
- The headache can precede, occur at the same time, or follow the aura with a free interval of less than 60 minutes.

Also, there should be no indication of an underlying structural pathology or if there is it should be ruled out by appropriate investigations. If organic disease is present, migraine attacks do not manifest for the first time in close temporal relation to the disorders (Silberstein 1995).

Treatment

The therapy of migraine headache is based on treatment of the acute attack and prevention of recurrent headaches.

Prevention

The need for a preventive approach is based on the frequency of the attacks (at least two per month or more), the duration or significant disability produced by the headache, or if patients experience prolonged auras with risk of permanent neurological deficits. Preventive treatment is also indicated in cases refractory to the acute treatment due to overuse or intolerable side effects.

Several medications have been used for migraine prevention, particularly beta-adrenergic blockers, antidepressants, calcium channel antagonists, antiserotonergic agents, anticonvulsants, nonsteroidal antiinflammatory drugs, and so on. Beta blockers have been extensively used for migraine prevention. Propranol, a nonselective beta blocker, can be started at a dose of 40 mg a day and gradually increased to a maximum of 240 mg a day. Adverse effects have been described such as depression, bradycardia, nausea, dizziness, impaired sexual function with impotence, and so on. Contraindications include congestive heart failure, asthma, insulin-dependent diabetes, and Raynaud's disease. Other beta blockers used in migraine prevention include atenolol, nadolol, metoprolol, and timolol.

The antidepressants have been widely used for migraine prevention, particularly tricyclics. Amitriptyline, the prototype, is considered a first line drug in patients who suffer from migraine and are depressed or have a sleep disorder, or in the treatment of tension headache and chronic daily headache. Adverse effects are characterized by dry mouth, blurred vision, sedation, weight gain, cardiac arrhythmias, urinary retention, sexual dysfunction, and so on. Tricyclic antidepressants should not be used in patients with glaucoma, heart block, or urinary retention. The dose of amytriptyline is individualized from 10 to 150 mg a day. Fluoxetine (Prozac) a selective serotonin reuptake inhibitor has also been used in migraine associated with depression with a dose that varies from 20 to 80 mg a day and is usually well tolerated except for the occurrence of agitation, anxiety, insomnia, and nausea in some cases.

Calcium channel blockers also need to be considered for prophylactic treatment of migraine, and verapamil has been considered particularly in patients with frequent migraine attacks with auras. The dose varies from 80 to 480 mg a day and usual side effects include constipation, edema of the hands and feet, and cardiac abnormalities.

Anticonvulsant medications represent an important treatment in migraine prevention. Valproic acid has been effective in preventing migraine with and without aura. Adverse effects include gastrointestinal symptoms, such as nausea and vomiting, anorexia, and also tremor, hair loss, and weight gain. Absolute contraindications are pregnancy and liver disease. Divalproex sodium is a stable coordination of sodium valproate and valproic acid in 1:1 molar ratio. The dose varies from 500 to 1000 mg a day. Other anticonvulsants include gabapentin (Neurontin), which has good tolerance and has been used in doses that vary from 300 to 1800 mg with different results. Side effects are drowsiness, dizziness, and, rarely, a rash. Topiramate (topamax) has also been utilized for migraine prevention with improvement in headache frequency in some studies. The dosage varies from 25 to 400 mg a day and adverse effects include fatigue, dizziness, paresthesias, nausea, and anorexia.

Serotonin antagonist drugs used for prophylaxis of migraine include methysergide and cyproheptadine, the latter particularly in pediatric cases. Side effects are gastrointestinal symptoms, drowsiness, and weight gain. Retroperitoneal, pulmonary, or endocardial fibrosis has rarely occurred in patients treated with methysergide.

Nonsteroidal antiinflammatory drugs, such as naproxen sodium, tolfenamic acid, mefenamic acid, ketoprofen, and aspirin, are also part of preventive treatment.

Acute Attack

The acute treatment of migraine is based on the use of several medications, some specific, such as triptans and ergot alkaloids, and some not specific, such as nonsteroidal antiinflammatory agents (naproxen, ketoprofen, diclofenac, and so on) or analgesics (aspirin, acetaminophen) and narcotic analgesics (codeine and meperidine).

Triptans are effective drugs for migraine and include sumatriptan and the new "second-generation triptans" — zolmitriptan, naratriptan, rizatriptan, eletriptan, almotriptan, and frovatriptan. They are considered 5-HT–receptor agonists with activation of both $5HT_{1B}$ and $5-HT_{1D}$. Their mechanism of action consists of vasoconstriction, inhibitory action on inflammatory substance released by trigeminal fibers, and inhibition of central pain processing. Sumatriptan has been widely used in the form of subcutaneous injection (6 mg), oral (25, 50, and 100 mg), nasal, and rectal preparations. Injectable sumatriptan (6 mg) has shown higher efficacy than any other form in some studies. The recommended dose is 6 mg subcutaneously that can be repeated without exceeding 2 doses within 24 hours. The oral administration can be repeated up to a dose of 200 mg within 24 hours. Adverse effects include injection site reactions, chest discomfort, a feeling of warmth, and paresthesias. Contraindications to the use of triptans are the presence of cardiac disorders, such as ischemic heart disease or uncontrolled hypertension, and cerebrovascular disorders. Patients with basilar or hemiplegic migraine should also avoid the use of triptans.

Ergot alkaloids are represented by ergotamine and its derivative dihydroergotamine. Ergotamine can be administered orally or through a suppository form during the early stage of the headache. Dihydroergotamine can be given intravenously for a rapid relief of pain in association with an antiemetic. Adverse effects include diarrhea, nausea, cramps, and paresthesias. Due to their strong vasoconstrictive effect, they are contraindicated in patients with coronary or other systemic vascular disorders, uncontrolled hypertension, renal or hepatic failure, and so on.

Cluster Headache

Vignette

A 50-year-old airline pilot was taken to the emergency room by his distressed wife in the middle of the night because of left orbital pain that lasted approximately 60 minutes and was so severe that it made him cry. In the emergency room conjunctival injection, edema of the left eyelid, ptosis, and miosis are noted. For the last six weeks, the pilot had experienced similar episodes and the pain had occurred suddenly without warnings. He had a history of hypertension and coronary artery disease and quit smoking two years ago.

Summary A 50-year-old man with several episodes of severe left orbital pain lasting approximately 60 minutes, associated with other signs: left conjunctival injection, edema, ptosis, miosis, and lacrimation.

Localization and Differential Diagnosis

The differential diagnosis includes primary and secondary headaches.

Among the primary headaches, cluster headache should be considered first. Its clinical features are represented by brief, intermittent episodes of excruciating unilateral pain localized in the orbital and retroorbital area usually on the same side that last from 15 minutes to 3 hours and occur from one every other day to a maximum of eight times a day (Nappi and Russell). The pain is associated with autonomic signs, such as lacrimation, miosis with a partial Horner's syndrome, conjunctival injection, rhinorrhea, and so on. The episodes of severe, intermittent left orbital pain and associated features experienced by the patient described in the vignette are highly suggestive of cluster headache.

Chronic and episodic paroxysmal hemicrania that manifests with brief episodes of severe unilateral pain localized in the frontotemporal area that recur frequently is also a consideration in the differential diagnosis. Paroxysmal hemicrania, which predominantly affects females as opposed to cluster headache that occurs mainly in males, typically presents with frequent daily attacks (more than five times a day) of shorter duration than cluster headache (5 to 45 minutes) (Goadsby). Signs of autonomic dysfunction also occur and the treatment of choice is indomethacin that causes a rapid relief of the pain.

Migraine headache can also be differentiated from cluster headache. Migraine patients complain of unilateral pain that sometimes extends to the opposite side, associated with nausea, vomiting, photophobia, and phonophobia, as well as focal neurological symptoms that may precede, accompany or follow the headache. Patients suffering from cluster headache have marked autonomic symptoms on the side of the pain, such as conjunctival injection, lacrimation, rhinorrhea, and so on, but nausea, vomiting, and signs of focal cerebral and brainstem neurological dysfunction are not usually observed.

Trigeminal neuralgia typically manifests with paroxysmal, brief attacks of intense electric-like pain that is not accompanied by focal neurological or autonomic symptoms. The pain is very short in duration lasting less than a minute, occurs in the distribution of one or more division of the trigeminal nerve, and can manifest spontaneously or be induced by stimulation of trigger areas localized on the skin or mucous membrane. Therefore, it can easily be differentiated from the typical attacks of cluster headache.

Cluster headache can also be secondary to an underlying intracranial organic pathology, such as space occupying and vascular lesions, trauma, and viral infections. Meningioma of the parasellar area, pituitary adenoma, vertebral artery aneurysm or dissection, head injury, facial injury, and so on have been described with symptomatic cluster headache. Patients usually present with clinical features that do not correspond to the ones commonly found in the typical cluster headache, and have more persistent pain that does not respond to the usual treatment and focal neurological findings other than Horner's syndrome.

Diagnostic Criteria

The International Headache Society has established some criteria for various types of cluster headache.

Cluster Headache

Cluster headache should be characterized by five or more episodes of severe, unilateral pain localized in the orbital, supraorbital, and/or temporal area of a duration that varies from 15 to 180 minutes if not treated and occurring at a frequency that varies from one every other day to eight per day. At least one sign of autonomic dysfunction should occur on the side of the pain, such as rhinorrhea, lacrimation, conjunctival injection, nasal congestion, ptosis, myosis, increased sweating in the forehead and facial area, and edema of the eyelid.

There should be no evidence of organic pathology.

Episodic Cluster Headache

Episodic cluster has been characterized as headache manifesting with periods that last seven days to one year separated by pain-free intervals lasting 14 days or more; cluster periods usually last between two weeks and three months. There should be two cluster periods or more with a duration that varies from seven days to one year (untreated), separated by remission of at least 14 days.

Chronic Cluster Headache

Chronic cluster headache is characterized by attacks that may last more than one year without remission or with remission of less than 14 days' duration. Also, there can be no remission phases for one year or more, or remissions lasting less than 14 days.

Diagnosis

The diagnosis of cluster headache is based on a comprehensive history and neurological examination and also on neuroimaging studies CT and MRI of the brain if atypical features are present and an underlying organic pathology needs to be ruled out.

Treatment

Therapy involves treatment of the acute attack and prevention of recurrent headache. The treatment of the acute attack consists of the use of 100 percent oxygen inhalation for 15 minutes at the onset of headache, sumatriptan, dihydroergotamine, instillation of lidocaine nasal drops, corticosteroids, and so on. Prophylactic treatment is usually prescribed in patients with frequent, severe attacks, particularly those suffering from chronic cluster headache.

The therapy includes several medications such as methysergide, which is preferred in younger patients and has several adverse effects including the rare retroperitoneal fibrosis, and ergotamine that can be given at bedtime to prevent nocturnal attacks, keeping in mind the contraindications in patients with cardiac and cerebral vascular disorders. Other medications include corticosteroids that can be very effective as a short treatment because the side effects prevent prolonged use.

Verapamil is now considered the treatment of choice for prevention of chronic and episodic cluster headache. The dose varies from 80 to 240 mg a day and more based on individual patients. Side effects are constipation, limb edema, and heart block. Lithium carbonate is also effective particularly in patients with chronic cluster headache but has side effects such as gastrointestinal symptoms, CNS toxicity with tremor, confusion, seizures, etc. and needs careful monitoring of the blood level. Valproic acid, gabapentin, and topiramate are also considered prophylactic agents.

Trigeminal Neuralgia

Vignette

A 44-year-old housewife has a four-week history of lancinating pain involving the right cheek occurring about 30 times a day and lasting several seconds. The pain is quite severe and often precipitated by chewing. There is no nausea, vomiting, or photophobia, but the husband volunteered and she confirmed tearing of the eyes without redness or nasal congestion. General, physical, and neurological examinations are normal.

Summary A 44-year-old woman with right facial pain that occurs 30 times a day, of brief duration (several seconds), without other associated symptoms. Neurological examination is normal.

Differential Diagnosis

The differential diagnosis includes disorders characterized by facial pain. Trigeminal neuralgia needs to be considered first due to its features of abrupt, paroxysmal, excruciating pain described as a stabbing, electric-like sensation localized in the distribution of one or more divisions of the trigeminal nerve (usually the second and/or third division) of very brief duration (from seconds to less than 2 minutes). The pain can be triggered by touch or movements of the face, such as when talking or eating. In order to make a diagnosis of trigeminal neuralgia there should not be any focal deficit, particularly any facial area of sensory loss or any abnormality of the corneal reflex unless prior surgery has been obtained.

Postherpetic neuralgia, which is related to acute herpes zoster infection, tends to affect the ophthalmic division of the trigeminal nerve, which is not commonly involved in trigeminal neuralgia. The characteristics of the pain are described as a constant burning, sharp, itchy sensation, without a remitting pattern typical of trigeminal neuralgia.

Other neuralgic syndromes include glossopharyngeal neuralgia and atypical facial pain. Glossopharyngeal neuralgia is less common and has a different distribution of pain from trigeminal neuralgia, manifesting with paroxysmal attacks of severe stabbing or electric shock-like sensation localized in the posterior part of the tongue and tonsil area that recurs many times a day and lasts one minute. The pain can be precipitated by chewing, talking, coughing, swallowing, or yawning. The distribution of pain represents an important factor in the differentiation from trigeminal neuralgia. Atypical facial pain is characterized by a constant, unilateral pain of different intensity that does not follow any anatomical distribution. The pain does not occur in combination with any sensory abnormality.

Cluster headache manifests with severe, unilateral, excruciating pain of longer duration (15 to 180 minutes according to the International Headache Society Criteria) than the typical attacks of trigeminal neuralgia (seconds to less than two minutes) and associated with significant autonomic features. Conjunctival injection, lacrimation, and nasal congestion are accompanying signs of cluster headache. A partial Horner's syndrome may also manifest.

Trigeminal neuralgia may be indicative of structural lesions, such as tumors, aneurysms, infections, or demyelinating disorders. Impaired sensation, other cranial nerve involvement, and corneal reflex abnormalities may suggest an underlying organic pathology.

Treatment

The medical management of trigeminal neuralgia is based on the use of pharmacological agents such as carbamazepine, phenytoin, valproic acid, and baclofen, with carbamazepine being the first line of treatment. Gabapentin, lamotrigine, and oxycarbazepine have also been used with varying results. Surgical techniques have different approaches, from alcohol or glycerol injection to micro-vascular decompression that removes aberrant blood vessels from the trigeminal nerve root, to stereotactic radiosurgery.

Facial Palsy: Ramsey Hunt Syndrome

Vignette

A 62-year-old dry cleaning worker started complaining of severe pain and unpleasant loudness in his left ear. During the next 24 hours he became unable to close his left eye and noticed an unusual taste sensation on the tip of his tongue. In the ER, the neurology resident noticed a complete left facial paralysis and redness and tenderness of the left ear canal. The rest of the cranial nerves were normal as well as motor and sensory functions. His previous history was significant for heart disease and diabetes and he was fearful that he'd suffered a stroke.

Summary A 62-year-old man with left facial paralysis. Associated findings are severe left ear pain, redness, and tenderness; hyperacusia (unpleasant loudness); and taste dysfunction.

Localization

The first consideration is that this is a lower motor neuron lesion because the entire left face is affected. Taste dysfunction over the anterior two thirds of the tongue and hyperacusis (abnormal loudness of sounds due to paralysis of the stapedius muscle) help localize the lesion.

Lesions involving the facial nerve within the facial canal proximal to the exit of the nerve to the stapedius muscle can explain the ipsilateral facial paralysis, taste dysfunction over the anterior two thirds of the tongue, and hyperacusis. When the geniculate ganglion is affected, pain in the region of the eardrum may occur (Brazis).

Differential Diagnosis

In the differential diagnosis, disorders to be considered are idiopathic facial paralysis (Bell's palsy) and secondary processes affecting the facial nerve, such as infections, tumors, and trauma.

Bell's palsy, characterized by a nonprogressive peripheral facial paralysis, has been linked to different etiological processes particularly involving a viral inflammatory-immune mechanism. Some studies point to a herpes simplex virus-I infection. The presentation is usually acute and predisposing factors include diabetes, hypertension, or pregnancy. Infectious and parainfectious disorders causing facial paresis include herpes zoster cephalicus (Ramsey Hunt syndrome), acute inflammatory demyelinating polyradiculopathy (Guillain-Barré syndrome), infectious mononucleosis, Lyme disease, and others (chickenpox, mumps, influenza, HIV, leprosy, mucormycosis, and so on).

Ramsay Hunt syndrome (RHS) caused by herpes zoster virus infection, is characterized by excruciating ear pain accompanied by a vescicular eruption involving the external canal and pinna that can precede, accompany, or follow the onset of the facial paralysis. The ear can become red and tender. The paralysis is often severe and complete and postherpetic neuralgia may occur. The patient in the vignette with ear redness and tenderness and complete left VII nerve peripheral palsy may well represent a case of RHS. The diagnosis does not present difficulty in the presence of the typical skin rash. Oral acyclovir is the preferred treatment.

Facial weakness can be an important manifestation of Guillain-Barré syndrome and Lyme disease where it is often bilateral. In GBS cardinal features include symmetrical proximal weakness and hypo-areflexia. Lyme disease is also characterized by generalized weakness, fatigue, headache, fever, and so on.

Infectious mononucleosis rarely is responsible for unilateral, recurrent, or bilateral facial paralysis.

Complicated infections of the middle ear with involvement of the petrous apex, particularly in children, can be responsible for the so-called Gradenigo's syndrome characterized by severe ear pain and involvement of multiple cranial nerves, such as the ophthalmic division of the trigeminal nerve, the abducens, and facial nerve.

Primary and metastatic tumors may cause facial nerve dysfunction along its course but usually there are other signs and symptoms that suggest a more widespread involvement of other organs and neurological structures. Nuclear and fascicular pontine lesions involving the facial nerve due to vascular processes or tumors also affect other structures and cause long tract signs and gaze abnormalities.

Cerebello-pontine angle lesions, such as acoustic neuromas, facial neuromas, meningiomas, or metastatic processes, can cause facial nerve dysfunction in combination with other signs and symptoms, such as hearing loss, vertigo, tinnitus, diminished corneal reflex, and facial hypoesthesia.

Other causes of facial nerve abnormality include trauma, vasculitis, granulomatous disorders, and so on.

References

Painful Ophthalmoplegia

Adams, R.D. and Victor, M. Principles of Neurology, ed. 5. New York: McGraw-Hill, 1208–1209, 1993.

Cases Records of the Massachusetts General Hospital. Case 3. N. Engl. J. Med. 229–238, 1986.

Glaser, J.S. Neuroophthalmology, ed. 2. Philadelphia: J.B. Lippincott, 382–418, 1990.

Inzucchi, S.I. and Brine, M.L. Pituitary apoplexy. Neurology MedLink, Arbor, 1993–2001.

Laskowitz, D. et al. Acute visual loss and other disorders of the eyes. Neurol. Clin. North Am. 16:323–352, 1998.

Newman, N.J. Third, fourth, and sixth nerve lesions and the cavernous sinus. In: Albert D.M. and Jacobiec, F.A. (eds.). Principles and Practice of Ophthalmology, Vol. 4, Philadelphia: W.B. Saunders, 2444–2469, 1994.

Subdural Hematoma

Adams, R.D. and Victor, M. Craniocerebral trauma. In: Principles of Neurology, ed. 5. New York: McGraw-Hill, 749–775, 1993.

Lindsay, K.W. et al. Neurology and Neurosurgery, ed. 2. Edinburgh: Churchill Livingstone, 233–234, 1991.

Stein, S.C. et al. Acute subdural hematoma; Chronic subdural hematoma. Neurobase MedLink, Arbor, 1993–2000.

Woodruff, W.W. Fundamentals of Neuroimaging. Philadelphia: WB Saunders, 121–156, 1993.

Migraine and Cluster Headaches

Bogousslavski, J. et al. Opercular cheiro-oral syndrome. Arch. Neurol. 48:658–661, 1991.

Campbell, J.K. and Fumihiko, S. Migraine: Diagnosis and differential diagnosis. In: Olsen, J. et al. (eds.). The Headache. New York: Raven, 1993.

Edwards, K.R. Migraine Prevention. In: Drug therapies for prevention of migraine and treatment of painful diabetic neuropathy: A review and update for neurologists. April 2001.

Engel, J. Jr. Seizures and Epilepsy. Philadelphia: F.A. Davis, 145–146, 1989.

Freitag, F.G. Medical management of cluster headache. Kudrow, L. Clinical symptomatology and differential diagnosis of cluster headache. Silberstein, S.D. et al. Clinical symptomatology and differential diagnosis of migraine. Kunkel R.S. Medical management of acute migraine episodes. In: Tollison, C.D. et al. Headache: Diagnosis and Treatment. Baltimore: Williams & Wilkins, 197–204, 185–189; 59–75; 85–106, 1993.

Goadsby, P.J. Cluster and other short-lived headaches. American Academy of Neurology, 53rd Annual Meeting, Philadelphia, May 5–11, 2001.

Kudrow, L. Clinical symptomatology and differential diagnosis of migraine. In Tollison C.D. et al. Headache: Diagnosis and Treatment. Baltimore: Williams & Wilkins, 185–189, 1993.

Kunkel, R.S Medical management of acute migraine episodes. In: Tollison C.D. et al. Headache: Diagnosis and Treatment. Baltimore: Williams & Wilkins, 85–106, 1993.

Marks, D.R. and Rapoport, A.M. Diagnosis of migraine. In: Mathew, N.T. Cluster Headache. Semin. Neurol. 17:303–312, 313–323, 1997.

Mathew, N.T. Cluster headache. Semin. Neurol. 17:313–323, 1997.

Nappi and Russell. In: Olesen, J. et al. (eds.) The Headache. New York: Raven, 263–275, 277–281, 577–589, 1993.

Silberstein, S.D. Headache and facial pain. Continuum, Vol. 1, No. 5, Nov. 1995.

Silberstein, S.D. Migraine preventive treatment. American Academy of Neurology, 53rd Annual Meeting, Philadelphia, May 5–11, 2001.

Silberstein, S.D. et al. Clinical symptomatology and differential diagnosis of migraine. In: Tollison, C.D. et al. Headache: Diagnosis and Treatment. Baltimore: Williams & Wilkins, 59–75, 1993.

Varelas, P.N. et al. Uncommon migraine subtypes and their relation to stroke. Neurologist 5:135–144, 1999.

Trigeminal Neuralgia

Brazis, P.W. et al. Localization in Clinical Neurology, ed. 2. Boston: Little Brown, 189–202, 1990.

Gallagher, R.M. Drug Therapy for Headache. New York: Marcel Dekker. 255–273, 1991.

Silberstein, S.D. and Lipton, R.B. Headache and Facial Pain. Continuum, Vol. 1, No. 5, Nov. 1995.

Silberstein, S.D. and Young, W.B. Headache in the elderly. American Academy of Neurology, 52nd Annual Meeting, San Diego, 2000.

Zakizzewska, J.M. Trigeminal Neuralgia. Major Problems in Neurology, Vol. 28. Philadelphia: W.B. Saunders, 1995.

Facial Palsy

Brazis, P.W. et al. Localization in Clinical Neurology, ed. 2. Boston: Little Brown, 203–218, 1990.

Biller, J. Practical Neurology. Philadelphia: Lippincott Raven, 148–154, 1997.

Glaser J.S. Neuroopthalmology, ed. 2. Philadelphia: J.B. Lippincott, 239–278, 1990.

Russel, J.W. Bell's palsy. Neurobase MedLink, Arbor, 1993–2001.

12
Adult Seizures, Neuro-otology, and Sleep Disorders

New Onset Seizures in Adults

Vignette

A 43-year-old real estate broker, while playing golf, had a generalized tonic-clonic seizure witnessed by a friend. In the last three months he had a few episodes of lightheadness and on one occasion had experienced a feeling of floating and turning in space. He had a history of heavy alcohol abuse in his 20s but no current medical problems and was not taking any medication. In the emergency room he was postictal. Pupillary and corneal reflexes were normal. He withdrew all four extremities to pain.

Summary A 43-year-old man with history of a generalized convulsion and a few episodes of lightheadedness, including "feeling of floating" on one occasion. He had a history of heavy alcohol abuse 20 years earlier. The examination shows a postictal state without lateralizing signs.

Localization

This patient had a generalized convulsion most likely preceded by partial complex seizures. Therefore the discussion centers around new onset of seizures in a middle-aged man without any other apparent neurological symptoms. The first consideration is to distinguish between structural and nonstructural lesions.

Differential Diagnosis

When discussing the differential diagnosis, it is important to consider that in a 43-year-old man a first seizure, even when there is no apparent focal onset, raises concern about an underlying structural abnormality. Cerebral neo-plasm should be ruled out first on the list of possibilities because they often are responsible for late onset epilepsy. Depending on the population, brain tumor may represent the most frequent single cause of new onset epilepsy in adults between ages 35 and 55 and a major cause of seizures in the elderly (Ettinger). Seizures, focal or generalized, may be the first and presenting symptom particularly of an underlying slow-growing tumor, such as low grade astrocytoma or oligodendrogliom, in more than half of the patients. Meningioma can also present with seizures as an early sign due to irritation of adjacent cortex. Tumors that infiltrate widely, such as glioblastoma, on the other hand, tend to present with progressive neurological deterioration, focal cerebral symptoms, signs of increased intracranial pressure and cerebral edema. Brain metastases that usually derive from carcinoma of the lung, breast, kidney, and melanoma can commonly manifest with new onset of seizures. Parenchymal metastasis may present as multiple lesions located at the gray-white corticomedullary junction (but can also be solitary) with a tendency to hemorrhage; all factors that increase susceptibility to seizures.

Vascular malformations are very important entities to consider, particularly arteriovenous malformations and cavernous angiomas. Seizure is the presenting symptom in patients with AVM in 30 percent of the cases (Adams and Victor). Cavernous angiomas can also be complicated by seizures and according to Ettinger in 40 to 70 percent of the cases seizures are the presenting symptom usually in the third or fourth decade of life.

Cerebrovascular disorders, ischemic and hemorrhagic, are responsible for new onset of seizures particularly in the elderly. According to Edwards they account for one third of symptomatic epilepsies. Patients with cortical involvement are at risk and embolic strokes can particularly be complicated with seizures. Intraparenchymal hemorrhages other than hemorrhagic infarctions can manifest with seizures within 48 hours of the acute insult (Ettinger).

123

Infections are an important part of the differential diagnosis of new onset seizures. Meningitis, encephalitis, postinfectious encephalomyelitis, brain abscess, and granulomas can be associated with seizures, usually in combination with signs and symptoms of neurological and systemic involvement (not present in the vignette).

Other causes include developmental anomalies such as cortical dysplasias, as well as cortical sclerosis and eterotopias. Mesial temporal sclerosis is the pathological characteristic commonly associated with temporal lobe epilepsy in both children and adults.

Traumatic head injury, particularly if the trauma is associated with loss of consciousness lasting more than 24 hours or with skull fracture, can also be associated with new onset of seizures immediately following the trauma or several weeks or months after the head injury. The patient of the vignette did not have any history related to a prior trauma.

Nonstructural causes of seizures include toxic and metabolic disturbances. Seizures can be due to alcohol withdrawal and also to alcohol intoxication.

Metabolic abnormalities (hyponatremia, hypocalcemia, hepatic encephalopathy, hypoxia, uremia) can precipitate epileptic seizures and need cautious investigation.

The first step in evaluating a presumed seizure is determining if it was indeed a seizure versus a nonepileptic or other event that imitates epilepsy.

Conditions that need to be differentiated are syncope (cardiac and noncardiac), hypoglycemia, sleep disorders, movement disorders, transient ischemic attacks, transient global amnesia, and so on. Psychogenic seizures, hyperventilation, panic attacks, and malingering also enter the differential diagnosis.

If it is determined that the ictal event is epileptic, then the patient can be diagnosed with epilepsy if there is a recurrence of the episode.

The history represents an essential part of the diagnosis and should focus on a careful description of the aura if present, and the ictal and postictal periods. Other characteristic features include the frequency of the event, age of onset, triggering and exacerbating factors, and past medical history, including social and family history. The next step is to determine if the disorder is primary or secondary to an underlying treatable pathology.

Diagnosis

Neuroimaging studies are important in order to rule out a structural abnormality. MRI is the study of choice, particularly for detection of low grade tumors, vascular malformations, or mesial temporal sclerosis. Other imaging studies include positron emission tomography, which may show areas of hypometabolism in patients with epilepsy. Single photon emission computed tomography that measures cerebral blood flow can demonstrate areas

of hypoperfusion. Magnetic resonance spectroscopy also can help detect epileptic foci.

The EEG remains the most important diagnostic test for epilepsy, particularly in detecting interictal abnormalities. A routine normal study does not exclude the possibility of epilepsy and can be complemented by activation procedures such as hyperventilation and photic stimulation. Laboratory tests are also useful, such as complete blood count including differential white cell and platelet count, electrolytes, calcium, and liver and renal function tests. Lumbar puncture should be obtained when a CNS infection needs to be excluded.

Treatment

See next section.

Temporal Lobe Seizures

Vignette

An 18-year-old student started experiencing dizziness, a feeling of nausea, and butterflies in his stomach. He was then found unconscious and incontinent of urine by his roommate. In the emergency room he was lethargic. The neurological and physical examination was otherwise unremarkable. His past medical history indicates that he had suffered complicated febrile seizures during infancy. There was no history of alcohol or drug ingestion. Family history was unremarkable.

Summary An 18-year-old male experiencing dizziness, epigastric sensation, and one episode of loss of consciousness with urinary incontinence. Past medical history is significant for complicated febrile seizures. Neurological examination is not focal.

Localization

Localization demands consideration of whether the event in the vignette represents a seizure or a nonepileptic event.

If the event was a seizure, dizziness, nausea, and butterflies in the stomach could represent an "aura, which can provide evidence of a focal seizure onset." Epigastric sensations are the most common temporal lobe auras and include nausea, butterflies in the stomach, or a rising epigastric sensation (Luciano). The epigastric aura can derive from electrical stimulation of the amygdala or hippocampus but also of the mesial and orbitofrontal regions.

Special consideration needs to be given to mesial temporal lobe epilepsy (MTLE). Complicated febrile convulsions during infancy and early childhood are strongly associated with MTLE. Complicated febrile seizures are described as seizures lasting longer than 30 minutes, multiple separate seizures during the same febrile illness, or seizures with transient postictal hemiparesis (French et al.). Mesial temporal sclerosis (MTS) has also been associated with encephalitis, head injury, and birth trauma.

Hippocampal sclerosis is considered the pathological feature most commonly associated with TLE in both children and adults.

Differential Diagnosis

The differential diagnosis brings into consideration other focal lesions associated with partial epilepsy, such as tumors (hamartomas, dysembryoplastic neuroepithelial tumors, gangliogliomas, and oligodendrogliomas); vascular malformations (arteriovenous malformations and cavernous angiomas), developmental migration abnormalities (cortical dysplasias, gray matter heterotopias), and so on.

Conditions that imitate epilepsy, such as syncope, transient ischemic attacks, toxic or metabolic disorders, migraine, and so on, should also be excluded.

Recurrent abdominal pain or periodic syndrome presents with symptoms of abdominal pain, nausea, and vomiting that recurs for several days and weeks in school-aged children, needs to be differentiated from abdominal epilepsy in which condition the events are associated with altered level of consciousness, automatism, and abnormal EEG.

Other disorders include cyclic vomiting, which is associated with migraine headache (Morrell).

Clinical Features and Diagnosis

Temporal lobe epilepsy is the most frequent symptomatic epilepsy, because more than 50 percent of partial epilepsy orginates in the temporal lobe (Luciano). The age of presentation varies greatly but usually occurs in late childhood to early adult life.

Auras are commonly described and consist of different types of phenomena, such as emotional, autonomic, psychic, olfactory, gustatory, visual, distortion of memory function, dreamy state, and so on. Emotional auras are represented by fear, anger, anxiety, terror, and, less likely, joy and pleasure. Autonomic phenomena include feelings of nausea, butterflies in the stomach, and a rising sensation moving from the abdomen to the throat. Psychic phenomena consist of dreamy state, dissociation, feeling of déjà vu (illusion of familiarity), and jamais vu (illusion of unfamiliarity).

Illusions and hallucinations can be visual, olfactory, or gustatory and present with visual distortion of shape, size, color, and distance; formed visual hallucinations; unpleasant olfactory sensation; auditory distortions of sounds; or simple and complex auditory hallucinations, such as ringing, buzzing, voices, or music. The auras indicate activation of an area of cortex by a limited electrical discharge representing simple partial seizures (Luciano) and usually last seconds to minutes.

Auras can present in isolation or be accompanied by complex partial seizures. Complex partial seizures, characterized by altered level of consciousness often with automatic behavior, predominate in temporal lobe epilepsy. Automatism occurs in 50 to 100 percent of temporal lobe seizures during the ictal or postictal phases (Luciano). Temporal lobe epilepsy has been divided into medial (more common) and lateral temporal lobe syndromes (Devinsky).

Oroalimentary automatisms, which consist of lip smacking, chewing, swallowing, and pursing lips, are the most common in MTLE. Other automatisms are gestural, verbal, ambulatory, and so on (Williamson). Mesial temporal sclerosis is considered the pathological abnormality most frequently identified in TLE in both children and adults. A strong association has been reported between complex, prolonged febrile seizures during infancy and early childhood and the occurrence of MTLE (French). Other risk factors for MTLE include infections, such as meningitis and encephalitis, and head trauma (Devinsky). Lateral TLE is associated with low-grade tumors, cortical dysplasia, trauma, and infections (Devinsky).

EEG studies may show an interictal pattern of unilateral or independently bilateral anterior temporal spike discharges, unilateral focal sphenoidal, midtemporal, and temporal slowing. The discharges are seen more frequently during sleep and with special scalp and sphenoidal electrodes. MRI of the brain may help to detect hippocampal sclerosis in MTLE.

Treatment

Conventional Therapy

Carbamazepine, indicated for partial and tonic clonic seizures, is available for oral administration in conventional and extended-release preparations. The drug is metabolized in the liver and has a peak plasma concentration that occurs in 4 to 12 hours. The therapy is started in low doses (100 to 200 mg a day) with weekly increments up to an effective dose of 800 to 1600 mg in divided doses to generate serum drug level in most laboratories of 8 to 12 mg/ml. Dosing recommended for children is 5 to 20 mg/kg/day. Adverse effects include signs of neurotoxicity, such as double vision, nystagmus, incoordination, and drowsiness, which are dose-related, leukopenia, skin rashes, elevation of liver enzymes, and rare idiosyncratic reactions (Stevens-Johnson syndrome).

Phenytoin is used for partial and generalized tonic clonic seizures and can be administered orally, intravenously, and intramuscularly as fosphenytoin. The drug is started at a dose of 300 mg a day that requires 5 to 7 days to reach a therapeutic serum level of 10 to 20 mg/ml or can be started more rapidly with a loading dose of 10 to 20 mg/kg IV at 25 to 50 mg/min. Phenytoin is metabolized in the liver. Neurotoxic drug-related side effects include nystagmus, ataxia, dizziness, and so on. Chronic adverse effects are represented by hirsutism, gingival hyperplasia, peripheral neuropathy, osteomalaria, and folate deficiency.

Valproic acid, a broad-spectrum medication, is indicated in primary generalized tonic-clonic seizures, partial seizures, and typical and atypical absence and atonic and myoclonic seizures. It is also available as extended-release preparation and injection. The effective dose is 15 to 25 mg/kg/day in adults and 10 to 30 mg/kg/day in children in order to reach a therapeutic plasma concentration of 50 to 120 mg/ml. Adverse effects include nausea, gastrointestinal symptoms, weight gain, menstrual irregularities, tremor, trompocytopenia, hair loss, hepatitis, and pancreatitis.

Ethosuximide has been effective in the treatment of absence seizures, typical and atypical, and is given in a dose of 750 to 1500 mg/day in adults. Effective plasma concentrations are 40 to 100 mg/ml. Side effects include nausea, vomiting, anorexia, headache, and drowsiness.

Phenobarbital has been used for control of partial and generalized tonic-clonic seizures. It is available in capsule, elixir, tablets, and injection. The usual adult dose is 90 to 180 mg a day with an effective plasma concentration of 15 to 40 mg/ml. Adverse effects include sedation, agitation, and depression.

New Therapies

Felbamate is used as monotherapy and add-on therapy for partial onset seizures and primary generalized tonic-clonic seizures in adults age 14 and older. It has been also used as adjunctive therapy in children with Lennox-Gastaut syndrome. The effective dose varies from 1800 to 4800 mg daily in adults and 15 to 45 mg/kg/day in children. Adverse effects include anorexia, headache, nausea, insomnia, and fatigue, and severe idiosyncratic side effects are represented by aplastic anemia and liver failure.

Gabapentin, approved as adjunctive therapy of partial seizures in patients age 12 and older, has dosages that vary from 1800 to 3600 mg/day and no significant drug interactions or idiosyncratic side effects. Adverse effects usually consist of drowsiness, fatigue, and headache.

Lamotrigine is indicated as adjunctive therapy in patients with partial seizures and generalized seizures associated with Lennox-Gastaut syndrome. The usual dose in adults varies from 200 to 400 mg/day. Side effects include skin rash with an increased risk in patients receiving valproic acid, diplopia, somnolence, headache, and ataxia.

Tiagabine is effective as add-on therapy for partial seizures. The dosage ranges from 32 to 56 mg daily. Side effects include dizziness, somnolenceasthenia, and nervousness.

Topiramate has been used as an add-on therapy for treatment of partial and secondary generalized tonic-clonic seizures, particularly those that fail to respond to other drugs. The usual adult dose is 200 to 400 mg/day. Adverse effects include fatigue, dizziness, gastrointestinal upset, emotional lability, and so on.

The efficacy of vigabatrin against partial seizures has been indicated in multiple clinical trials in adults and children.

Status Epilepticus

Vignette

A 39-year-old homeless man was witnessed by a policeman to collapse and have a seizure while on a street corner. He then experienced two more seizures 15 minutes after arriving in the emergency room and was noted to have held up his left arm, which started jerking, before he developed the tonic-clonic seizures. On examination he was unresponsive to verbal and painful stimuli, with sluggish pupils and bilateral upgoing toes. No past medical history could be obtained.

Summary A 39-year-old man with repetitive tonic-clonic seizures without recovery of consciousness between seizures.

Localization

The vignette clearly indicates a clinical case of status epilepticus, particularly generalized tonic-clonic status epilepticus with partial onset and secondary generalization. This is the most frequent and alarming type and represents a neurological emergency. Seventy to eighty percent of patients with tonic-clonic status have a partial onset (partial motor, postural, or controversive head and eye mevements) (Walsh). The patient described in the vignette has no known previous medical history that may help to identify the possible etiology. Therefore, this is a discussion of all the possible causes of convulsive status epilepticus.

In patients with prior history of epilepsy, status epilepticus can be precipitated by noncompliance or withdrawal from antiepileptic medications. Other factors that can precipitate this situation are drug and alcohol abuse and withdrawal, a new anticonvulsant regimen, sleep deprivation, fever, intercurrent infections, metabolic abnormalities (e.g., hypoglycemia, hypocalcemia, and hyponatremia), hyperosmolarity due to hyperglycemia, hepatic and renal failure, and so on. Status epilepticus may be precipitated by an acute cerebral insult, such as a cerebrovascular accident (ischemic or hemorrhagic), infections (meningitis, encephalitis), head trauma, anoxic encephalopathies, brain tumors, and so on. In children, frequent causes of status epilepticus are cerebral infections.

Systemic complications can occur from tonic-clonic status epilepticus resulting in brain damage and death. They include metabolic, autonomic, renal, and cardiorespiratory complications.

Metabolic abnormalities are represented by lactic acidosis, hypoxia, hypercapnea, hypoglycemia (due to depletion of glycogen stores and hyperinsulinemia), hyponatremia, and hyperkalemia.

Autonomic complications include increased body temperature (due to profuse muscular activity), abnormal cerebrovascular autoregulation leading to cerebral edema, electrolyte and fluid loss, increase in sweat, salivation, and so on.

Renal complications include acute renal insufficiency and myoglobinuria due to rhabdomyosis.

Cardiopulmonary complications are represented by cardiac arrhythmia, hypotension, pulmonary edema, and so on.

Treatment

The treatment of status epilepticus begins with the ABC that includes supporting airways and maintaining blood pressure and circulation. Clinical and electrical seizures should be stopped as soon as possible to prevent systemic complications.

The recommendation of the Epilepsy Foundation of America's working group on status epilepticus is that intravenous benzodiazepines, diazepam, or lorazepam should be used first, followed by intravenous phenytoin or intravenous phenobarbital if those are not effective in stopping the status.

Willmore suggests a dose of 0.1mg/kg lorazepam given at 2 mg/min up to 4 mg total dose or 0.2 mg/kg of diazepam at 5 mg/min up to 20 mg maximum that can be administered again after 5 minutes if seizures persist. Phenytoin is given next at a loading dose of 20 mg/kg phenytoin no faster than 50 mg/min in adults and 1 mg/kg/min in children, always monitoring cardiac status and blood pressure. Fosphenytoin may be administered at 150 phenytoin-equivalents/min as a safe substitute for phenytoin. An additional dose can also be administered if the seizures are not controlled. Another choice is phenobarbital 20 mg/kg IV at 60 mg/min. If status persists, anesthesia with pentobarbital, midazolam, or propofol; intubation; ventilation; and vasopressors will be required.

Neuro-Otology and Sleep Disorders: Meniere's Syndrome

Vignette

A 56-year-old cleaning woman with a previous medical history of hypertension and migraine, started experiencing severe episodes of sudden spinning of the surroundings, imbalance, and vomiting lasting over one hour. During the third attack she complained of a feeling of pressure on the right ear, a bothersome high-intensity roaring sound that subsided over a few days, and decreased hearing. A couple of times she suddenly fell to the ground as though being pushed and hit her head on the concrete without losing consciousness. On neurological examination, there was a right beating nystagmus. The Weber test lateralized to the left and the Rinne test was positive bilaterally. Motor, sensory, and coordination examinations were normal.

Summary A 56-year-old woman with history of recurrent, severe vertigo associated with vomiting. Other symptoms include pressure on the right ear, tinnitus, hearing loss, and two episodes of what seem to be drop attacks. Neurological examination showed right beating nystagmus and right sensorineural hearing loss. Previous history included hypertension and migraine.

Localization

First it must be determined if the vertigo is due to a central, peripheral, or systemic cause. Vertigo can occur as a result of pathology involving the labyrinthine structures or vestibular nerves, or may be due to central causes involving the brainstem or cerebellum. Peripheral disorders manifest with recurrent attacks of spontaneous vertigo associated with signs of auditory impairment, such as tinnitus, fullness in the ear, and hearing loss. Nausea and vomiting can also be prominent findings. Nystagmus that tends to fatigue and is inhibited by visual fixation is typically unidirectional, horizontal in type, with a rotatory component.

Lesions involving the brainstem and cerebellum are characterized by vertigo that does not occur in isolation but is accompanied by other signs and symptoms of neurological dysfunction. Balance is often severely affected and auditory symptoms are not common. Nystagmus in central lesions is a significant finding and has certain characteristics, such as fatigue, can be unidirectional or bidirectional, and is worsened by visual fixation.

Systemic disorders causing vertigo are due to endocrine, metabolic, or hematologic diseases and will also be discussed in this section.

The patient in the vignette exhibits signs of peripheral involvement characterized by severe recurrent vertigo, tinnitus, and hearing loss. The two episodes of sudden falling to the ground without loss of consciousness can occur with disorders of the labyrinth (typically, Meniere's disease) or may be observed in vascular disorders, such as vertebrobasilar insufficiency causing drop attacks typically in older patients with known risk factors for cerebral ischemia. Patients with Meniere's disease describe a feeling of being pushed or shoved to the ground, often noting an illusion of movement of the environment just before the fall (Baloh). Drop attacks attributed to other causes typically result in a slumping to the ground due to a sudden loss of tone in the lower extremities (Baloh). Other causes of sudden loss of muscle tone include atonic seizures and cataplectic attacks in narcolepsy.

Differential Diagnosis

Benign positional vertigo is characterized by brief recurrent episodes of paroxysmal vertigo associated with nystagmus lasting less than a minute and precipitated by changes in head position. Auditory function is not affected and the nystagmus has characteristics of being transient, fatigues rapidly, and is unidirectional. The vertigo is also fatigable and is abolished with repetition of the maneuver. This disorder is clearly not a consideration in the patient described in the vignette who had experienced episodes of prolonged vertigo, vomiting, hearing loss, and tinnitus.

Vestibular neuronitis presents with acute onset of severe vertigo, nausea, and vomiting without any sign of auditory dysfunction. Nystagmus is invariably present with its quick phase beating to the opposite side of the vestibular dysfunction. A history of upper respiratory or other viral infection can often be elicited by the patient and symptoms only last several days and gradually subside. This syndrome with its characteristic symptoms can also be excluded in the patient described in the vignette.

Acute and recurrent peripheral vestibulopathy is characterized by frequent attacks of vertigo without signs of auditory dysfunction in older people over the course of months to years.

Ototoxic drugs such as antibiotics of the group of the aminoglycosides (streptomycin, gentamycin, amikacin), salicylates, anticonvulsants, and so on can be responsible for damage to the labyrinths. Symptoms are usually bilateral and include vertigo, tinnitus, disequilibrium, hearing loss often accompanied by nausea, vomiting, and poor balance. There is no mention in the vignette to any prior use of ototoxic drugs.

Meniere's disease, characterized by recurrent episodes of vertigo associated with tinnitus, a sensation of fullness in the ear, and fluctuating hearing loss can explain the symptoms in the vignette. The sudden falling spells described as a feeling of being pushed to the ground suggest a sudden stimulation of the otolithic membrane of the utricle, saccule, or both, from the increased intralabyrinthine pressure (Baloh).

Infections can be associated with dysfunction of the labyrinth and produce signs and symptoms that mimic Meniere's disease. In particular, neurosyphilis can cause episodes of vertigo and hearing loss.

In the differential diagnosis, other disorders may be considered. The patient described in the vignette had a history of migraine headache. Vertigo can often accompany migraine pain occurring before or during the headache but also as a migraine equivalent not associated with headache. Migraine equivalents can manifest as recurrent attacks of vertigo in children that later on may develop symptoms of migraine, as well as in adults, particularly women. The vertigo can be accompanied by nausea, vomiting, nystagmus, disequilibrium, and phonophobia but without other signs of auditory dysfunction.

Migraine and attacks of Meniere's disease can also occur in the same patient. Migraine should be suspected if there is a long history of recurrent attacks of vertigo without auditory or neurological symptoms and a possible positive family history. Basilar migraine, which is a type of complicated migraine, can present with vertigo, tinnitus, and auditory dysfunction, but the symptoms also include ataxia, diplopia, visual field defects, dysarthria, and signs of posterior fossa abnormalities that are transient and followed by severe throbbing headache.

Cerebellopontine angle tumors are also part of the differential diagnosis of the vignette but they are usually characterized by progressive hearing loss, tinnitus, and signs of cranial nerve and cerebellar involvement rather than recurrent attacks of vertigo.

Cerebrovascular disorders, in particular vertebrobasilar ischemia, can be responsible for recurrent episodes of vertigo due to involvement of the vestibular nuclei and their connections. Vertigo does not usually occur in isolation but is accompanied by other neurological symptoms of posterior circulation compromise such as dysarthria, diplopia, weakness, sensory loss, and ataxia. The vertigo usually is of sudden onset, associated with nausea, vomiting, and nystagmus that changes direction in different head position and is not inhibited by visual fixation. Patients have risk factors for cerebrovascular disorders or a history of heart disease. Typical disorders include the lateral medullary syndrome due to occlusion of the vertebral or PICA artery and presenting with symptoms of vertigo, nausea, vomiting, ipsilateral eye and facial pain, Horner's syndrome, contralateral limb hypoesthesia, dysmetria, and so on, and the lateral pontomedullary syndrome, caused by ischemia in the territory of the AICA and manifesting with vertigo, nausea, vomiting, nystagmus, tinnitus, unilateral hearing loss, ipsilateral facial paralysis, and ipsilateral ataxia.

Multiple sclerosis can be associated with vertigo in the initial episode or during relapse (Matthews et al.). Other central signs such as cerebellar dysfunction, diplopia, and ophthalmoplegia can help pinpoint the correct diagnosis.

Finally, Cogan's syndrome can be mentioned for completion. It manifests with symptoms of vertigo, hearing loss, and interstitial keratitis and is due to a vasculitic process.

In summary, after all the possibilities have been considered, Meniere's disease remains the preferred diagnosis.

Clinical Features

Meniere's disease typically presents with recurrent attacks of vertigo, a sense of fullness in the ear, tinnitus, and hearing loss. The vertigo occurs suddenly lasting from minutes to several hours and can reach such an intensity that the patient becomes unable to stand or ambulate. When it gradually lessens, a feeling of imbalance and dizziness can be experienced for several days. Nausea and vomiting are also associated symptoms, as well as tinnitus described as a roaring or hissing sound. Nystagmus can be observed during the acute episode and is horizontal with a rotary component. Past pointing and lateral propulsion are to the side of the lesion (Victor and Adams). During the attack, the patient tends to lie with the involved ear uppermost, afraid that any movement will make the vertigo worse. Auditory dysfunction is an important feature of Meniere's disease and is characterized by fluctuating sensorineural hearing loss that is unilateral in 80 to 90 percent of cases with a severe deficit in half the patients (Drachman).

Patients with Meniere's disease can also experience sudden episodes of falling that have been defined as otolithic catastrophes and are described as a sudden push or shove to the ground often associated with an illusion of environmental tilting (Baloh). These attacks need to be differentiated from drop attacks due to other causes. They are due to a sudden stimulation of the otolithic membranes of the utricle, saccule, or both.

Diagnosis

The diagnosis of Meniere's disease depends on the clinical history of the attacks and the audiologic findings of fluctuating sensorineural low tone loss. Word recognition is usually preserved and brainstem auditory evoked responses are normal.

Treatment

The treatment consists of symptomatic therapy of the acute episodes and prevention of recurrent attacks with a diet based on salt restriction and the use of diuretics. During an acute attack of Meniere disease, bed rest is recommended. Promethazine, which is effective for relieving the acute vertigo, nausea, and vomiting, should be taken at the beginning of the symptoms.

Narcolepsy

Vignette

A 28-year-old maintenance worker was brought to your attention after being fired because he had frequently been found asleep at work. He had experienced a few years of sleepiness during the day with refreshing naps, frequent awakening at night, and nightmares while falling asleep, consisting of terrifying visual hallucinations. He also describes several episodes of knee buckling and rubbery feelings in his legs. Twice, after verbal confrontations, he fell to the ground without losing consciousness. Other times he had to lean momentarily against the wall for support. General physical and neurological examinations were normal.

Summary A 28-year-old man with excessive daytime sleepiness, frequent awakening at night, visual hallucinations, and falling spells without loss of consciousness. The examination is normal.

Localization and Differential Diagnosis

The category of disorders to be considered is sleep disorders. Also in the differential diagnosis, the falling spells without loss of consciousness or drop attacks should be considered.

Sleep disorders, according to the international classification, are divided into dyssomnias, parasomnias, and sleep disorders associated with medical and psychiatric conditions. Dyssomnias are disorders manifesting with excessive sleepiness or symptoms of insomnia. Parasomnias are characterized by abnormal behavior, such as sleepwalking, sleep terror, movements such as rhythmic movement disorder, nocturnal leg cramps, sensations, or other phenomena, such as sleep bruxism, and sleep enuresis that manifest during sleep but are not associated with insomnia or excessive sleepiness (Aldrich). Sleep disorders caused by medical and psychiatric disturbances are associated with the appropriate etiology.

The clinical case described in the vignette, therefore, is a case of sleep disorder included in the category of the dyssomnias. Some characteristic findings described help the diagnosis:

- Excessive daytime sleepiness with refreshing naps.
- Disrupted sleep at night with frequent awakening and

hallucinations that can be vivid and distressing when falling asleep.
- Sudden loss of muscle tone without loss of consciousness, precipitated by emotional states.
- Normal neurological examination.

These clinical symptoms strongly suggest the diagnosis of narcolepsy with cataplexy. The International Classification of Sleep Disorders characterizes narcolepsy as a disorder of unknown etiology that manifests with excessive daytime sleepiness and is associated with cataplexy and other abnormal manifestations of REM sleep, such as sleep paralysis and hypnagogic hallucinations.

The differential diagnosis primarily includes sleep apnea.

Obstructive sleep apnea manifests with excessive daytime sleepiness, unrefreshing sleep or insomnia, and often loud snoring. The main clinical feature is represented by recurrent episodes of complete (apnea) or partial (hypopnea) cessation of breathing during sleep despite continued effort to breathe (Chervin). The site of airway narrowing is in the upper airway, between the caudal region of the soft palate and the epiglottis (Chervin). Obstructive sleep apnea manifests during periods of both REM and NREM sleep and preferentially affects middle-age obese males. Narcolepsy usually has its onset in younger patients sometimes during adolescence and can typically be associated with cataplexy. Also, narcoleptics usually benefit from naps, feeling refreshed, while patients with sleep apnea feel tired and unrefreshed in the morning and can experience a choking sensation or breathing difficulty on awakening and often a morning headache.

Nocturnal polysomnography is the test of choice for sleep apnea and may demonstrate the episodes of apnea-hypopnea, arterial oxygen desaturation, and disturbed sleep pattern.

A central sleep apnea is characterized by the absence of respiratory effort and therefore the absence of airflow during sleep (Guilleminault and Robinson). This disorder may affect patients with brainstem lesions involving the medulla. Other causes include degenerative and metabolic disorders, encephalitis, Creutzfeld-Jacob disease, amyotrophic lateral sclerosis, poliomyelitis, and so on.

Idiopathic hypersomnolence starts in young patients with symptoms of protracted somnolence with unrefreshing naps and without the occurrence of cataplexy. Sleep laboratory investigations help differentiate this disorder from narcolepsy.

Kleine-Levine syndrome, which usually affects adolescent boys, is also characterized by excessive sleep with episodes of prolonged diurnal hypersomnia lasting from days to weeks and recurring few times a year, associated with overeating and altered libido.

Excessive daytime hypersomnolence can also be a manifestation of periodic limb movement disorder that often causes insomnia.

Neurological disorders associated with hypersomnolence include degenerative disorders such as Parkinson's disease and Alzheimer's disease, vascular disorders such as thalamic infarction, infections such as encephalitis, structural lesions such as tumors, and trauma.

Cataplexy, which is characterized by a sudden loss of muscle tone triggered by excitement or emotion and with preserved consciousness needs to be differentiated from other disorders. These include drop attacks due to vertebrobasilar ischemia; seizures, atonic and gelastic (in the latter ictal laughing may be associated with a fall); periodic paralysis; and myasthenia gravis. The associated clinical features, duration of the attacks, and precipitating events usually point to the correct diagnosis.

Clinical Features

Narcolepsy is a neurological disorder that manifests with excessive daytime sleepiness, cataplexy, and pathological manifestations of REM sleep. Excessive daytime sleepiness is an important clinical feature and at times becomes irresistible for the patient, manifesting during different situations such as standing, driving, eating, and even during a conversation. Naps are felt refreshing and sometimes associated with dreams.

Cataplexy manifests with sudden loss of muscle tone precipitated by emotions or excitement. Laughing, fear, and rage can be provocative factors. Consciousness is preserved and the duration of the episode is less than a few minutes. The severity of the cataplectic attack varies from knee buckling, feeling weak, dropping of the arms, sagging of the face, to complete fall to the ground.

Sleep paralysis, manifested by inability to move for a few seconds or minutes while falling asleep at night or upon awakening, is another manifestation of narcolepsy and can occur with hypnagogic and hypnopompic hallucinations. The hallucinations can be simple or complex, are most commonly visual and involving people or animals. Abnormal sleep pattern with frequent awakening is also an important characteristic.

Narcolepsy affects both sexes and manifests in young patients usually in the second decade of life. There is a strong association with the human leukocyte antigen DRw15.

Diagnosis

The diagnosis is confirmed by the multiple sleep latency test (MSLT), which demonstrates REM sleep at sleep onset or within 15 minutes thereafter (sleep onset REM or

SOREM) (Bassetti and Aldrich). Narcolepsy can be easily diagnosed when cataplexy and more than two sleep onset REM periods are noted on MSLT. Other sleep disorders can complicate narcolepsy such as sleep apnea, two periodic limb movements of sleep, and so on.

Treatment

The treatment of narcolepsy revolves around patient and family education, inclusion of a few naps during the day, avoidance of sleep deprivation, and the use of stimulants to treat sleepiness. The most commonly used stimulants are methylphenidate (Ritalin), dextroamphetamine (Dexedrine) and pemoline (Cylert). Tricyclic antidepressants are the first line treatment for cataplexy and sleep paralysis.

References

New-Onset Seizures in Adults/Temporal Lobe Epilepsy

Adams, R.D. and Victor, M. Principles of Neurology, ed. 5. New York: McGraw-Hill, 728–734, 1993.

Devinsky, O. Diagnosis and treatment of temporal lobe epilepsy. Rev. Neurol. Dis. Vol. 1, Winter 2004.

Edwards, J.C. Seizure types: Epilepsy Syndromes, Etiology and Diagnosis. CNS Spectrum 6:750–755, 2001.

Ettinger, A.B. Structural causes of epilepsy. In: Epilepsy. II: Special Issues. Neurol. Clin. 12:41–56, 1994.

Fischer, J.H. and Habib, M. Guide to antiepileptic agents. CNS News, Special Edition, Vol. 5, 2003.

French, J.A. et al. Characteristics of mesial temporal lobe epilepsy: I. Results of history and physical examination. Ann. Neurol. 34:774–787, 1993.

Hamati-Haddam, A. et al. Epilepsy diagnosis and localization in patients with antecedent childhood febrile convulsions. Neurology 50:917–922, 1998.

Luciano, D. Partial seizures of frontal and temporal origin. Neurol. Clin. 11:805–834, 1993.

Luders, H.O. Epilepsy: Comprehensive Review and Case Discussions. London: Martin Dunitz, 2001.

Mattson, R.H. An overview of the new antiepileptic drugs. Neurologist (Suppl.) 4:S2–S10, 1998.

Morrel, M.J. Differential diagnosis of seizures. In: Epilepsy. I: Diagnosis and Treatment. Neurol. Clin. 11:737–754, 1993.

Muro, G.J. and Karis, J.P. Neuroimaging. In: Temporal Lobe Epilepsy. CNS Spectrum 2:31–42, 1997.

Wieser, H.G. Temporal lobe epilepsies. In: Handbook of Clinical Neurology. Vol. 73: The Epilepsies, Part II. New York: Elsevier, 53–96, 2000

Williamson, P.D. Mesial temporal lobe epilepsy. MedLink, Arbor, 1993–2000.

Status Epilepticus

Leppik, I.E. Status epilepticus. In: The Treatment of Epilepsy: Principles and Practice. Wyllie, E. (ed.). Philadelphia: Lea and Febiger, 678–685, 1993.

Luders, H.O. Epilepsy: Comprehensive Review and Case Discussions. London: Martin Dunitz, 327–333, 2001.

Scholtes, F.B.J. Status epilepticus. In: Handbook of Clinical Neurology. Vol. 73, The Epilepsies, Part II. New York: Elsevier, 317–341, 2000.

Sirven, J.I. Management of status epilepticus. American Academy of Neurology, 53rd Annual Meeting, Philadelphia, May 5–11, 2001.

Walsh, G.O. and Delgado-Escueta, A.V. Status Epilepticus. In: Epilepsy. I: Diagnosis and Treatment. Neurol. Clin. 2:835–856, 1993.

Willmore, L.J. Epilepsy emergencies: The first seizure and status epilepticus. In: Wilder, B.J. Management of epilepsy: Consensus conference on current clinical practice. Neurology 51(Suppl 4):S34–S38, 1998.

Meniere's Syndrome

Adams, R.D. and Victor, M. Principles of Neurology, ed. 5. New York: McGraw-Hill, 247–269, 1993.

Baloh, R.W. Drop attacks in Meniere's syndrome. Ann. Neurol. 28:384–387, 1990.

Baloh, R.W. et al. Neurotology. Continuum, Part A. 2:55–85, 1996.

Brazis, P.W. et al. Localization in Clinical Neurology. Boston: Little Brown, 219–237, 1990.

Drachman, D.A. Dizziness and vertigo. American Academy of Neurology, 51st Annual Meeting, Toronto, 1999.

Matthews, et al. McAlpine's Multiple Sclerosis. New York: Churchill Livingstone, 1991.

Pfaltz, C.R. Controversial Aspects of Meniere's Disease. New York: Thieme, 1986.

Narcolepsy

Aldrich, M. Narcolepsy. American Academy of Neurology, 51st Annual Meeting, Toronto, 1999.

American Sleep Disorders Association: ICSD—International Classification of Sleep Disorders: Diagnostic and Coding Manual. Diagnostic Classification Steering Committee, Thorpy, M.J. (Chairman). Rochester, MN: American Sleep Disorders Association, 1990.

Bassetti, C. and Aldrich, S. Narcolepsy. Neurol. Clin. 14:545–571, 1996.

Chervin, R.D. and Guilleminault, C. Obstructive sleep apnea and related disorders. Neurol. Clin. 14:583–609, 1996.

Fry, J.M. Current issues in the diagnosis and management of narcolepsy. Neurology 50 (Suppl. 1):S1–S48, 1998.

Guilleminault, C. and Robinson, A. Central sleep apnea. Neurol. Clin. 14:611–628, 1996.

Shapiro, C.M. ABC of Sleep Disorders. London: BMJ, 1993.

13
Multiple Sclerosis

Multiple Sclerosis

Vignette

During the past six months a 22-year-old student experienced several episodes of sudden stabbing pain in both cheeks, especially around her eyes. The pain was severe and debilitating, making her unable to talk for a few seconds. For the last two months her gait has been unsteady and cautious, at times veering to the left. She has also complained of dizziness, described as "severe spinning" for a few minutes, which did not improve with eye closing. One year ago she suffered painful loss of vision in her left eye, which partially resolved within 1 week. She had no history of smoking, alcohol, or drug abuse. Her mother had migraine headache. The neurological examination indicates a normal mental status. The right pupil promptly constricts on illumination. As the light is rapidly moved to the left, the left pupil dilates. Mild left hemiparesis is also noted. Gait is ataxic.

Summary A 22-year-old woman experiencing several episodes of pain in the cheeks, unsteady gait, vertigo, and left visual loss that partially recovered. Neurological examination shows a left afferent pupillary defect, left hemiparesis, and ataxic gait.

Localization

It is important to localize the lesion and determine whether it is focal, multifocal, or diffuse. A multifocal lesion is represented by two or more focal lesions distributed randomly. In the vignette presented, the patient clearly has multifocal lesions disseminated in space and time. Therefore we can identify pyramidal signs (left hemiparesis), cerebellar signs (gait ataxia), vestibular dysfunction (vertigo), trigeminal neuralgia (stabbing pain in the cheeks), and optic nerve dysfunction (left painful visual loss, afferent pupillary defect).

Differential Diagnosis

Several categories of neurological disorders can be considered in the differential diagnosis of multifocal pathology, including

- Demyelinating disorders: multiple sclerosis.
- Infectious and inflammatory disorders: acute disseminated encephalomyelitis, HIV, Lyme disease, systemic lupus erythematosus, Sjögren syndrome.
- Vascular disorders: cerebral vasculitis, multiple emboli, familial cavernous hemangiomas.
- Cerebral malformations: Chiari malformation.
- Space-occupying lesions: primary lymphoma of the brain, multiple metastases.
- Hereditary disorders: leukodystrophies, mitochondrial disorders.

In a young adult presenting with focal neurological deficits separated in both time and space, a demyelinating disorder such as multiple sclerosis (MS) ranks high on the list of possible diagnoses.

Trigeminal neuralgia in multiple sclerosis is much more often bilateral (Matthews) and occurs approximately in 1 percent of patients and usually at an earlier age than the idiopathic form.

Corticospinal tract involvement is part of the initial attack of MS in 32 to 41 percent of patients (Miller). Lower extremities weakness seems more common than upper extremities involvement and can be unilateral.

Cerebellar involvement is also common in multiple sclerosis and is indicated by the manifestations of ataxia, incoordination, intention tremor, dysarthria, and so on.

Cerebellar ataxia as an early sign can predict a bad prognosis without significant remission (Matthews).

Vertigo can occur during the initial attack of MS or during relapse.

A relative afferent pupillary defect such as the one described in the vignette suggests optic nerve pathology and consists of a relative decrease in pupillary constriction to light stimulation of the affected eye.

It is important to discuss the differential diagnosis. Other conditions that can be disseminated in space and sometimes in time may simulate MS. Infectious, postinfectious, and inflammatory disorders are important considerations.

Acute disseminated encephalomyelitis (ADEM) can be easily ruled out from the vignette. This disorder is characterized by widespread manifestations that reflect involvement of multifocal areas such as cerebrum, brainstem, cerebellum, optic nerve, and spinal cord. A history of upper respiratory or other viral infections or immunization precedes the onset of neurological symptoms, characterized by fever, headache, meningeal signs, altered consciousness, convulsions, ataxia, myoclonus, paraplegia, sphincteric dysfunction, and so on. Children are preferentially affected more than adults. Varicella and unidentified upper respiratory tract viral causes are probably the major preceding infections causing ADEM in North America (Munsat). A mortality up to 20 percent has been reported (Matthews) and neurological sequelae in surviving cases vary from spinal cord dysfunction to mental retardation and epilepsy.

The relapsing form of ADEM can simulate MS and sometimes creates diagnostic difficulties. Also confusing is when MS presents with an acute fulminating form.

The examination of the CSF may show increased IgG and myelin basic protein in both disorders but oligoclonal bands are less commonly found in ADEM. The MRI of the brain shows multifocal white matter lesions hyperintense on T_2 and does not clearly differentiate between MS and ADEM.

Other infections and inflammatory disorders also need to be considered.

Lyme disease is an important part of the differential diagnosis because it can simulate MS, particularly when it presents with signs of multifocal cerebral and spinal cord dysfunction (encephalomyelitis). On the other hand, the most common presentation in Lyme disease is that of a meningoencephalitis (Paty and Ebers) and it is very unlikely that such an infection would manifest with a typical MS-like picture characterized by isolated episodes of CNS dysfunction separated by months or years (Miller). In Lyme disease, the history of prior living or visiting an endemic area, erythema migrans when demonstrated, extraneurological and systemic manifestations, such as arthritis, carditis, generalized malaise, fatigue, and so on, positive serology, and CSF studies can help make the correct diagnosis.

Systemic lupus erythematosus (SLE) can simulate MS and present some diagnostic difficulties when the neurological symptoms precede the signs of systemic involvement. Lupus could be confused with MS when it presents with signs of optic neuritis combined with spinal cord dysfunction (Matthews). The most common manifestations of cerebral involvement in SLE are usually psychiatric, such as psychosis, depression, delusions, and hallucinations (Aminoff). Seizures, aseptic meningitis, and movement disorders rather than signs suggestive of white matter dysfunction are also described. Laboratory studies of immune function will complete the diagnosis.

Sjögren's syndrome, characterized by xerostomia, xerophtalmia, and arthritis, can rarely affect the nervous system (less than 10% of patients) (Aminoff).

Behçet's disease can present with multifocal cerebral symptoms but usually the typical ocular lesions and oral and genital ulcers are antecedent or accompany the neurological symptoms. Occasionally, though, they can occur later (Matthew). Neurological signs and symptoms are seen in 4 to 29 percent of patients (Aminoff). Signs of central nervous system involvement include hemiparesis, ataxia, seizures, pseudobulbar palsy, spinal cord dysfunction and can manifest a fluctuating course mimicking MS.

Sarcoidosis can also be responsible for a multifocal neurological pathology with involvement of the optic nerve, brainstem, cerebral hemispheres, and spinal cord, but only rarely these are the first signs and some typical features such as diabetes insipidus, hydrocephalus, and peripheral neuropathy not expected with MS help the differential diagnosis. Also, sarcoidosis more commonly than MS may cause anosmia, facial palsy, deafness, and progressive optic atrophy (Matthew). Sarcoidosis is a systemic disorder that affects several organs, particularly lymphonodes, lungs, skin, eyes, salivary glands, and so on, and a positive diagnosis is based on the demonstration of the characteristic noncaseating granuloma.

AIDS also needs to be ruled out because it can cause widespread neurological involvement usually associated with other systemic manifestations.

Central nervous system vasculitis that is restricted to the CNS without systemic manifestations can cause multifocal neurological signs but is a rare disorder, and headache and changes in mental status are usually prominent. The diagnosis is based on angiographic findings and brain biopsy.

Cerebrovascular disease, particularly multiple emboli, can be part of the differential diagnosis of lesions disseminated in space and time. The vignette does not suggest any risk factors for embolic stroke, which in a young person are usually represented by cardiac disorders, either congenital or acquired. Other risk factors for ischemic or hemorrhagic events are also not indicated in the vignette (vasculopathies, coagulopathies, Moya Moya, pregnancy, puerperium, use of illicit drugs, oral contraceptive medications, hematological disorders, such as antithrombin III, protein C and S deficiency, and antiphospholipid antibody syndrome, sickle cell anemia, and so on).

Cerebral malformations such as Arnold-Chiari malformation can present with multiple neurological signs disseminated in space and referable to the cerebellum, upper cervical cord, and brainstem but some clinical features are characteristics such as pain in the occipital cervical and upper limb area, hydrosyringomyelia with dissociated sensory loss, nystagmus, predominantly vertical, and so on. The diagnosis can be difficult and MS should be ruled out in those patients presenting with progressive cerebellar and limb ataxia, spastic weakness, dysarthria, nystagmus, and so on.

Neoplastic disorders (multiple metastases, primary CNS lymphoma, remote effect of carcinoma such as paraneoplastic cerebellar degeneration with limbic encephalitis and optic neuritis) are obviously and easily ruled out from the vignette, but are mentioned because they can occasionally resemble MS presenting with neurological signs and symptoms disseminated in space and time.

Finally, we will very briefly consider hereditary disorders, such as leukodystrophies, mitochondrial disorders, and dominantly inherited ataxias. Adrenoleukodystrophy typically presents during childhood and rarely can be confused for MS. Adrenomyeloneuropathy that manifests in young adults can have signs of spinal cord dysfunction usually in combination with peripheral neuropathy and adrenal insufficiency.

Mitochondrial disorders can have multifocal involvement, but typically include signs of myopathy, peripheral neuropathy, exercise intolerance, unexplained headache and vomiting, hearing loss, dysmorphic features, and so on that may point to the correct diagnosis.

The hereditary spinocerebellar ataxias are readily distinguished from multiple sclerosis by their chronic progression, insidious onset, family history, symmetrical distribution, and associated abnormalities, neurological and nonneurological such as reflex loss, skeletal deformities, heart dysfunction, and so on.

Diagnosis

Several diagnostic criteria have been used to classify MS into clinically definite, probable, or possible. The clinical diagnosis of definitive MS is based on the age of presentation (10 to 59 years according to Poser) (The Washington Committee criteria); two attacks separated in time and space or two attacks with one clinical and one paraclinical evidence of lesion (where paraclinical indicates abnormal findings on neuroimaging studies, evoked potentials, and urodynamic studies).

Laboratory Data

The examination of the cerebrospinal fluid can support the diagnosis of MS and demonstrate characteristic, but not specific, abnormalities, which can also be observed with other pathology. Cell count may show a mononuclear pleocytosis (10 to 50 mm^3). Red blood cell and glucose content are normal. The total protein level can be mildly elevated, but an abnormally high level (over 100 mg/dl) may be suspicious of pathology other than MS.

There is an increased level of immunoglobulins in the CSF, primarily IgG, which represent over 13 percent of the total proteins in 70 percent of clinically definite MS (Paty and Ebers).

The IgG index, which is an indication of IgG production in the CSF, is determined by the ratios of IgG and albumin in the CSF and serum. The presence of oligoclonal bands, which is characterized by the demonstration of two or more distinct IgG bands in the gamma region of the electrophoresis, is found in 85 to 95 percent of clinically definite MS (Paty and Ebers). Oligoclonal bands are not specific for MS but can be detected in patients with acute and chronic infections, such as meningitis and encephalitis, and also chronic neuropathies, sarcoidosis, and so on. The myelin basic protein content and antibodies to myelin basic protein are nonspecific diagnostic tests and have been used in some laboratories as an indication of active disease.

Magnetic resonance imaging is a very important test for detecting MS abnormalities and can demonstrate high-intensity periventricular lesions on T$_2$-weighted images of different sizes from a few millimeters to centimeters, and Gd-DTPA enhancement with inflammatory activity. MRI criteria that are highly indicative of MS as described by Rudick include the presence of more than four white matter lesions equal or larger than 3 mm or three lesions and one adjacent to the ventricles, lesions having a diameter of 6 mm or more, ovoid lesions bordering the ventricles, lesions involving the corpus callosum or brainstem, and ring-like enhancing lesions with Gd-DPTA.

Some basic laboratory tests, such as CBC, ESR, ANA, and B$_{12}$ are always obtained to rule out other pathology. In selective cases, specific laboratory screening tests are performed such as Lyme titer, HIV, HTLV-1, antineuronal antibodies, thyroid function tests, very-low-chain fatty acids, and so on. Evoked potentials (VER, BAER, SEPs) are still obtained in many laboratories.

Treatment

The treatment of MS is one of the most important issues in neurology and a fundamental oral board question. It can be easily classified into treatment of acute relapse and treatment of prevention of relapses and accumulation of deficits.

Treatment of Acute Relapse

A relapse is defined as the occurrence of a new neurological deficit or the exacerbation of a preexisting deficit of at least 24 hour's duration and not caused by other pathology. The use of intravenous steroids in acute relapse is particularly indicated in patients whose exacerbation creates a significant neurological impairment. Intravenous methyl prednisolone is administered over five days at a dose of 1000 mg/day, followed by a 12-day prednisone taper (60 mg/day for four days, 40 mg/day for four days, 20 mg/day for four days). Adverse effects of the chronic use of steroids are well known.

Prevention of Relapses

The prevention of relapses is based on the use of interferon-beta that includes three preparations interferon beta-1b (Betaseron) and two interferon beta-1a (Avonex and Rebif). Other prophylactic agents include glatiramer acetate (Copaxone) and mitoxantrone (Novantrone). Interferon beta-1b has demonstrated a reduction of 30 percent in clinical relapses and decreased MRI disease activity. The dose in 250 mcg injected subcutaneously every other day. Common adverse effects include flu-like symptoms (fever, myalgia, sweating and chills), headache, depression, injection site reactions, menstrual abnormalities, decreased white cell and platelet counts, and liver enzymes elevation.

Avonex has shown to reduce the frequency of the attacks and also has demonstrated a reduction of gadolinium GD enhancing lesions on MRI. The injection is given once a week intramuscularly in a dose of 30 mcg. Adverse effects are similar to Betaseron but skin reactions are not observed. Rebif is given three times a week subcutaneously at doses of 22 or 44 mcg. Side effects are comparable to those of Avonex.

Glatiramer acetate (Copaxone) has demonstrated a decrease in relapse rate of 29 percent. It is administered at a dose of 20 mg daily subcutaneously. Common side effects include injection site reactions, such as erythema and swelling, and systemic postinjection reactions, such as anxiety, palpitations, chest tightness, and shortness of breath, lasting less than one hour.

Mitoxantrone (Novantrone) has immunomodulating effects by suppressing humoral activity and acting on T and B cells (Arnason and Wojcik). It reduces the frequency of clinical relapses and the neurological disability in patients with secondary progressive, progressive relapsing, or worsening relapsing-remitting MS (Kaba). The dose has been established as 12mg/m^2 every 3 months. Adverse effects include nausea, hair loss, amenorrhea, and bone marrow suppression.

Optic Neuritis

Vignette

A 35-year-old social worker woke up with right retroorbital pain and blurry vision. The pain increased with eye movements, particularly in extreme of gaze. On examination visual acuity was 20/20 on the left and 20/80 on the right. Funduscopic and visual field tests were normal. Swinging flashlight test showed a 2+ Marcus Gunn pupil on the right. The rest of the neurological examination was unremarkable. A few days later, her vision seemed to worsen, especially after physical activity.

Summary A 35-year-old woman with right orbital pain, diminished vision worsened by exercise, and right afferent pupillary defect on examination.

Localization

Acute or subacute visual loss can be caused by optic neuritis, ischemic vascular disease, or increased intracranial pressure.

Optic neuritis is characterized by acute or subacute unilateral visual loss associated with pain that increases with eye movements and precedes the onset of visual symptoms. The visual impairment progresses rapidly over one to two weeks and then starts improving over the next month. The presence of a relative afferent pupillary defect (RADP), also termed a Marcus Gunn pupil, characterized by an abnormal response to light stimulation is commonly observed. Uthoff's phenomenon, characterized by worsening of vision with exercise, fatigue, stress, or increased body temperature can be noticed during the recovery stage of optic neuritis (Matthews). In the retrobulbar form of optic neuritis, funduscopic examination is normal or will show some pallor of the disk if prior episodes of demyelination have occurred. Visual function shows a generalized involvement of the visual field or a large central scotoma.

The vignette clearly describes a case of optic neuritis but other causes of unilateral visual loss need to be also considered in the differential diagnosis.

Optic neuritis is an inflammatory disorder of the optic nerve and represents the initial manifestation of multiple sclerosis in up to 20 percent of cases (Hogancamp and Noseworthy).

It is an important feature of Devic's disease characterized by bilateral optic nerve and spinal cord involvement, and clinically by sudden and complete visual loss first in one eye and then in the other, associated with paresthesias and weakness that progress to paraparesis and tetraparesis.

Infectious and inflammatory disorders can also be responsible for optic neuritis, particularly bacterial, viral, and parasitic infections. Syphilis, tuberculosis, toxoplasmosis, *Borrelia burgdorferi,* and viral encephalitides (measles, mumps, chickenpox, infectious mononucleosis, herpes zoster, CMV, HIV, HTLV-I) can be responsible for a clinical picture of optic neuritis. Immune-mediated inflammatory disorders include systemic lupus erythematosus, Sjögren's syndrome, Behçet's disease, and ulcerative colitis.

Differential Diagnosis

In the differential diagnosis of acute or subacute visual loss, several conditions need to be considered:

- Ischemic optic neuropathy.
- Compressive and infiltrative lesions.
- Hereditary optic atrophies.
- Toxic and metabolic disorders.

Ischemic optic neuropathy, which usually affects the prelaminar portion of the optic nerve, is called anterior ischemic optic neuropathy and can be arteritic and nonarteritic. The nonarteritic form, which affects older patients particularly with hypertension, diabetes, and arteriosclerosis, is characterized by painless visual loss, maximal at onset, altitudinal field defect, and swelling of the optic disk. The arteritic form occurs in the elderly and is characterized by headache and systemic symptoms, such as fatigue, myalgia, arthralgia, elevated sedimentation rate, and previous episodes of amaurosis fugax.

Infiltrative and compressive lesions involving the optic nerve or the orbit, pituitary gland, and parasellar structures, such as tumors (gliomas, meningiomas), infections, inflammatory processes, and thyroid ophthalmopathy, can be responsible the occurrence of progressive visual loss, usually in combination with other signs and symptoms, such as proptosis, ophthalmoparesis, and so on.

Hereditary optic neuropathies include Leber's optic neuropathy, which affects young individuals, particularly males, in the second and third decades of life and is characterized by maternal transmission and sudden, progressive, painless loss of central vision affecting first one eye and weeks to months later the other.

Optic neuropathies associated with nutritional deficiencies and toxic agents, such as B_1 and B_{12} deficiency, tobacco, alcohol, isoniazide, and ethambutol, usually manifest with a subacute, bilateral, central visual loss.

Diagnosis

Neurological and ophthalmological consultations, including visual field evaluation, are the first steps in the diagnostic workup. Blood tests, including cell count and differential, ESR chemistry panel, VDRL, Lyme titer, ANA, ACE, and so on, are usually obtained. A chest x-ray and CSF studies are important in selective cases to exclude CNS and systemic infections. MRI of the brain assumes a primary role in the diagnosis of multiple sclerosis and to exclude a compressive lesion.

Treatment

The optic neuritis treatment trial study group determined several guidelines for the management of acute optic neuritis. There is a consensus that in patients presenting with the typical manifestations of optic neuritis, such as subacute onset of painful unilateral visual loss that improves within four weeks, blood tests, CXR and CSF studies are of limited value. Oral prednisone is not recommended because according to the study it did not show any efficacy in improving visual outcome and caused an increased rate of new episodes of optic neuritis (Kaufmann). MRI of the brain needs to be considered, particularly as a predictor of MS development. Treatment with high doses of IV methylprednisolone has been recommended if the MRI study is highly suggestive of a demyelinating disorder consistent with multiple sclerosis or if a rapid recovery of vision is desired.

Syringomyelia and Syringobulbia

Vignette

A 22-year-old nurse's aide was in excellent health until six months ago when she fell on a wet floor in a supermarket, striking her head. Two days later she started complaining of vertigo, right hand numbness, and severe headache. She felt unsteady and had the impression that objects in her vision were jumping back and forth. After a prolonged coughing bout, she developed more vertigo, diplopia, and slurred speech. On neurological examination the aide was alert and cooperative. The right pupil was 2 mm and the left was 4 mm briskly reactive. A slight right ptosis was identified. She had marked rotatory nystagmus when looking down and the tongue deviated to the left. DTR were brisk in the lower extremities and could not be elicited in the upper extremities where fasciculations were noted. Pinprick sensation and temperature were decreased on both arms. Gait was mildly spastic. She had a stiff neck and the hairline was low.

Summary A 22-year-old woman with the following neurological symptoms that started after a fall:

- Vertigo.
- Right hand numbness.

- Headache.
- Unsteady gait.
- Jumpy vision.

After a bout of severe coughing (that implies the Valsalva's maneuver) the symptoms worsened, with

- Increased vertigo.
- Diplopia.
- Dysarthria.

The neurological examination shows

- Pupillary anisocoria with right ptosis.
- Tongue deviated to the left.
- Rotatory downbeat nystagmus.
- Areflexia of the upper extremities and fasciculations.
- Hyperreflexia of both lower extremities.
- Hypoesthesia to pain and temperature on both upper extremities.

Localization

Localization of the lesions causing the abnormalities described in the vignette include the brainstem and the cervical cord. The patient in the vignette has signs and symptoms significant for an intrinsic brainstem lesion, predominant on the left.

The description of jumpy objects in front of the patient's vision describes oscillopsia. Oscillopsia is defined as the false illusion of back and forth movements of the environment created by the repeated transit of images of stationary objects across the retina (Glaser). The onset of oscillopsia and vertigo suggests a brainstem problem (Barnett et al.).

Rotatory nystagmus may indicate a localization to the medullary area. Downbeat nystagmus in the primary position is characteristic of lesions in the medullary cervical area, such as syringobulbia, Chiari's malformation, basilar invagination, and so on (Adams and Victor).

The involvement of the hypoglossal nerve in the medulla is suggested by the ipsilateral tongue deviation to the left.

The signs suggesting a cervical localization can be summarized as follows:

- Right Horner's syndrome is indicated by pupillary anisocoria (right 2 mm, left 4 mm) and right ptosis. This is caused by involvement of the ciliospinal center of Budge with C8–T2 lesions.
- Areflexia and fasciculations of the upper extremities indicate segmental involvement of the anterior horn cells at the level of the lesion.
- Segmental dissociated anesthesia to pain and temperature at the level of upper extremities is caused by involvement of the decussating fibers of the spinothalamic tract.

- Hyperreflexia and spasticity of the lower extremities are due to corticospinal tract involvement.

Once the lesion is localized (in this case, the intrinsic brainstem and cervical cord area) then diagnosis and differential diagnosis need to be considered.

Differential Diagnosis

In the differential diagnosis, important consideration needs to be given to syringomyelia and syringobulbia that can be associated with malformations and developmental anomalies or can be secondary to other pathology such as tumors and trauma.

Intramedullary tumors present some diagnostic difficulty in the differentiation from a syringomyelic process because they can be associated with central cord cavitation. According to Foster, the highest percentage of cavitation occurring with tumors is in cases of von Hippel-Lindau disease or von Recklinghausen's disease.

Extramedullary neoplasms usually manifest with radicular pain, signs of spinal cord compression, and involvement of the dorsal column without sensory dissociation. The combination of upper and lower motor neuron signs and dissociated sensory loss are more suggestive of an intramedullary cord lesion.

Foramen magnum tumors need special consideration because of the difficulties in the differentiation from syringomyelia and syringobulbia.

Neurofibromas (schwannomas or neurilemmomas) and meningiomas are the most common types of tumors in this location (Adams and Victor).

Foramen magnum tumors can have a variety of symptoms that include neck and suboccipital pain and stiffness, progressive spastic weakness, hand atrophy, sensory changes, and, rarely, findings indicative of posterior column dysfunction or a syringomyelia-type of sensory dissociation. Lower cranial nerve palsies can occur as well as downbeat nystagmus, Horner's syndrome, and cerebellar ataxia.

Syringomyelia complicating spinal trauma usually manifests months or even longer after the initial injury and is a rare event.

Among the congenital anomalies, Chiari's malformation, characterized by caudal localization of the cerebellar tonsils below the foramen magnum, and other malformations can be associated with syringomyelia and syringobulbia, therefore creating diagnostic difficulties in separating the effects of the two disorders.

Chiari's malformation can present with signs of brainstem and cerebellar compression such as downbeat nystagmus, tongue atrophy, hoarse voice, dysarthria, ataxia, and symptoms and signs of hydrosyringomyelia.

Other malformations, such as basilar invagination of

the skull or basilar impression (platybasia), may simulate the symptoms of syringomyelia and may coexist with this process.

ALS is easily ruled out by the sensory loss described in the vignette.

Multiple sclerosis may mimic syringomyelia, but hyporeflexia and fasciculations are unlikely in MS.

The mention in the vignette of low hairline may suggest a developmental lesion at the craniovertebral junction.

Treatment

The treatment is based on the appropriate cause.

Transverse Myelitis

Vignette

A 42-year-old lawyer started complaining of numbness and tingling involving the bottom of her left foot one week ago. The tingling then traveled to her left leg and lower trunk. Two days later, she woke up feeling numbness in her right foot and had some difficulty judging bladder fullness. She had fallen twice after catching her toes on a curbstone and was complaining of mild chest pain. Her past medical history was unremarkable. She was recently on a week's vacation to Mexico where she experienced some mild diarrhea. On examination, her mental status and cranial nerves were normal. Abdominal reflexes were absent. Knee and ankle jerks were brisk and the left toe upgoing. There was decreased vibration of both great toes. Gait was spastic.

Summary   A 42-year-old woman with progressive numbness, unsteady gait, bladder dysfunction, chest pain, signs of bilateral upper motor neuron lesion with lower extremities hyperreflexia and left Babinski; hypoesthesia to vibration on both toes.

Localization

The vignette clearly localizes to the spinal cord. Involvement of the spinal cord is manifested with spastic weakness, paresthesias, numbness, and bladder dysfunction. Chest pain can occasionally be neurological in origin and can suggest disease of the corresponding level of the spinal cord, nerve root, or, rarely, peripheral nerve.

Differential Diagnosis

Among the diagnostic possibilities leading to progressive subacute myelopathy, which is the case described in the vignette, several categories of disorders, such as demyelinating, infectious, inflammatory, vascular, neoplastic, nutritional, hereditary, and degenerative need to be mentioned.

Subacute spinal cord dysfunction is often a manifestation of multiple sclerosis but other causes, such as structural and compressive disorders, need to be excluded, such as tumor, malformations, or herniated disks causing cord compression. A careful history is necessary, particularly when other clinical signs and symptoms of multiple sclerosis are not apparent.

Several infectious disorders are responsible for causing myelopathy, such as bacterial, viral, fungal and parasitic diseases. Spinal syphilis, tuberculous myelitis, Lyme disease, schistosomiasis, cryptococcosis, herpes infections, AIDS, and HTLV-I are just some of the many responsible agents.

Noninfectious inflammatory disorders, such as systemic lupus erythematosus, also need to be considered in the differential diagnosis because SLE is a well-known cause of transverse myelitis. Spinal cord symptoms may be steadily progressive, recurrent or, more commonly, rapid or sudden, with little tendency to remission (Matthews). In 40 percent of the patients, myelopathy precedes the diagnosis of SLE, but most cases have evidence of multiple organ system dysfunction at the time of presentation (Aminoff).

Other collagen vascular disorders, which can be easily ruled out, are Sjögren's syndrome, mixed connective tissue disease, and so on.

Vascular diseases of the spinal cord (ischemic or hemorrhagic) can present with spastic weakness and can be caused by thrombotic occlusion, trauma, vascular malformations, or coagulopathies. Ischemic disease of the spinal cord most commonly involves the territory of the anterior spinal artery and causes acute onset of weakness (instantaneously or over an hour or two and commonly more rapidly than the other myelopathies) (Adams and Victor). Spastic weakness, dissociate sensory loss with involvement of pain and temperature, and sparing of vibration and position sense below the level of the lesion, and sphincteric abnormalities are characteristic.

Vascular malformations of the spinal cord are another important consideration in the differential diagnosis.

Compressive myelopathies due to abscess or tumor (extramedullary or intramedullary) are also included in the differential diagnosis. Nutritional deficiencies, particularly vitamin B_{12} deficiency, can present as a myelopathy.

The hereditary forms that need attention are hereditary spastic paraplegia (easily excluded in this vignette because of the lack of suggestive family history) and the leukodystrophies (also excluded by the lack of other associated symptoms, such as a positive family history, a demyelinating neuropathy, prominent behavioral change or dementia or marked autonomic dysfunction).

References

Multiple Sclerosis/Transverse Myelitis

Adams, R.D. and Victor, M. Principles of Neurology, ed. 5. New York: McGraw-Hill, 1993.

Aminoff, M.J. Neurology and General Medicine. New York: Churchill Livingstone, 389–411, 1989.

Arnason, B.G.W. and Wojcik, W.J. Multiple sclerosis: An update. Progr. Neurol. Dec. 2000.

Burks, J.S. and Johnson, K.P. Multiple Sclerosis: Diagnosis, Medical Management and Rehabilitation. New York: Demos, 127–138, 2000.

Guttman, B.W. and Cohen, J.A. Emerging therapies for multiple sclerosis. Neurologist 2:342–55, 1996.

Kaba, S.E. Multiple sclerosis: A review of the disease and available treatments. CNS News Special Edition 5:96–101, 2003.

Lublin, F. Current topics in multiple sclerosis. American Academy of Neurology, 50th Annual Meeting, Minneapolis, April 25–May 2, 1998.

Matthews, W.B. (ed.). McAlpine's Multiple Sclerosis, ed. 2. New York: Churchill Livingstone, 1991.

Miller, A. Diagnosis of multiple sclerosis. Semin. Neurol. 18:309–316, 1998.

Munsat, T.L. Demyelinating and immune diseases. Continuum, Part A. 8–81, 1994.

Noseworthy, J.H. Multiple sclerosis clinical trials: Old and new challenges. Semin. Neurol. 18:377–388, 1998.

Paty, D.W. and Ebers, G.C. Multiple Sclerosis. Philadelphia: F.A. Davis, 1998.

Rudick, R.A. Multiple sclerosis and its masquerades. Diagnostic dilemmas: Making the diagnosis of multiple sclerosis. American Academy of Neurology, 52nd Annual Meeting, San Diego, 2000.

Tselis, A.C. and Lisak, R.P. Multiple sclerosis therapeutic update. Arch. Neurol. 56: 277–280, 1999.

Optic Neuritis

Glaser, J.S. Topical diagnosis: Prechiasmal visual pathways. In: Neuroophthalmology, ed. 2. Philadelphia: J.B. Lippincott, 83–170, 1990.

Hogancamp, W.E. and Noseworthy, J.H. Optic neuritis. In: Current Therapy in Neurologic Disease. ed. 5. St. Louis: Mosby, 170–175, 1997.

Kaufmann, D. The optic nerve. American Academy of Neurology, 52nd Annual Meeting, San Diego, 2000.

Litwak, A.B. Optic disk edema. In: Blaustein, B.H. Ocular Manifestations of Neurologic Disease. St. Louis: Mosby, 153–174, 1996.

Matthews, W.B. et al. McAlpine's Multiple Sclerosis, ed. 2. Edinburgh: Churchill Livingstone, 79–93, 1991.

Munsat, T.L. and Mancall, E.L. Demyelinating and immune diseases. Continuum, Part A. 77–82, 1994.

Paty, D.W. and Ebers, G.C. Multiple Sclerosis. Philadelphia: F.A. Davis, 229–256, 1998.

Purvin, V. Optic neuropathies for the neurologist. Semin. Neurol. 201:97–110, 2000.

Reder, A.T. Optic neuritis. Neurobase MedLink, Arbor, 1993–2000.

Sedwick, L.A. Optic neuritis. Neurol. Clin. 9:97–114, 1991.

Syringomyelia and Syringobulbia

Adams, R.D. and Victor, M. Principles of Neurology, ed. 5. New York: McGraw-Hill, 1993.

Barnett, H.J.M. et al. Syringomyelia. Philadelphia: W.B. Saunders, 1973.

Brazis, P.W. et al. Localization in Clinical Neurology, ed. 2. Boston: Little Brown, 1990.

Case records of the Massachusetts General Hospital. Case 3. N. Engl. J. Med. 316:150–157, 1987.

14
Neurological Complications of Systemic Disorders

Wegener's Granulomatosis

Vignette

A 56-year-old writer started complaining of frontal headache, depression, decreased hearing, and transient double vision. Her speech had become dysarthric and a right facial paralysis was noted. For the last three months she had experienced weight loss, fatigue, generalized malaise, recurrent bloody cough, and several episodes of rhinitis and epistaxis. On neurological examination, she exhibited a right third and sixth nerve palsy, right facial weakness, and a bilateral sensorineural hearing loss, worse on the right.

Summary A 56-year-old writer with history of headache, depression, hearing loss, and diplopia. Neurological examination shows a right third, sixth, seventh, and bilateral eighth nerve lesion. Systemic symptoms include weight loss, fatigue, generalized malaise, bloody cough, and epistaxis.

Localization

The neurological localization of multiple cranial nerve dysfunction in the patient presented in the vignette points to a process extrinsic to the brainstem. Lesions extrinsic to the brainstem tend to affect adjacent cranial nerves, which often occur in succession, and are painful, without crossed sensory and motor paralysis, which is usually typical of an intramedullary lesion (Adams and Victor).

Differential Diagnosis

Infectious, inflammatory, neoplastic, and vascular processes can be the causative factors.

Chronic meningoencephalopathies such as those due to pneumococcal, tubercular, cryptococcal, mycoplasmal,

and treponemal infections can cause multiple cranial neuropathies usually in combination with headache, altered mentation, seizures, meningeal signs, and so on.

Granulomatous disorders, such as sarcoidosis, may affect multiple cranial nerves, particularly the seventh, second, and eighth. Patients usually have a history of systemic sarcoidosis but if there is no known history the diagnosis can be challenging.

Inflammatory disorders (vasculitis), typically Wegener's granulomatosis, may manifest with involvement of multiple cranial nerves in combination with systemic symptoms. Neurologic involvement is attributed to contiguous extension of the granulomas and to systemic vasculitis. Contiguous extension of the granulomas is responsible for cranial neuropathies in the middle and posterior fossa. Wegener's granulomatosis preferentially involves the optic, abducens, and facial nerves (Swanson). Sensorineural hearing loss can also be present due to cochlear involvement and in combination with a conductive component (Swanson). Systemic symptoms of Wegener's granulomatosis include sinusitis, fever, headache, fatigue, generalized malaise, joint pain, rhinitis, cough, and hemoptysis (Burnett). Pulmonary and renal complications are also common.

Primary and metastatic tumors at the base of the skull can be responsible for multiple cranial neuropathies. They include, for example, nasopharyngeal tumors, lymphoma, leukemia, and breast carcinoma.

Meningeal carcinomatosis that complicates systemic cancer typically involves multiple cranial nerves, often bilaterally, but is also accompanied by headache and signs indicative of intracranial hypertension.

Clinical Manifestations

Wegener's granulomatosis is a systemic vasculitis that predominantly involves the pulmonary, upper respiratory, and renal systems. The neurological complications include, in particular, peripheral neuropathy, which is the most common neurological manifestation (Swanson), and cranial neuropathies. Mononeuritis multiplex is the most frequent pattern but a distal symmetrical sensorimotor peripheral neuropathy can also occur (Swanson).

Cranial neuropathy tends to preferentially affect the optic, abducens, and facial nerves unilaterally (Swanson). Conductive and sensorineural hearing loss have also been described, as well as headache, external ophthalmoplegia, myelopathy, and myopathy. Cerebrovascular accidents, ischemic and hemorrhagic seizures, and meningitis can also occur rarely.

Diagnosis

The diagnosis is based on laboratory studies that include

- Increased ESR and C-reactive protein.
- Neutrophilic leukocytosis.
- Normocytic and normochromic anemia.
- Increased blood urea, nitrogen, and creatinine.
- Presence of antibodies to proteinase 3 in greater than 90 percent of patients with active disease that are highly specific (Burnett).
- CSF examination is usually normal.

Neuroimaging studies, in particular MRI, may demonstrate aspecific white matter lesions and meningeal enhancement.

The prognosis is severe in untreated or ineffectively treated patients.

Treatment

The management is based on the use of oral cyclophosphamide (2 mg/kg/day) and oral prednisone (1 mg/kg/day).

Neurological Complications of Rheumatoid Arthritis

Vignette

A 62-year-old retired firefighter had a history of neck pain and occipital headache for one year. He also noted bilateral arm weakness and leg stiffness associated with numbness, and paresthesias of his hands and feet. Neurological examination showed 4/5 weakness of the upper extremities, hyperreflexia, and bilateral upgoing toes. There was decreased vibration in the upper and lower extremities. Gait was spastic. Past medical history was significant for diabetes and long-standing rheumatoid arthritis.

Summary A 62-year-old man with history of neck pain and occipital headache experiencing bilateral arm weakness and leg stiffness. The examination shows weakness of the upper extremities, hyperreflexia, Babinski's signs, spastic gait, and sensory loss. The past medical history is significant for diabetes and long-standing rheumatoid arthritis.

Localization and Differential Diagnosis

The localization is in the cervical spinal cord and is due to a process causing progressive cervical myelopathy.

The differential diagnosis of a progressive myelopathy includes several considerations and the causes have been described in a different section of this book. In the following list, a summarized differential diagnosis is provided:

Compressive and neoplastic disorders
- Cervical spondylosis or disk disease causing cord compression.
- Extramedullary and intramedullary tumors.
- Paraneoplastic syndromes.
- Epidural or paraspinal abscess, hematoma.

Degenerative disorders
- Progressive lateral sclerosis: ALS variant with only upper motor neuron signs.

Infectious/postinfectious disorders
- Viral (HIV, HSV, HTLV-I/II).
- Bacterial (syphilis, tuberculoma).
- Fungal (cryptococcoma, coccidiomycosis).

Inflammatory disorders
- Systemic lupus erythematosus.
- Sarcoidosis.
- Rheumatoid arthritis.

Demyelinating disorders
- Multiple sclerosis.
- Devic's syndrome.

Vascular disorders
- Spinal cord infarction.
- Arteriovenous malformations.

Nutritional/toxic
- B_{12} and folate deficiency.
- Lathyrism.
- Chronic cyanide intoxication.

In the clinical case presented, great consideration needs to be given to the possibility of compressive myelopathy, particularly because a well-recognized syndrome is cervical myelopathy associated with rheumatoid arthritis. Damage to the cervical spine in RA generally involves the atlantoaxial complex and the subaxial spine. Proliferation of synovial tissues damaging the bone, ligaments, and cartilage, is responsible for the occurrence of atlantoaxial subluxations (Barr). The occipitoatlantoaxial junction is particularly involved in the rheumatoid process. The three most common lesions that result in cervical instability are atlantoaxial subluxation, followed by basilar invagination, and subaxial subluxation, or a combination of these three conditions (Rawlins et al.). The initial manifestation is usually pain localized in the neck and occipital area, which is present in 40 to 80 percent of patients (Rawlins et al.).

Clinical Features

The patients may complain of numbness and paresthesias of the upper and lower extremities, generalized weakness, and gait disturbances. Signs of compressive myelopathy manifest with progressive spastic tetraparesis, hyperreflexia, bilateral upgoing toes and sphincteric dysfunction. Lhermitte's sign, characterized by a sensation of electric shock traveling down the spine and triggered by sudden neck movements, can be observed. Lower cranial nerve involvement with dysphagia and dysphonia can rarely occur, particularly with vertical subluxation.

Respiratory compromise can affect patients with severe medullary compression. Sudden death can complicate severe medullary compression and be preceded by premonitory signs, such as weakness in both hands, occipital headache, dysphagia, nausea, and incontinence (Bruyn).

Signs of vascular compromise such as vertebrobasilar insufficiency with vertigo, nausea, nystagmus, ataxia, drop attacks, and so on, or signs of anterior spinal artery ischemia with weakness, atrophy, and hyporeflexia have also been described.

Diagnosis

The diagnosis is based on the constellation of signs and symptoms, x-rays of the neck, and MRI studies. Anterior AAS is considered if the distance between the posterior-inferior aspect of the anterior arch of the atlas and the most anterior point of the odontoid process is >2.5mm in females, and >3.0 mm in males (Chang and Paget). A distance of 10 mm or more suggests that there is compression of the spinal cord (Bruyn and Markusse).

Treatment

The treatment is conservative if neurological deficits are not observed. Surgical intervention with posterior fusion by internal fixation of C1–2 for anterior AAS, occiput C2 for vertical subluxations, and posterior fusion of the involved cervical vertebrae for subaxial subluxations is indicated if the pain is refractory to treatment or if there are symptoms of progressive myelopathy (Chang and Paget).

Other Complications

Other neurologic complications of rheumatoid arthritis include

- Entrapment neuropathies, particularly carpal tunnel syndrome, ulnar neuropathy at the elbow, and tarsal tunnel syndrome.
- Peripheral neuropathies due to vasculitis that can present as distal sensory neuropathy, sensorimotor neuropathy, and mononeuritis multiplex.
- Myopathy caused by disuse atrophy secondary to pain from synovitis but also may be iatrogenic (Chang).
- Central nervous system involvement due to cerebral vasculitis (rarely observed).

Neurological Complications of Malabsorption

Vignette

A 22-year-old medical student started experiencing diarrhea, abdominal pain, and vomiting for the last two months, with a 20-pound weight loss. He had unremarkable past medical history and denied any recent traveling outside the country. Initial tests, including HIV and toxic screen, were negative. The mother had severe Crohn's disease. Neurological examination showed mild memory loss, some dysarthria, bilateral horizontal nystagmus, ataxia myoclonus, Babinski's signs, and loss of pain and temperature below the knees.

Summary A 22-year-old man experiencing abdominal symptoms with nausea, vomiting, pain, diarrhea, and weight loss for two months in association with neurological abnormalities.

Localization

The patient has neurological findings indicating involvement of multiple systems such as cerebellum, corticospinal tract, and peripheral nerves. The history is highly significant for a systemic disorder characterized by diarrhea, abdominal pain, vomiting, and weight loss, and the neurological symptoms seem to be related to complications of malabsorption.

Several intestinal disorders, hereditary or acquired, can be responsible for malabsorption, in particular, celiac disease, Whipple's disease, inflammatory bowel disease, infective gastroenteritis, amyloidosis, abetalipoproteinemia, disaccharidase deficiency, and so on. Neurological complications of malabsorption may cause a wide constellation of signs and symptoms with involvement of the central and peripheral nervous systems.

Wernicke's encephalopathy, due to thiamine deficiency that affects chronic alcoholics but also patients with severe vomiting and malabsorption due to gastrointestinal disturbances, is characterized by ophthalmoplegia, nystagmus, ataxia, and altered mentation with a global confusional state (Adams and Victor).

Vitamin E deficiency due to prolonged malabsorption can be associated with spinocerebellar degeneration, peripheral neuropathy, and retinitis pigmentosa. Vitamin B_{12} deficiency that occurs in pernicious anemia and affects patients with gastric and ileal resection and other disorders of malabsorption manifests with ataxia, hyperreflexia, proprioception loss, unsteady gait, and behavioral abnormalities.

Celiac disease, characterized by small bowel dysfunction and gluten intolerance, can be associated with neurological complications that include internuclear ophthalmoplegia, cerebellar ataxia, hyperreflexia, tremor, and cognitive impairment.

Inflammatory bowel disease can also have neurological complications, in particular, acute or chronic inflammatory demyelinating polyneuropathy, thromboembolic disease, myelopathy, and so on.

Whipple's disease is a rare disorder that affects multiple systems and considered to be caused by an infectious etiology. Extraneurological manifestations include abdominal pain, diarrhea, steatorrhea, joint pain, and lymphadenopathy. Neurological manifestations are the presenting symptoms in a minority of patients. The most common feature is dementia (Aminoff). Other symptoms include cerebellar ataxia, myoclonus, supranuclear ophthalmoplegia, seizures, and some unique features, such as oculomasticatory and oculofacial-skeletal myorhythmia. The diagnosis is based on biopsy of the jejunal mucosa that demonstrates macrophages filled with PAS-positive granules. CSF and brain parenchyma may also show PAS-positive hystiocytes. The treatment is based on the use of antibiotics and steroid medications.

Neuroleptic Malignant Syndrome

Vignette

A 25-year-old artist with history of bipolar disorder was admitted to the hospital after manifesting acute psychotic behavior. Ten days after being started on haloperidol, he was found febrile, rigid, and diaphoretic. On examination he was stuporous and had generalized hyperreflexia.

Summary A 25-year-old man treated with haloperidol for psychosis, who developed fever, rigidity, hyperreflexia, and stupor.

Localization and Differential Diagnosis

There should be no doubt that the patient in the vignette manifests signs and symptoms related to exposure to a dopamine receptor–blocking agent (haloperidol). This typically represents the neuroleptic malignant syndrome (NMS). The main features of NMS are elevated temperature, signs of extrapyramidal involvement, and autonomic instability (Addonizio and Susman).

Hyperthermia is an important feature of NMS and can reach dangerous levels. Rigidity also occurs in the majority of patients, often associated with tremor and dystonia. Autonomic instability, defined by Addonizio and Susman as the third cardinal feature, is characterized by hypertension or unstable blood presssure, tachycardia, diaphoresis, incontinence, profuse sweating and so on. Altered level of consciousness manifests with agitation, confusion, delirium, and obtundation.

Addonizio and Susman established a diagnosis of "definite" neuroleptic malignant syndrome if temperature was above 99° F, severe rigidity or tremor was present, and three of the following seven minor criteria also occurred:

- Tachycardia (above 100 beats per minute).
- Diaphoresis.
- Leukocytosis (above 10,800 cells/mm³).
- Increased level of creatinine phosphokinase.
- Hypertension.
- Changes in mental status with confusion.
- Incontinence.

Other disorders enter in the differential diagnosis of the patient described.

Malignant hyperthermia, characterized by severe rigidity, hyperpyrexia, tachycardia, rhabdomyolisis, and marked increases in CPK and myoglobin, occurs after anesthetic and not neuroleptic exposure.

Lethal catatonia is a rare disorder characterized by altered consciousness, rigidity, fever, and autonomic dysfunction, and may simulate neuroleptic malignant syndrome, sometimes creating some diagnostic difficulties, in particular because neuroleptic medications can also worsen the symptoms of lethal catatonia.

Heat stroke can also complicate treatment with neuroleptics manifests with fever, altered sensorium, confusion, tachycardia, excessive breathing, hypotension, and so on. In the majority of the patients, there is no sweating and muscles are flaccid rather than rigid.

Other disorders may mimic NMS, but are usually distinguished by clinical or laboratory parameters. They include infections of the central nervous system, acute dystonic reaction, tetanus, and so on.

Diagnosis

The clinical history of neuroleptic exposure is an important point of the diagnosis. Several tests, including complete blood count, chest x-ray, urinalysis, blood and urine cultures, and toxicology screen, should be performed to exclude any source of infection or toxic exposure. CSF studies are part of the workup, particularly if meningitis or encephalitis is suspected. In NMS, CPK is often markedly elevated and leukocytosis is usually observed.

Fatal complications are attributed to pneumonia or renal failure secondary to myoglobinuria (Friedman).

Treatment

Treatment is based on prompt diagnosis and discontinuation of the neuroleptics, pulmonary care, and vigorous hydration to prevent complications, such as rhabdomyolysis-induced renal failure. Amantadine, bromocriptine, levodopa, pancuronium, or dantrolene sodium, alone or in combination, have been used for treatment of rigidity with varying results.

Vitamin B$_{12}$ Deficiency

Vignette

A 62-year-old street vendor started complaining of numbness and paresthesias of his feet and unsteady gait over the course of one year. His balance seemed particularly poor when attempting to walk in the dark or across uneven ground. He had a history of Crohn's disease and had been anemic all his life. He was a resident of a shelter and had stopped using alcohol five years prior. On examination he was irritable and forgetful. There was markedly decreased vibration sense and proprioception in the toes and mild distal weakness. Diffuse hyperreflexia and absent ankle jerks were noted. Gait was moderately ataxic.

Summary A 62-year-old man with history of numbness, paresthesias, and unsteady gait. The neurological examination shows an irritable, forgetful man with sensory loss, mild distal weakness, and gait ataxia in combination with hyperreflexia and absent ankle reflexes.

Localization and Differential Diagnosis

The symptoms described in the vignette indicate involvement of the peripheral nerve (sensory loss to vibration and proprioception, sensory ataxia, absent ankle jerks) as well as involvement of the spinal cord (diffuse hyperreflexia). In addition, behavioral changes (irritability, forgetfulness) are described. Other important elements are the history of Crohn's disease, anemia, and previous use of alcohol.

The combination of symmetrical sensory loss and dis-

tal loss of reflexes with long tract motor signs indicates a syndrome of combined system degeneration with peripheral neuropathy. Subacute combined degeneration is usually due to vitamin B$_{12}$ deficiency.

Vitamin B$_{12}$ deficiency, characterized by distal paresthesias, sensory loss particularly to proprioception and vibration, hyperreflexia associated with absent ankle reflexes, and cognitive and behavioral abnormalities, can well explain the symptoms of the patient described in the vignette. In addition, the history of Crohn's disease that, as cause of malabsorption, can lead to vitamin B$_{12}$ deficiency, increases the possibility of this diagnosis.

In the differential diagnosis, other causes of combined system degeneration with neuropathy should be considered. These include infections such as HIV, HTLV-1 associated myelopathy, neurosyphilis, and so on, hereditary neurometabolic disorders (adrenomyeloneuropathy), paraneoplastic sensory neuronopathy, and so on.

Multiple sclerosis may simulate some of the manifestations of vitamin B$_{12}$ deficiency but the pattern of presentation is usually asymmetrical and there is never involvement of the peripheral nervous system.

Diabetes and toxic neuropathy, due to chronic alcohol abuse, are in the differential diagnosis of vitamin B$_{12}$ deficiency, but other characteristics, such as corticospinal tract abnormalities, mental or visual abnormalities, and laboratory investigations, help point to the most likely possibility.

Clinical Features

Vitamin B$_{12}$ deficiency, which is caused by lack of intrinsic factor in the parietal cells of the gastric mucosa (pernicious anemia) or by malabsorption from a variety of causes (Crohn's disease, Whipple's disease, tuberculosis, tropical sprue, surgical resection of the distal ileum, and so on) may present with hematological, neurological, psychiatric and gastrointestinal manifestations.

Neurological symptoms include numbness and paresthesias, sensory loss particularly to proprioception and vibration, ataxia, increased reflexes often with hyporeflexia or areflexia of the ankle jerk, and so on. Behavioral and cognitive dysfunction varies from depression, irritability, and memory impairment to dementia. Optic atrophy can occur but is rare.

The hematological manifestations are characterized by macrocytic anemia with hypersegmentation of neutrophil nuclei and megaloblastic changes in the bone marrow. Gastrointestinal symptoms consist of glossitis, gastritis, and so on.

Diagnosis

Electrophysiological studies demonstrate evidence of a predominantly sensorimotor axonal neuropathy. Cobalamine levels are decreased in the serum but it is important to obtain serum or urine levels of methylmalonic acid and total homocysteine that increase in patients with cobalamine deficiency.

Treatment

The treatment consists of intramusclular injections of cyanocobalamin.

Neurological Complications of Diabetes

Vignette

A 75-year-old man started complaining of numbness and tingling in the lower extremities and burning pain involving the bottom of the feet, particularly at night. He also started experiencing dizziness and lightheadness when suddenly standing from a lying position, impotence, and profuse sweating after eating. His medical history included hypertension and diabetes for over 10 years. He was recently diagnosed with lung cancer treated with chemotherapy. Neurological examination shows mild weakness of foot dorsiflexion and absent reflexes in the legs. Sensation was decreased to pain, temperature, and vibration, more than proprioception below the knees.

Summary A 75-year-old man experiencing paresthesias and pain in the lower extremities together with autonomic symptoms. The neurological examination shows evidence of mild distal weakness, sensory loss, and absent reflexes in the lower extremities. Medical history is significant for diabetes, hypertension, and lung cancer treated with chemotherapy.

Localization and Differential Diagnosis, and Diagnosis

The localization is the motor unit, in particular the peripheral nerve, with suggestion of a distal symmetrical sensorimotor neuropathy with autonomic symptoms.

Several neuropathies are associated with painful paresthesias. These include, in particular, idiopathic sensory polyneuropathy and neuropathy secondary to diabetes mellitus. In both conditions the pain is symmetrical and worse in the feet.

Idiopathic sensory neuropathy is a chronic disorder of unknown cause that affects individuals in the sixth or seventh decade of life and is characterized by painful dis-

tal paresthesias due to small-fiber involvement with slow, proximal progression.

Diabetic neuropathy can certainly explain the symptoms manifested by this patient, characterized by spontaneous burning pain in the feet, sensory loss to pain, temperature, and vibration, mild distal weakness, and lower extremity hyporeflexia. The history of long-standing diabetes also supports the diagnosis.

Other causes of painful neuropathy include vasculitic neuropathies characterized by painful dysesthesia and a pattern of multiple mononeuropathy that progresses in a stepwise distribution. Systemic symptoms of anorexia, fatigue, weight loss, and arthralgia are often accompanying signs.

Amyloidosis should be considered in patients presenting with symptoms of painful neuropathy and autonomic dysfunction but it is relatively rare. In amyloid neuropathy, sensory symptoms occur early and are characterized by distal dysesthesias. Patients describe the pain as lancinating, burning, excruciating, and so on.

Toxic agents and drugs (e.g., arsenic, thallium, taxol, thalidomide) can be associated with painful neuropathies and are related to the use of the offending agent.

Other causes of painful neuropathies include malnutrition, particularly due to chronic alcohol ingestion. HIV neuropathy can also be responsible for painful distal paresthesias. Genetic disorders include, for example, Fabry's disease, which is responsible for spontaneous attacks of distal limb pain.

In the clinical case described in the vignette, consideration must be given to the fact that the patient was recently diagnosed with lung cancer which may suggest the paraneoplastic neuropathies. The most common underlying neoplasm is small-cell cancer of the lungs. Patients may present with a predominant autonomic neuropathy, severe sensory neuronopathy, demyelinating polyradiculopathy, or vasculitic neuropathy (Mendell).

Diabetic Neuropathy

Diabetes can frequently be complicated by peripheral neuropathy that manifests with several distinct types. Among them, the most common presentation of diabetic neuropathy is the distal symmetrical sensory or sensorimotor polyneuropathy that particularly correlates with the duration of diabetes. Clinical features include progressive distal sensory loss, sometimes associated with painful paresthesia. The sensory loss spreads in a length-related pattern involving the legs and even the hands in a typical stocking/glove distribution. A mild distal weakness can accompany the sensory loss and deep tendon reflexes can be reduced or absent, particularly at the ankle. Signs of autonomic involvement include postural hypotension, resting tachycardia, impotence, bladder dysfunction with atony, and so on.

The pathological basis for this neuropathy is a distal axonopathy of dying-back type (Comi). Electrophysiological studies show evidence of a predominantly axonal neuropathy.

Diabetic autonomic polyneuropathy is characterized by severe autonomic dysfunction, usually in combination with the distal symmetrical peripheral neuropathy. A particularly disabling symptom is orthostatic hypotension. Other features include erectile dysfunction, diarrhea or constipation, incontinence, pupillary abnormalities, and so on.

Pseudotabetic diabetic neuropathy manifests with sensory ataxia, severe joint position, sense impairment, and autonomic manifestations.

Diabetic neuropathic cachexia is characterized by severe painful paresthesias associated with marked weight loss.

Diabetic focal and multifocal neuropathies affect cranial and peripheral nerves and can also present with the picture of mononeuritis multiplex. The third and sixth cranial nerves are most often affected in diabetes mellitus and there is typical pupillary sparing. In the extremities, median, ulnar, peroneal, and lateral femoral cutaneous nerves are particularly susceptible to compression.

Diabetic amyotrophy is characterized by low back pain and asymmetrical proximal weakness and atrophy and usually affects older patients often with poorly controlled diabetes.

Treatment

The treatment of diabetic neuropathy is based on glucose control and symptomatic management of pain and autonomic manifestations.

References

Wegener's Granulomatosis

Adams, R.D. and Victor, M. Principles of Neurology, ed. 5. New York: McGraw-Hill, 1170, 1993.

Aminoff, M.J. Neurology and general medicine. New York: Churchill Livingstone, 389–411, 1989.

Burnett, M.E. Wegener's granulomatosis. Neurobase MedLink, Arbor, 2000.

De Groot, K. et al. Standardized neurologic evaluations of 128 patients with Wegener granulomatosis. Arch. Neurol. 58: 1215–1221, 2001.

Jain, K.K. Multiple cranial neuropathies. Neurobase MedLink, Arbor, 1993–2000.

Moore, P.M. Inflammatory diseases. In: Feldman, E. (ed.). Current Diagnosis in Neurology. St. Louis: Mosby, 194–197, 1994.

Swanson, J.W. Neurological disorders in Wegener's granulomatosis. In: Aminoff, M.J. and Goetz, C.G. (eds.). Handbook of clinical neurology. Vol. 27: Systemic diseases, Part II. New York: Elsevier, 173–189, 1998.

Rheumatoid Arthritis

Barr, W.G. Neurologic complications of rheumatoid arthritis: Identifying clinical features of nerve involvement. Advan. Immunother. Dec. 2000.

Bruyn, G.AW. and Markusse, H.M. Nervous system involvement in rheumatoid arthritis. In: Aminoff, M.J. and Goetz, C.G. (eds.). Handbook of Clinical Neurology. Vol. 27: Systemic diseases, Part III. New York: Elsevier, 15–33, 1998.

Chang, D.J. and Paget, S.A. Neurologic Complications of rheumatoid arthritis. In: Rheum. Dis. Clin. North Am. 19: 955–973, 1993.

Nakano, K.K. et al. The cervical myelopathy associated with reumatoid arthritis: Analysis of 32 patients with 2 postmortem cases. Ann. Neurol. 3:144–151, 1978.

Paget, S.A. and Erkan, D. Case studies: Neurologic complications of rheumatoid arthritis. Advan. Immunother. Dec. 2000.

Rawlins, B.A. et al. Rheumatoid arthritis of the cervical spine. Rheum. Dis. Clin. North Am. 24:55–65, 1998.

Neurological Complications of Malabsorption

Abarbanel, J.M. and Osimani, A. Neurological manifestations of malabsorption. In: Aminoff, M.J. and Goetz, C.G. (eds.). Handbook of Clinical Neurology. Vol. 26: Systemic Diseases, Part II. New York: Elsevier, 224–238, 1998.

Adams, R.D. and Victor, M. Principles of Neurology, ed. 5. New York: McGraw-Hill, 1993.

Aminoff, M.J. Neurology and General Medicine, New York: Churchill Livingstone, 1989.

Arce, E.A. and Paulson, G.W. Blepharospasm and vertical ophthalmoparesis as presenting symptoms in Whipple's disease: Report of a case. Neurologist 5:33–36, 1999.

Carpenter, D. Whipple's disease. Semin. Neurol. 5:4 275–277, 1985.

Louis, E.D., et al. Diagnostic guidelines in central nervous system Whipple's disease. Ann. Neurol. 40:561–568, 1996.

Perkin, G.D. and Murray-Lyon, I. Neurology and the gastrointestinal system. J. Neurol. Neurosurg. Psychiatry 65:291–300, 1998.

Neuroleptic Malignant Syndrome

Addonizio, G. and Susman, V.L. Neuroleptic Malignant Syndrome: A Clinical Approach. St. Louis: Mosby, 1991.

Aminoff, M.J. Neurology and General Medicine. New York: Churchill Livingstone, 513–514, 1989.

Friedman, J.H. Neuroleptic malignant syndrome and other neuroleptic toxicities. In: Feldman, E. Current Diagnosis in Neurology. St. Louis: Mosby. 382–384, 1994.

Friedman, J.H. Neuroleptic malignant syndrome. Neurobase MedLink, Arbor, 1993–2000.

Vitamin B$_{12}$ Deficiency

Bosque, P.J. Vitamin B$_{12}$ deficiency. Neurobase MedLink, Arbor, 1993–2000.

Cole, M. Neurological manifestations of vitamin B$_{12}$ deficiency. In: Handbook of Clinical Neurology. Vol. 26: Systemic Disease, Part II. New York: Elsevier, 367–405, 1998.

Feldmann, E. Current Diagnosis in Neurology. St. Louis: Mosby, 202–205, 1994.

Johnson, R.T. and Griffin J.W. Current Therapy in Neurologic Disease, ed. 5. St. Louis: Mosby, 356–358, 1997.

Mendell, J.R. Peripheral neuropathy. Continuum, Part A 1:56–59, 1994.

Mendell, R.J. et al. Diagnosis and Management of Peripheral Nerve Disorders. New York: Oxford University Press, 532–538, 2001.

Neurological Complications of Diabetes

Bird, S.J. and Brown, M.J. The clinical spectrum of diabetic neuropathy. Semin. Neurol. 16:115–122, 1996.

Comi, G. and Thomas, P.K. Neurological Complications of Diabetes. Clin. Neurosci. 4:341–345, 1997.

Dumitru, D. et al. Electrodiagnostic Medicine, ed. 2. Philadelphia: Hanley & Belfus, 2002.

Mendell, J.R. et al. Peripheral neuropathies. Continuum, Part A, 1:68–74, 1994.

Mendell, J.R. et al. Diagnosis and Management of Peripheral Nerve Disorders. New York: Oxford University Press, 373–399, 2001.

15
Toxic and Metabolic Disorders

Wernicke-Korsakoff Syndrome

Vignette

A 68-year-old man was found by the police wandering at the airport confused, disheveled, and actively confabulating. In the emergency room, he seemed malnourished and had low-grade fever. He knew his name, but could not tell the date or place. He could not remember three items after five minutes. He did not recall his birthday or his mother's name. He identified the patient in the next bed as his father and seemed to recognize people whom he never saw before. On examination, he had normally reactive pupils. On attempted lateral gaze to each side, the adducting eye moved only a few degrees medial to the midline. There was a coarse nystagmus of the abducting eye. Motor and sensory examinations were normal. Ankle jerks were absent bilaterally. Gait was wide-based ataxic.

Summary A 68-year-old man disoriented, confused, hallucinating, with both anterograde and retrograde amnesia, bilateral internuclear ophthalmoplegia, absent ankle jerks, and ataxic gait.

Localization

Confusion is attributed to bilateral cerebral dysfunction. The amnestic disorder may localize to lesions affecting the diencephalon and mesencephalon, particularly the medial dorsal nucleus of the thalamus and the hippocampal formation (Adams and Victor).

Differential Diagnosis

The first consideration among the clinical features described in the vignette is the severe amnestic syndrome with confabulations. The differential diagnosis includes several categories, but the patient found confused with severe memory loss and typical neurological findings could represent a clear example of the Wernicke-Korsakoff syndrome, which is due to thiamine deficiency. The causes include primarily chronic alcohol abuse but also severe vomiting, gastric and other malignancy, and chronic systemic disorders.

In the differential diagnosis of the case presented, consideration also needs to be given to other etiologies:

- Vascular disorders, such as bilateral posterior cerebral artery CVA that can manifest with severe amnesia, agitation, and delirium but also cortical blindness.
- Infections, such as herpes encephalitis, that cause acute mental status changes and hallucinations.
- Paraneoplastic limbic encephalitis.

Clinical Features

Wernicke's disease is characterized by typical neurological findings that include nystagmus, ophthalmoplegia, imbalanced gait with ataxia, and mental status changes. Korsakoff psychosis is defined by Adams and Victor as an abnormal mental state in which memory and learning are affected out of proportion to other cognitive functions in an otherwise alert and responsive patient.

Ocular abnormalities include nystagmus, which can be horizontal and vertical, and ophthalmoplegia that involves the abducens nerve with bilateral lateral rectus paralysis. Conjugate gaze paralysis, particularly horizontal, ptosis, and internuclear ophthalmoplegia are other ocular findings described in patients with Wernicke's syndrome.

Unsteady gait with ataxia of varying degree of severity is also commonly found, as well as signs of peripheral nerve dysfunction such as pain, paresthesias, and reflex and sensory loss.

Mental status changes present in Wernicke's encephalopathy include apathy, drowsiness, inattention, confusion, stupor, and so on. Korsakoff's amnestic syndrome that can represent the initial manifestation of WKS is characterized by prominent retrograde and anterograde amnesia (the latter more severe) which in some patients is associated with confabulations. The diagnosis of Korsakoff's amnestic state also includes other aspects of mental functions, such as an alert and responsive patient who is aware of his or her surroundigs and does not show an inappropriate social behavior (Adams and Victor).

The hallmarks of the disorder are

- Retrograde amnesia: Inability to recall events and other information that had been acquired over a period of many months or years before the onset of the illness.
- Anterograde amnesia: Inability to secure new information by learning or forming new memories.
- Confabulations: Falsifications of memory. Patients tend to fill in blanks in their memory with material that they fabricate.

Delirium Tremens

Vignette

A 55-year-old construction worker became confused two days after undergoing total right knee replacement. The neurology resident called by a concerned orthopedic attending noticed that the patient was agitated and uncooperative and he was pointing around the room as if he was seeing people or objects that were not present. He was tremulous and tachycardic. Otherwise the neurological examination was not focal.

Summary A 55-year-old man with changes in mental status two days after undergoing surgery for right knee replacement.

Differential Diagnosis, Diagnosis, and Treatment

Several syndromes can be associated with delirium and acute confusional state, particularly in hospitalized patients. These include systemic infections causing bacteremia, septicemia, and pneumonia, or infections localized to the central nervous system, such as meningitis, encephalitis, and so on.

Metabolic and endocrine abnormalities are an important consideration, in particular hypo/hyperosmolality, hypo/hypernatremia, hypercalcemia, hypoglycemia, hepatic and uremic encephalopathy, and so on.

Other etiologies include trauma, particularly complicated by subdural hematoma, intracranial hemorrhages, transient ischemic attacks, hypertensive encephalopathy,

multiple emboli, and drug and alcohol intoxication and withdrawal.

Considering the case presented in the vignette, acute confusion with tremulousness and visual hallucinations beginning two days after admission to the hospital is highly suspicious of delirium tremens. Delirium tremens manifests acutely several days after alcohol withdrawal. Typical symptoms include confusion, agitation, tremor, diaphoresis, insomnia, delusions, visual hallucinations, and marked sympathetic hyperactivity with hyperthermia, tachycardia, pupillary dilatation, tremor, nausea, vomiting, diarrhea, profuse sweating, and so on.

Associated electrolyte abnormalities, hyperthermia, and dehydration with circulatory collapse can be fatal (Miles and Diamond). In the majority of cases, the episode lasts less than 72 hours and resolves.

The treatment is based on the correction of fluid and electrolyte abnormalities. Withdrawal symptoms and agitation are treated with the use of benzodiazepines.

Toxemia of Pregnancy

Vignette

A 32-year-old female recent Pakistani immigrant started experiencing visual difficulties and became completely blind after a few hours. Her previous history was significant for 34 weeks of gestation and poor prenatal care. In the emergency room she appeared drowsy and was complaining of headache. Blood pressure was 150/100. Pupils were 3 mm and normally reactive. Funduscopic examination was normal, with spontaneous venous pulsation. She did not blink to threat. The rest of the neurological examination was normal.

Summary A 32-year-old woman 34 weeks pregnant, hypertensive, experiencing acute bilateral visual loss and drowsiness.

Localization

The localization points to a postchiasmatic lesion. The normal pupillary reactions and normal ophthalmoscopic findings are characteristic of cortical blindness.

Differential Diagnosis and Diagnosis

Several disorders can be associated with cortical blindness, such as vascular, infectious, toxic, metabolic, neurodegenerative, traumatic, and so on.

The patient described in the vignette is a pregnant woman with hypertension. This suggests the very important possibility of preeclampsia or eclampsia as a causative factor. Blindness can be a complication of severe preeclampsia and eclampsia and may last several days, rapidly resolving after delivery. The problem usually is caused by multiple microhemorrhages and microinfarcts occurring in the occipital lobe (Arias).

Cortical blindness can also be caused by vascular disorders involving the posterior circulation, in particular embolic or thrombotic occlusion of the posterior cerebral arteries or basilar artery.

Infectious processes include meningitis, encephalitis such as Creutzfeld-Jacob disease, AIDS, subacute sclerosing panencephalitis, and so on.

Metabolic and toxic causes include hypoglycemia, uremia, carbon monoxide poisoning, mercury, ethanol intoxication, and so on.

Degenerative causes of cortical blindness include metachromatic leukodystrophy, Leigh's disease, mitochondrial disorders, and so on.

Finally, a transitory form of cortical blindness may be the consequence of head trauma, particularly in children. Basilar migraine can also manifest with transitory cortical blindness.

Preeclampsia is characterized by hypertension, proteinuria, edema, and headache after 20 weeks of gestation. Eclampsia is characterized by the occurrence of generalized tonic-clonic seizures in women with preeclampsia. Eclampsia occurs antepartum in 46.3 percent, intrapartum in 16.4 percent, and postpartum in 37.3 percent of cases (Arias).

Visual hallucinations, usually streaks of light, often precede the onset of eclamptic convulsions (Donaldson in Devinsky et al.). Visual hallucinations and cortical blindness are due to involvement of the occipital area. Other neurological signs include hyperreflexia and occasionally clonus.

The management includes magnesium sulfate for seizure prevention, control of severe hypertension, and fluid restriction to prevent worsening of cerebral edema.

References

Wernicke-Korsakoff Syndrome

Adams, R.D. and Victor, M. Principles of Neurology, ed. 5. New York: McGraw-Hill, 851–858, 1993.

Case Records of the Massachusetts General Hospital. Case 33. N. Engl. J. Med. 503–508, 1986.

Miles, M.F. and Diamond, I. Neurological complications of alcoholism and alcohol abuse In: Aminoff, M.J. and Goetz, C.G. (Eds.). Handbook of Clinical Neurology, Vol. 26. New York: Elsevier, 339–365, 1998.

Victor, M. et al. The Wernicke-Korsakoff Syndrome. Philadelphia: F.A. Davis, 1989.

Delirium Tremens

Adams, R.D. and Victor, M. Principles of Neurology, ed. 5. New York: McGraw-Hill, 912–915, 1993.

Miles, M. and Diamond, I. Neurological complications of alcoholism and alcohol abuse. In: Handbook of Clinical Neurology, Vol. 26. New York: Elsevier, 340–345, 1998.

Tasman, A. et al. Psychiatry, Vol. 1. Philadelphia: W.B. Saunders, 917–921, 1997.

Toxemia of Pregnancy

Arias, F. Practical Guide to High-Risk Pregnancy and Delivery, ed. 2. St. Louis: Mosby, 183–210, 1992.

Cunningham, F.G. et al. Blindness associated with preeclampsia and eclampsia Am. J. Obstet. Gynecol. 172:1291–1298, 1995.

Devinsky, O. et al. Neurological Complications of Pregnancy. New York: Raven, 25–33, 1994.

Goodlin, R.C. et al. Cortical blindness as the initial symptom in severe preeclampsia. Am. J. Obstet. Gynecol. 147:841–842, 1983.

Hinchey, J. et al. A reversible posterior leukoencephalopathy syndrome. N. Engl. J. Med. 334:494–500, 1996.

Rowland, L. Merritt's Textbook of Neurology, ed. 8. Philadelphia: Lea and Febiger, 896–897, 1989.

16
Pediatric Epilepsy

Neonatal Seizures

Vignette

A 2-day-old baby girl, while being changed by her mother, became less responsive and started experiencing jerking movements of the left arm, followed by right leg jerking. When the nurse was called to the bedside she noticed that the right arm instead was jerking. The baby was the product of a full-term pregnancy of a 38-year-old mother. Labor lasted 48 hours and the baby was delivered by midforceps. There was no family history of neurological disorders.

Localization

Cortical: Is this episode a seizure?

Differential Diagnosis and Diagnosis

Seizures represent the most important manifestation of neurological dysfunction in the newborn. Neonatal convulsions usually present with a focal or multifocal pattern particularly compared to seizures of older children and adults (Rust and Volpe in Dodson and Pellock). Seizures in the newborn are less organized, therefore generalized tonic-clonic and absence seizures are not commonly encountered. The age-dependent clinical and EEG features in neonates are due to the immaturity of cortical organization and myelination (Holmes). It is not always an easy task to distinguish a possible seizure activity from other phenomena that can represent normal movements or behavior or from abnormal movements of different etiology. Abnormal paroxysmal recurrent behavior, motor or autonomic manifestations, should be considered a possible seizure.

Volpe classified neonatal seizures into subtle, clonic, tonic, and myoclonic, further classified as focal, multifocal, or generalized. Clonic seizures can be classified as focal or multifocal. Focal clonic seizures are characterized by rhythmic unilateral jerking movements involving the face or one limb that can spread to involve other body parts on the same side without affecting consciousness. Focal clonic seizures can be associated with an underlying structural abnormality such as a focal cerebrovascular lesion (ischemic or hemorrhagic) but may also accompany diffuse encephalopathies such as hypoxic-ischemic or metabolic (Rust and Volpe in Dodson and Pellock). The EEG findings may be consistent with focal ictal sharp wave discharges and interictal focal slowing or background attenuation.

Multifocal clonic seizures are manifested by jerking movements that shift randomly from one body part to another, ipsilaterally and contralaterally in a nonjacksonian pattern, and are often associated with metabolic causes of brain dysfunction such as hypocalcemia or with hypoxic-ischemic encephalopathy. Multifocal rhythmic discharges and interictal slowing can be observed on the EEG study.

Subtle seizures are described by Rust and Volpe as paroxysmal abnormal manifestations more often observed in premature babies that involve the motor or autonomic function or the behavior and that cannot be categorized as tonic, clonic, or myoclonic seizures. They are characterized by repetitive facial movements, such as sucking, chewing, drooling, eye blinking, fixation of gaze, eye deviation, and so on, or other motions of the extremities such as pedaling and boxing-like movements, and so on. These manifestations have not been consistently associated with EEG abnormalities, according to Mizrahi and Kellaway. Only tonic deviation of the eye has been consistently associated with seizure activity.

Tonic seizures can be classified as focal or generalized. Focal tonic seizures, often observed in hypoxic-ischemic encephalopathy, manifest with protracted flexion or extension of an extremity or of axial muscle groups and are usually associated with epileptiform discharge.

Generalized tonic seizures can simulate decerebrate or decorticate posturing with sustained hyperextension of the limbs or tonic flexion of the upper extremities with extension of the lower extremities (Rust and Volpe). They can be observed in premature neonates often in association with structural brain lesions such as intraventricular hemorrhage. Mizrahi and Kellaway proposed the possibility that they may consist of a brainstem release phenomenon partly because of the poor response to anticonvulsant medications.

Myoclonic seizures present with sudden brief rapid jerks of muscle groups. They can be distinguished into focal, multifocal, or generalized, and are associated with metabolic abnormalities, hypoxia, or structural brain lesions.

Apneic spells rarely represent seizure activity in the absence of other abnormal phenomena.

Etiology

Rust and Volpe differentiated between early- and late-onset convulsions based on the time of presentation during the first three days of life or after that period.

In terms of etiology, they considered the most common cause of early seizures that occur during the first 3 days being hypoxic-ischemic encephalopathy. Prenatal indicators may be represented by intrauterine growth retardation and decreased fetal movements. Postnatal signs consist of low Apgar scores, jitteriness, lethargy, obtundation, increased intracranial pressure, and so on. Metabolic causes such as hypoglycemia, hypocalcemia, hyponatremia, and hypernatremia can also be responsible for early neonatal seizures as well as drug withdrawal, particularly heroin, methadone, sedative-hypnotics, and alcohol.

Cerebrovascular lesions, such as infarction or hemorrhage (subarachnoid, subdural, intracerebral), congenital and postnatal brain infections, and so on, can also represent the pathology underlying early neonatal seizures.

After 72 hours, inborn errors of metabolism, especially aminoaciduria represent an important consideration (Fenichel).

Evaluating a neonate with seizures requires attentive documentation of the family and prenatal history, and a careful examination of the infant.

Laboratory investigations, particularly serum electrolytes, glucose, calcium, magnesium, and phosphorus, are important in order to rule out a metabolic dysfunction. EEG is valuable as a diagnostic instrument and also in term of prognosis. Holmes divides the ictal patterns into four basic types: focal ictal pattern with normal background activity, focal ictal pattern with abnormal background, focal monorhythmic periodic patterns of different frequencies, and multifocal ictal pattern. Neuroimaging (CT, MRI) studies are important for the detection of structural abnormalities, and lumbar puncture should be considered highly in order to rule out infections.

Further investigations may be needed in selected cases if the possibility of an inborn error of metabolism or a disorder of mitochondria or peroxisomes is suspected. These tests include serum amino acids, lactate, ammonia, very-long-chain fatty acids, and urine test for organic acid screen.

It is not an easy task to differentiate between epileptic and nonepileptic phenomena. Rust and Volpe mention several observations that can be made to facilitate the distinction, such as stimulus sensitivity of the nonepileptic behavior, its suppression or elimination by gentle passive restraint, and the absence of associated autonomic phenomena. Some of the neonatal movements and behaviors that need to be distinguished from seizures include

- Jitteriness or tremulousness characterized by rhythmic movements of flexion and extension may simulate clonic activity but the flexion-extension phases have the same amplitude and duration and can be precipitated by tactile, proprioceptive, or auditory stimuli. Jitteriness can be a benign phenomenon but can also be associated with hypoxic and metabolic encephalopathies, drug intoxication and withdrawal, and intracranial hemorrhage.
- Benign neonatal sleep myoclonus manifests with bilateral asymmetrical myoclonic jerks that occur during sleep and are not stimulus sensitive. Such movements stop when the infant is awakened. EEG shows normal activity.
- Other nonepileptic phenomena include nonspecific and random movements of the extremities, spontaneous sucking movements, head rolling, body rocking, and so on. Hyperreflexia has been defined as an exaggerated startle response to a sudden stimulus in otherwise healthy infants.

Treatment

The correction of a possible metabolic abnormality is an important part of the management. Phenobarbital and phenytoin are the first line treatment in neonatal seizure. The half-life of these drugs is prolonged in the neonate compared with the adult. Phenobarbital is recommended in an initial loading dose of 20 mg/kg, and a maintenance dose of 3 to 4 mg/kg/day. Serum levels between 16 and 40 mcg/ml are required to obtain a good therapeutic response. Phenytoin can be administered at a loading dose of 15 to 20 mg/kg. The duration of therapy is based on the risk of developing recurrent seizures (Volpe).

Infantile Spasms and Tuberous Sclerosis

Vignette

A 2-year-old girl was brought to your attention because of aggressive behavior, emotional lability, poor social interaction, hyperactivity, and generalized convulsions. At the age of 5 months she started experiencing unusual spells, during which time she would drop her head and raise her arms several times while awakening. During the examination she was uncooperative, not verbal and, did not follow commands. Cranial nerves, motor, and sensory examinations were normal. Gait revealed a clumsy child, but not clear ataxia. Several pale patches on the dorsum of her left hand and on her back were noted. Family history was unremarkable.

Summary A 2-year-old girl with behavioral and cognitive abnormalities and generalized convulsions. Past medical history includes unusual spells consisting of head dropping and arm elevation at 5 months. Cutaneous findings are described as pale patches on the dorsum of left hand and back.

Localization and Differential Diagnosis

The first concern is to determine whether the unusual spells of neck flexion and arm extension represent epileptic seizures or nonepileptic paroxysmal events.

Considering epileptic seizures or syndromes with onset occurring during the first year of life and presenting as brief flexor or extensor contraction of the muscles of the neck, trunk, or extremities, the differential diagnosis may initially include infantile spasms.

The vignette describes a child with clear developmental delay and behavioral disturbances in association with seizures and cutaneous manifestations (pale patches). The presence of pale patches or hypopigmented macules, particularly in combination with infantile spasm, may support a diagnosis of tuberous sclerosis (TS). Tuberous sclerosis is a hereditary neurocutaneous disorder transmitted with an autosomal dominant pattern and affecting multiple organs, resulting in a variety of clinical symptoms. Signs of neurological dysfunction include seizures, mental retardation, and behavioral abnormalities. Seizures are the most common presenting complaint in 84 percent of patients of all ages, and in more than 95 percent of all infants (Griesemer).

Infantile spasms are particularly common in the first year of life. Later on, most patients will experience other types of generalized convulsion or focal seizures.

Infantile Spasms

Spasms are characterized by clusters of sudden, briefly sustained movements (Dulac et al.). They can involve the flexor or the extensor muscles and affect the axial and/or appendicular musculature.

Motor spasms have been divided into flexor, extensor, and mixed-type based on the predominant feature. The mixed flexor-extensor is considered the most common type (Holmes) and is characterized by axial flexion and arm extension and abduction. Spasms may manifest with different intensity, from slight nodding movements to violent flexion of the axial musculature and the extremities, and usually follow a crescendo-decrescendo pattern. They commonly present in clusters, particularly when the infant awakens or is falling asleep, rarely occurring in isolation, and can be accompanied by autonomic phenomena, such as increased sweat, pupillary dilatation, alteration in respiration, and so on. Age of onset is in the first year of life, usually usually between 5 and 7 months of age.

The EEG is significantly abnormal and represents the most important confirmatory test for the diagnosis. Hypsarrhythmia has been defined as the interictal EEG pattern most commonly associated with infantile spasms, particularly during the early stages. It is represented by the appearance of a disorganized irregular and chaotic background pattern presenting with high-voltage slow waves and spikes occurring randomly, particularly during nonREM sleep, and with a posterior predominance. In REM sleep, the recording becomes less chaotic. The hypsarrhythmic pattern can be identified in the younger infant and tends to evolve over time to a more organized background. The most common ictal EEG pattern associated with infantile spasms is a generalized slow-wave transient, followed by an abrupt attenuation of background activity in all regions (Dulac et al.).

Infantile spasms can be idiopathic when no apparent cause can be discovered or symptomatic due to various prenatal, perinatal, or postnatal factors. Among the symptomatic group, tuberous sclerosis is an important consideration because it can initially present with infantile spasm. Other disorders that can manifest with infantile spasms include neurofibromatosis, agenesis of the corpus callosum, and metabolic diseases, such as aminoacidopathies, Krabbe's disease, neonatal adrenoleukodystrophy, maple syrup urine disease, and pyridoxine dependency. Postnatal causes comprise hypoxia, trauma, and infection. West's syndrome refers to the combination of infantile spasms, mental retardation, and significant EEG abnormalities.

Differential Diagnosis

Seizure disorders presenting during first year of life that need to be differentiated from infantile spasms particularly include

- Early onset Lennox-Gastaut syndrome.
- Benign myoclonic epilepsy.
- Severe myoclonic epilepsy.
- Early infantile epileptic encephalopathy.

Lennox-Gastaut syndrome typically presents between 3 and 6 years of age but cases manifesting at an earlier age of onset have also been described (Fejerman in Dulac et al.). Atonic seizures and atypical absence are characteristic of Lennox-Gastaut syndrome, but tonic seizures can create a diagnostic problem. The EEG findings of LGS, consisting of slow spike and wave discharges occurring at a frequency of approximately 1.5 to 2.5 Hz and superimposed on a slow background pattern, can also be less typical in early-onset cases and therefore create some confusion.

Benign myoclonic epilepsy occurs in children who are neurologically normal between 4 months and 2 years of age and is characterized by brief myoclonic jerks causing head dropping and outward movements of the arms with flexion of the legs. Ictal EEG recording shows a generalized 3-Hz spike and wave or polyspike and wave discharge, and the background EEG activity is usually normal.

Severe myoclonic epilepsy is characterized by onset during the first year of life with febrile clonic seizures and later generalized myoclonic seizures. Other features include a positive family history in many cases, progressive mental deterioration, and poor response to anticonvulsant treatment. EEG shows evidence of bilateral spike-wave and polyspike-wave discharges.

Early infantile epileptic encephalopathy presents early in life, during the first weeks, and is characterized by spasms involving the flexor or extensor muscles, intractable seizures, and marked neurological deterioration, and a possible association with West's syndrome. EEG recordings show a pattern of burst suppression.

Infantile spasms also need to be differentiated from paroxysmal phenomena that occur during the first year of life but are not epileptic. These may include

- Recurrent abdominal pain (colic).
- Benign sleep myoclonus presents with jerking movements of the limbs that occur during sleep and are associated with a normal EEG.
- Startle disease (also called hyperreflexia) is an autosomal dominant disorder manifesting during the first year of life of rare occurrence and characterized by episodes of stiffness, hypertonia, and jerking movements provoked by auditory or tactile stimuli. The interictal EEG remains normal and major and minor

forms of the disorder have been described based on the severity of the symptoms.

- Benign myoclonus of early infancy affects normal infants between 4 and 9 months of age with clusters of myoclonic or tonic contractions of the limbs or axial musculature. It may simulate infantile spasm but the neurological examination, EEG and developmental history are normal.
- Exaggerated Moro reflex and attacks of opisthotonos may also simulate infantile spasms but usually occur in patients with spastic tetraparesis from severe leukomalacia (Fejerman in Dulac et al.).
- Paroxysmal choreothetosis is a familial disorder characterized by attacks of dystonia or choreoathetosis induced by sudden movement or startle in older children usually, after the first year of life. EEG remains normal.

Treatment

The treatment of infantile spasms is based on the use of ACTH or prednisone that may result in marked improvement or discontinuation of the seizures and cessation of the hypsarrhythmic pattern (Dulac et al.). There is no consensus on which dose is more effective or how long the treatment should be continued. Some authors recommend a dose of ACTH of 150 U/m^3 given intramuscularly for 4 weeks duration followed by progressive tapering off to a complete discontinuation or minimal effective dose. Other physicians prefer smaller doses due to the side effects of the medication, such as metabolic abnormalities, hypertension, cushingoid features, and so on.

Prednisone is suggested at a dose of 2 to 3 mg/kg/day orally for 2 to 6 weeks followed by progressive tapering. Vigabatrin is now regarded by many specialists as the drug of choice for infantile spasms, particularly in patients carrying the diagnosis of tuberous sclerosis. Infants with spasms may need up to 150 mg/kg/day (Brodie and Schachter). Adverse effects include drowsiness, agitation, hyperactivity, facial edema, and visual field dysfunction with constriction.

Other treatments include high-dose pyridoxine (100 to 300 mg/kg/day) that has shown some benefits in selected cases (Dulac et al.).

Epilepsy surgery can be utilized in selected cases with medically refractory seizures when a focal lesion can be identified.

The prognosis of children with infantile spasms remains unfavorable, particularly in cases where a degenerative brain process is present. More than half of children diagnosed with infantile spasms will develop other types of seizures, such as Lennox-Gastaut syndrome (Dulac et al.).

Tuberous Sclerosis

Tuberous sclerosis is a hereditary autosomal dominant neurocutaneous disorder linked to chromosomes 9q34 and 16p13.3 (Griesemer). It is characterized by involvement of multiple organs, particularly the skin, brain, heart, and kidney. Neurological manifestations include particularly seizures, which are the most common symptom of the disease, and occur at any time after birth (Swaiman). Infantile spasms have been reported to be the presenting symptom in up to 69 percent of patients with TS (Curatolo in Dulac et al.) and usually manifest between 4 and 7 months of age. Later on, other seizure types occur, particularly in mentally retarded children, including focal and generalized tonic, clonic, myoclonic, and akinetic seizures. Recurrent seizures can be refractory to treatment and difficult to control.

Varying degrees of cognitive and behavior abnormalities can manifest, such as mild to severe mental retardation, hyperactivity, aggressiveness, autistic traits, and so on. According to Curatolo, infants with parietotemporal and frontal tumors more commonly manifest autistic features.

Intracranial tumors, such as giant cell astrocytoma, can also be discovered and cause hydrocephalus due to obstruction of the foramen of Monro and signs of increased intracranial pressure.

Neuropathological findings associated with tuberous sclerosis include primarily cortical tubers and subependymal nodules. Cortical tumors are characterized by areas of disorganized gliotic brain tissue located in the cerebral hemispheres. Subependymal nodules, defined as candle-dripping in appearance, are calcified lesions located in the ventricular wall.

Subependymal giant cell astrocytoma and disorders of myelination are also described.

The dermatological features of TS typically include ("adenoma sebaceum," which is usually recognized after the first year and manifests as a red papular rash that can present in patches or in a butterfly-shaped configuration on or around the nose, cheeks, chin, and malar regions. Areas of hypopigmentation (oval or leaf-shaped) over the trunk and limbs but also involving the scalp hair or eyelashes can be discovered early and be already apparent at birth. Ocular lesions such as hamartomas of the retina or the optic nerve are also part of the tuberous sclerosis complex. Cardiac lesions typically include rhabdomyomas that can be responsible for cardiac failure. Renal angiomyolipomas that can be multiple are another important feature of this disorder.

Diagnosis

Tuberous sclerosis should be highly considered in infants with developmental abnormalities and hypopigmented areas of the skin and should become the preferred diagnosis if infantile spasms occur in association with the skin lesions and intellectual impairment. Adenoma sebaceum in children tend to manifest on the face, typically in a butterfly distribution. Neuroimaging studies, particularly

computed tomography, can show multiple areas of calcification in the subependymal region. TS is considered an autosomal dominant disorder but spontaneous mutations also manifest without a prior family history.

Absence Seizures

Vignette

An 8-year-old girl was brought to your attention because of inattentiveness, poor concentration, poor school performance, daydreaming, clumsiness, and incoordination. Her teacher noticed that at times she would stop talking, become pale, and drop objects or stare at her hand. The perinatal, developmental, and medical history were unremarkable. The mother had a learning disability and depression. The father was a recovered alcoholic. Two siblings had learning disabilities and hyperactivity. The girl's general physical and neurological examination were normal.

Summary An 8-year-old girl with poor school performance and daydreaming, is noted to have episodes of pallor and to drop objects. Family history is significant for learning disability and alcohol abuse (father).

Localization, Differential Diagnosis and Diagnosis

In evaluating a young child presenting with poor school performance and episodes of daydreaming and unawareness of the surroundings, the consideration of a possible seizure disorder ranks high in the list of the causes.

The differential diagnosis of seizure disorder will particularly include absence and complex partial seizures. Nonepileptic manifestations that enter into consideration are daydreaming, hyperventilation, tics, and pseudoseizures.

The absence seizure is defined by Pearl and Holmes as sudden discontinuation of activity with loss of awareness, responsiveness, and memory, and an equally abrupt recovery (Pearl and Holmes in Dodson and Pellock). Typical attacks may be associated with other phenomena that can include motor behavioral and autonomic features. Particularly, sudden hypotonia can cause head nodding or dropping of objects. Autonomic phenomena may also occur and be responsible for sudden pallor and also increased heart rate, salivation, enlargement of the pupils, and so on.

Complex partial seizures, which are an important part of the differential diagnosis, can also present with decreased level of consciousness, staring spells, changes in muscle tone, automatic behavior, and autonomic phenomena. Complex partial seizures are usually more common than absence seizures, tend to have a longer duration and a less abrupt onset than absence seizures and may be preceded by an aura. If there is an aura and some degree of postictal impairment, such as drowsiness or confusion, the diagnosis points toward complex partial seizures (Pearl and Holmes).

Typical absence seizures are characterized by episodes of very short duration (5 to 15 seconds) without any postictal impairment, while complex partial seizures last more than one minute and may be followed by tiredness, fatigue, confusion, and so on. Occasionally, brief temporal lobe seizures may be clinically indistinguishable from more prolonged absences that show automatisms (Berkovic in Wyllie). In general, complex partial seizures originating in the temporal lobe last 1 to 2 minutes and rarely less than 30 seconds (Fenichel); and are accompanied by an aura, complex automatism, and postictal impairment. The EEG can clearly differentiate between these two types of seizures when positive.

Episodes of staring or daydreaming can sometimes simulate absence seizures and create some diagnostic difficulties. Daydreaming is characterized by vacant staring episodes that occur when the child is in a specific environment, such as a classroom setting, and can last longer than the typical absence seizures, which instead occur randomly and do not favor any specific environment. Absence seizures are usually of brief duration (5 to 15 seconds) and may occur during regular activities, such as when the child is talking, playing, and eating. They can be associated with postural changes and automatism, which are never observed during the daydreaming episodes. Daydreaming, as opposed to absence seizures, can be interrupted by a sudden stimulus.

Hyperventilation can simulate absence seizures but other symptoms usually occur, such as lightheadedness, breathing difficulties, numbness, paresthesias, and so on.

Tics can rarely be confused with absence seizures.

Finally, pseudoseizures need particular consideration and can manifest with abnormal behavior that can be repetitive and may indicate a need for seeking attention.

Absence Syndromes

A distinction between typical and atypical absence seizures needs to be made. Typical absence seizures that can be simple or complex when accompanied by other phenomena (motor, behavioral, and autonomic) are characterized by abrupt onset and cessation, brief impairment in consciousness without postictal confusion, and EEG findings consistent with generalized 3-Hz spike and wave discharges.

Atypical absence seizures can have longer duration and less sudden onset and cessation, and occur in children who are often retarded and exhibit other seizure types. EEG shows a generalized 1.5 to 2.5 slow spike and wave discharge, which can be irregular and more often asymmetrical.

Absence Seizures

Typical absence seizures manifest with brief episodes of impaired level of consciousness and unawareness that cause interruption of ongoing activities for several seconds and a blank facial expression (staring spell). Other phenomena may be associated, such as automatic behavior, change in muscle tone, clonic activity, and autonomic components.

According to Pearl and Holmes automatisms are the most common clinical accompaniment (Pearl and Holmes in Dodson and Pellock). Automatisms may consist of eyelid elevation and twitching, lip smacking, licking, swallowing, hand fiddling, and so on. Changes in muscle tone may manifest with head dropping or dropping objects from the hand due to hypotonia or to hypertonia of the flexor or extensor muscles. Clonic activity may consist of eye blinking or clonic contractions of the extremities. Autonomic phenomena consist of pallor, increased heart rate, salivation, and so on.

The typical EEG findings consist of generalized 3-Hz spike and wave discharges associated with normal background activity.

Epileptic syndromes with typical absence seizures include

1. Childhood absence epilepsy.
2. Juvenile absence epilepsy.
3. Juvenile myoclonic epilepsy.
4. Myoclonic absence epilepsy.

Childhood Absence Epilepsy

Childhood absence epilepsy (CAE) also called piknolepsy, which affects children between the ages of 3 and 8 years, preferentially girls, is characterized by a strong genetic predisposition. One third of patients have a family history of epilepsy and siblings of affected children have a 10 percent chance of experiencing seizures (Berkovic in Wyllie). Patients are neurologically intact.

The episodes are brief, lasting several seconds and tend to recur during the day and to abruptly terminate without any postictal impairment. Generalized tonic-clonic seizures can also occur but are infrequent.

The ictal EEG as we already described, shows generalized 3-Hz spike and slow wave complexes and the interictal pattern is normal or shows rhythmic posterior delta activity. Hyperventilation and photic stimulation can activate the discharge.

Therapeutical choices for absence seizures include

ethosuximide, valproate, and lamotrigine. The preferred drug for typical absence epilepsy when there is no history of other types of seizures, such as tonic-clonic, is ethosuximide, which is initially administered at a dose of 10 to 15 mg/kg/day and then maintained at 15 to 40 mg/kg/day once to three times a day in order to reach a target plasma level between 40 and 100 mcg/ml. Adverse effects are dose related and include gastrointestinal symptoms, such as nausea, vomiting, and decreased appetite. Headache, sedation, and behavioral dysfunction can also occur. Idiosyncratic side effects may be manifested with blood dyscrasia, lupus-like syndrome, and so on.

Valproate has been indicated in those children experiencing absence and generalized tonic-clonic seizures and can be used in combination with ethosuximide. The pediatric dose is 15 to 60 mg/kg/day two to four times a day with a lower dose at the beginning (15 to 20 mg/kg/day). The therapeutic plasma concentration ranges between 50 and 100 mcg/ml.

Adverse effects, which are dose related, include malaise, anorexia, GI symptoms, sedation, irritability, tremors, weight gain, and hair loss. Idiosyncratic effects include hepatic dysfunction, toxicity, thrombocytopenia, pancreatitis, and so on.

Lamotrigine has shown some efficacy in the management of absence seizures with a maintenance dose that ranges between 5 to 15 mg/kg/day starting at 0.6 mg/kg/day. If valproate is combined with lamotrigine the dose is reduced to 1 to 5 mg/kg/day with an initial dose of 0.1 to 0.2 mg/kg/day. Side effects include skin rash that can be severe and can occur more frequently in children, particularly when valproate is used in combination, nausea, drowsiness, and ataxia. Idiosyncratic reactions include severe skin rash, such as the Stevens-Johnson syndrome, and hepatic dysfunction.

Juvenile Absence Epilepsy

Juvenile absence epilepsy manifests around puberty, equally affecting both sexes, and is characterized by absence seizures and generalized tonic-clonic and myoclonic seizures, often experienced on awakening. The EEG pattern shows generalized spike and wave discharges, often faster than 3 Hz (4 to 5Hz).

Juvenile Myoclonic Epilepsy   (J m C)

Juvenile myoclonic epilepsy, also called impulsive petit mal, that manifests between 12 and 18 years of age is characterized by brief myoclonic jerks affecting preferentially the upper extremities that occur in the morning after the child awakens and can be precipitated by sleep deprivation, stress, fatigue, or alcohol. The myoclonic jerks may be subtle or severe and cause the dropping of objects from the hand or interfere with routine morning activities. Generalized tonic-clonic seizures can frequently occur, and absences are less common. EEG recording during the myoclonic seizures shows rapid 10- to 16-Hz spikes followed by irregular 1 to 3-Hz slow waves of varying amplitude.

Myoclonic Absence Epilepsy

Myoclonic absence epilepsy affects children between 2 and 12 years of age who are often mentally impaired and manifests with absence and bilateral myoclonic jerks involving muscles of the shoulders. The ictal EEG recording demonstrates generalized rhythmic 3-Hz spike or polyspike and slow wave discharges.

Febrile Seizures

Vignette

An 18-month-old girl was taken to the emergency room after a generalized tonic-clonic seizure. Her temperature was 103.5°F. Neurological examination was normal except for being postictal and lethargic. Developmental milestones were normal, and family history was unremarkable.

Summary An 18-month-old girl with history of one generalized tonic-clonic seizure associated with high temperature; normal developmental and family history.

Localization and Differential Diagnosis

The vignette describes a child experiencing a generalized tonic-clonic convulsion that manifested when she had high temperature. Several possibilities need to be considered in particular, if this represents a simple febrile seizure, which is a solitary, brief, isolated, and self-limited event triggered by the high temperature, or if instead there is an underlying brain infection, or if the generalized tonic-clonic convulsion indicates the onset of a seizure disorder triggered by the high temperature (Fenichel).

Febrile seizures that usually manifest in children between 6 months and 4 years of age are characterized by seizures that occur in association with fever, particularly early during the rise of the temperature, and represent the most common seizure disorder in young children (Nelson in Dodson and Pellock). In infants younger than 6 months, the possibility that the febrile seizure is associated with a brain infection needs to be cautiously investigated. A positive family history can often be found. The seizure usually manifests with a generalized tonic-clonic convulsion that tends to recur at the time of other febrile illness and is associated with common childhood infections involving the ear, or upper respiratory or gastrointestinal system. The risk of recurrence increases if the child is younger than 6 months at the time of the first febrile seizure.

Febrile seizures have been divided into simple and complex or complicated, based on the duration and associated symptoms. A simple febrile seizure is characterized by a convulsion of brief duration (less than 15 minutes), lack of focal neurological deficits, and manifesting in children who are neurologically normal. Complicated febrile seizures have a longer duration, can repeat during a 24-hour period, can be associated with focal deficits, and greatly increase the risk of further developing epilepsy. Other risk factors for a subsequent seizure disorder are neurological or developmental impairment prior to experiencing the first febrile seizure and parents or siblings with a seizure disorder.

Diagnosis

The evaluation of febrile seizures should include a careful history and neurological evaluation in order to recognize any possible focal neurological signs and also a cautious search for any source of fever and identification of brain infection suggestive of meningitis or of any electrolyte disturbance. Neuroimaging studies such as CT scanning or MRI need to be performed in children with focal neurological signs. A lumbar puncture should be promptly obtained when a meningitis is suspected by signs of meningeal irritation, lethargy, irritability, mental status changes, and bulging of the fontanelles. The decision to perform a lumbar puncture in patients who lack any signs of meningitis should otherwise be made by individual cases.

Treatment

The treatment of febrile seizures should be contemplated when:

- Febrile seizures are recurrent and prolonged (more than 15 min.) (complex).
- Focal neurological deficits are observed.
- Patients have an abnormal developmental or neurological status.

The medications include phenobarbital (15 to 30 mg/kg) or diazepam (0.33 mg/kg) every 8 hours. Adverse effects of phenobarbital include irritability, hyperactivity, sleep disturbances, rash, and so on. Diazepam can also be given rectally at the time of high temperature in susceptible children as a short-term prophylactic agent. Long-term treatment is based on the use of phenobarbital and valproic acid.

The prognosis remains favorable in most cases. It is important to clearly distinguish between febrile seizures, which are a benign entity, and epilepsy worsened by fever.

Juvenile Myoclonic Epilepsy

Vignette

A 15-year-old girl, while visiting her grandmother in Florida, experienced a generalized tonic-clonic seizure early in the morning. In the emergency room, except for a postictal lethargy, she was noted to be neurologically normal. CT scan of the brain and lumbar puncture ordered by a worried ER resident did not show any abnormality. There was no history of alcohol or drug abuse and all laboratory tests came back with normal values. Family history was negative. The mother noticed that the girl was at times very clumsy, especially in the morning, dropping objects or smearing her lipstick or toothpaste. She had noticed jerking movements of the head, neck, and upper arms that seem to occur only in the morning.

Summary A 15-year-old girl experiencing a generalized convulsion. The vignette also described jerking movements and clumsiness in the morning.

Localization, Differential Diagnosis, and Diagnosis

The description is of a generalized tonic-clonic seizure in a child with a history of previous myoclonic jerks particularly observed in the morning. The normal neurological examination represents an important point of the vignette.

Myoclonus is defined as a sudden brief, involuntary muscle contraction that can represent a seizure component or can be secondary to diffuse encephalopathy, such as metabolic, toxic, postanoxic, or viral, or can be a physiological response to startle or falling asleep. The vignette is a good representation of juvenile myoclonic epilepsy (JME).

Other conditions to be considered in the differential diagnosis are myoclonic absence and epilepsy with grand mal seizures on awakening.

Juvenile myoclonic epilepsy that accounts for 10 percent of all epilepsies (Serratosa and Delgado-Escueta in Wyllie) is a genetic disorder with an autosomal recessive trait characterized by myoclonic, tonic-clonic and absence seizures that occur particularly on awakening and involves patients between the ages of 12 to 18.

Myoclonic absence epilepsy is rare and manifests with absence and brief myoclonic jerks involving the upper extremities, particularly the proximal muscles, in children between the ages of 2 to 12 who are often mentally impaired and is also refractory to antiepileptic agents.

Epilepsy with grand mal seizures on awakening is characterized by generalized tonic-clonic seizures that occur particularly on awakening but without myoclonic seizures and affects the second decade of life.

The progressive myoclonic epilepsies can be easily excluded by the vignette. Their clinical manifestations include myoclonus; seizures, particularly generalized tonic-clonic but also clonic, myoclonic, and focal visual; progressive cerebral impairment; and cerebellar ataxia in combination with other signs of neurological dysfunction involving the pyramidal, extrapyramidal, visual, and sensory systems.

JME or "impulsive petit mal" (preferred diagnosis) is a genetic disorder linked to chromosome 6, which clinically manifests between ages 12 and 18 with various types of seizures, such as myoclonic, generalized tonic-clonic, and absence. Myoclonic jerks tend to involve preferentially the upper extremities and only occasionally the lower extremities and often interfere with the morning routine activities. They can occur as a single jerk or in clusters and have varying intensity, sometimes being so severe that they will cause objects to fall from the hand or cause the child to drop to the floor. Myoclonic jerks tend to manifest on awakening and are not associated with impairment of consciousness. The EEG recording is consistent with generalized 10- to 16-Hz polyspike discharges followed by slow waves. Generalized tonic-clonic seizures also can manifest after awakening and are triggered by sleep deprivation, alcohol, stress and fatigue. In JME, typical absence seizures can occur but are less frequent.

Treatment

The treatment of JME is based on the use of valproic acid, which usually provides good seizure control. Lamotrigine represents another therapeutic option.

Lennox-Gastaut Syndrome

Vignette

A 3-year-old boy started experiencing staring spells, neck stiffening, and head nodding episodes numerous times a day. He fell several times, injuring his face and head. His past medical history was significant for developmental delay, hyperactivity, and febrile convulsions treated with phenobarbital. An EEG obtained by his pediatrician showed diffuse slow spike and wave discharges. The neurological examination was significant for poor language skills with receptive and expressive dysfunction and a wide-based gait.

Localization and Diagnosis

The vignette describes a young patient with history of developmental delay and hyperactivity, experiencing a seizure disorder that started during early childhood. Several types of episodes ("seizures") are described: "neck stiffening," "head nodding," "staring spells," "falling." The EEG is also abnormal, showing diffuse slow spike and wave discharges. Neck stiffening can be part of a tonic seizure. Head nodding, head drops, and falling can be clinical manifestations of tonic, atonic, or myoclonic seizures. The vignette describes a patient with characteristic clinical and electrophysiological findings, which should bring into consideration atypical absence seizures and the Lennox-Gastaut syndrome.

The Lennox-Gastaut syndrome (LGS) is characterized by onset between 2 and 7 years of age, male predominance, a mixture of seizure types that are difficult to control, developmental delay, cognitive impairment, and typical EEG findings of slow spike and wave discharges superimposed on an abnormal background activity. Mental impairment and behavioral abnormalities are usually noted before the onset of the seizures but can also occur thereafter. Neurological symptoms may include hyperreflexia, hypotonia, and speech and coordination abnormalities. A prior history of West's syndrome is found in more than 30 percent of patients with LGS and symptomatic West's syndrome increases the risk of developing Lennox-Gastaut (Farrel in Wyllie).

Seizure types include tonic, atonic, myoclonic, generalized tonic-clonic, and atypical absence. Tonic seizures are particularly characteristic of LGS and also represent the most common type. They are usually brief and associated with altered consciousness, and can manifest with tonic contraction of the neck, face, and masticatory muscles, shoulder elevation, or increased tone in the upper and lower extremities, often provoking a sudden fall. Autonomic phenomena may be associated, such as facial flushing, salivation, tachycardia, pupillary dilatation, and respiratory dysfunction.

Myoclonic seizures manifest with brief recurrent twitches, particularly noted in the upper extremities but also involving face, trunk or lower limbs, that are not accompanied by altered consciousness. Atonic seizures may cause drop attacks due to loss of muscular tone or head and neck dropping. Generalized tonic-clonic seizures can also occur.

Atypical absence seizures, which are not characterized by the typical EEG recording of regular symmetrical 3-Hz spike and wave discharge but by an asymmetrical slow spike and wave pattern, usually last longer than the typical absences with gradual onset and termination, are not activated by hyperventilation or photic stimulation, and can be accompanied by myoclonic movements, automatisms, and autonomic phenomena.

TABLE 16.1. **Progressive Myoclonus Epilepsy**

Clinical manifestations are seizure disorder in association with myoclonus, progressive neurological deterioration, and ataxia.

Common PME	Clinical Features	Age at Onset (years)	EEG	Treatment
Unverricht-Lundborg disease (Bluntic)	Insidious onset; autosomal recessive inheritance; severe action myoclonus particularly on awakening associated with clonic or tonic-clonic seizures; ataxia and mild cognitive dysfunction.	9–13	Normal/slow background with paroxysmal activity consisting of brief generalized spike-wave discharges.	Valproate; clonazepam; phenobarbital.
Lafora body disease	Autosomal recessive inheritance disorder presenting with generalized tonic-clonic seizures; occipital seizures and severe myoclonus in association with progressive mental deterioration and neurological signs characterized by pyramidal signs, ataxia and involuntary movements. Typical inclusion bodies (Lafora bodies) are discovered in the sweat glands and liver and cerebral cortex.	6–19	Multifocal and generalized discharges and abnormal background.	Refractory to treatment.
Ceroid lipofuscinosis (Batten's diseases)	Late infantile form is characterized by generalized seizures and stimulus-sensitive myoclonus; ataxia; severe mental impairment; pyramidal and extrapyramidal involvement; and optic atrophy.	1–4	Focal and multifocal discharges and an abnormally slow interictal pattern.	Valproic acid, clonazepam.
	Juvenile form is characterized by visual loss due to retinitis pigmentosa; progressive mental deterioration; ataxia; pyramidal/extrapyramidal signs; acion myoclonus; and tonic-clonic and absence seizures.	4–14	Paroxysmal bursts of slow spike-wave discharges and abnormal background activity.	Valproic acid, benzodiazepines.
Mitochondrial encephalopathy with ragged red fibers	It is characterized by myoclonus generalized tonic-clonic seizures; progressive mental deterioration; ataxia; deafness; neuropathy; myopathy; pyramidal signs; and ragged red fibers on muscle biopsy.	5–12		Valproic acid, benzodiazepines, coenzyme Q.
Sialidosis	Type 1 due to deficiency of alpha-N-acetylneuraminidase; characterized by features of PME and includes severe stimulus-sensitive myoclonus; generalized tonic-clonic seizures; ataxia; cherry red spot on funduscopic examination; and a painful neuropathy.	8–15	Generalized spike-wave discharges.	Valproic acid, benzodiazepines.

The characteristic EEG findings of LGS are the slow 1.5 to 2.5 generalized spike and wave discharges predominantly in the frontal regions superimposed on an abnormal slow background activity.

Many etiologies have been identified in LGS, such as brain malformation and migration disorders, hypoxic-ischemic encephalopathy, brain infections, neurodegenerative disorders such as neuronal ceroid lipofuscinosis, tuberous sclerosis, neurofibromatosis, and so on. In primary cases, the etiological factor cannot be identified.

Neuroimaging studies and evaluation for metabolic diseases are an important part of the diagnostic workup.

The long-term prognosis of children with LGS is not favorable due to the difficulty to control the seizures and the association with cognitive impairment and developmental delay. Some factors may worsen the prognosis, such as younger children, a prior history of West's syndrome, recurrent intractable seizures, and frequent episodes of status epilepticus (De Vivo).

Differential Diagnosis

Lennox-Gastaut syndrome needs to be differentiated from the following conditions:

- Myoclonic astatic epilepsy of early childhood, which affects patients between the ages of 1 to 5 and has a strong familial predisposition. It is characterized by the presence of myoclonic-astatic seizures often in association with absence and generalized tonic-clonic seizures. Astatic seizures can manifest with head nodding or a sudden fall without loss of consciousness, often in association with myoclonic jerking movements that mainly involve the upper extremities and often precede the sudden loss of postural tone. Children can be neurologically normal at the onset of seizures or have signs of mental deterioration. The EEG shows a bilaterally synchronous 2- to 3-Hz slow spike waves discharge and a background exhibiting excessive abnormal theta activity.
- Primary generalized epilepsy such as childhood absence epilepsy can be differentiated by the clinical characteristics (described in this chapter) and typical EEG criteria.
- Electrical status epilepticus of sleep (ESES syndrome) manifests with persistent generalized slow spike wave-like discharges during non-REM sleep that disappear in waking state or REM sleep. Generalized and partial seizures occur during sleep. Atypical absences are observed during the day but tonic seizures are not experienced. Cognitive and behavioral abnormalities also frequently occur in these children, and seizures are self-limited and tend to disappear approaching puberty.
- Epilepsy with myoclonic absences, which has a mean age of onset of 7 years and affects preferentially males, is characterized by absence seizures associated with severe myoclonic jerks and tonic contractions. Children can be mentally impaired and the EEG recording shows generalized 3-Hz spike and wave discharges.
- Landau-Kleffner syndrome is a rare disorder of childhood characterized by acquired aphasia, epileptic partial and generalized seizures, and intellectual and behavioral deterioration. The EEG patterns are similar to LGS, but this disorder has a better long-term prognosis. The EEG shows paroxysmal discharges of slow spike wave activity activated during sleep and predominant over the temporal or temporo-parieto-occipital area.

Treatment

Lennox-Gastaut syndrome is often refractory to successful treatment. Valproic acid remains for most specialists the drug of choice but is often less than satisfactory and only partially effective. The risk of hepatotoxicity and liver failure are increased in younger children, particularly if the use of other anticonvulsant agents is required.

New antiepileptic drugs shown to have promising results in the treatment of LSG are lamotrigine, topiramate, and felbamate. Lamotrigine is well tolerated and should be started at a low dose (1 mg/kg/day) and increased slowly over two months, to the typical full dose of 5 to 10 mg/kg/day. If the child is also taking valproic acid, which interferes with lamotrigine, reducing the rate of metabolism and increasing the effective dose, lamotrigine should be started at 0.1 to 0.25 mg/kg/day and increased slowly over two months to 1 to 2 mg/kg/day. A rash can complicate the initial treatment and, in severe cases, bullous erythema multiforme, Steven-Johnson syndrome, and toxic epidermal necrolysis have been described. Common adverse effects include gastrointestinal symptoms, headache, tremor, and so on.

Topiramate also shows efficacy in the management of LGS. Starting dose is 1 mg/kg/day, increased over a few weeks to a full dose of 6 to 10 mg/kg/day. Adverse effects include sedation, fatigue, emotional lability, confusion, paresthesias, and so on.

Felbamate should not be used as a first line drug, but only after several medications have failed, due to the risk of aplastic anemia and liver failure.

Nonpharmacological treatment includes a ketogenic diet and surgical interventions such as corpus callostomy and vagal nerve stimulator. Corpus callostomy has been used to control drop attacks that may cause serious injuries to the child.

Benign Childhood Epilepsy with Centrotemporal Spikes

Vignette

An 8-year-old boy was found twice by his mother making a gurgling noise, unable to speak, and experiencing twitching of the right side of his face and drooling for two minutes while in bed at night. Immediately afterwards he was able to speak and interact normally. His past medical history was normal. There was no history of febrile seizures, head trauma, headaches, or behavior problems. Physical and neurological examinations were unremarkable.

Summary An 8-year-old previously healthy boy experiencing two brief episodes of right facial twitching, drooling, and inability to speak. Physical and neurological examinations are normal.

Localization and Differential Diagnosis

In order to localize and make a differential diagnosis, the category of the disorder must be determined. The two brief episodes in this healthy child may represent a paroxysmal event, typically a partial seizure. An important consideration is to differentiate benign partial epilepsy from epileptic seizures associated with diffuse cerebral dysfunction of different etiology or with an underlying structural process.

Among the benign partial seizure disorders, benign focal epilepsy of childhood with centrotemporal spikes should be considered first. It usually affects children between 3 and 13 years of age who have a normal developmental history and is characterized by focal seizures and EEG recording showing frequent centrotemporal spikes.

The seizures usually occur at night and are associated with somatosensory, motor, and autonomic phenomena involving the face, mouth, tongue and throat. These include paresthesias of the tongue, lips, or inner cheeks; motor manifestations that consist of tonic or tonic-clonic activity of one side of the face and, less commonly, arm and leg; guttural sounds; arrest of speech; and drooling from increased salivation. The seizures last 1 or 2 minutes and consciousness is not impaired. Nocturnal hemifacial convulsions can become secondarily generalized, particularly in younger children.

Affected children are otherwise healthy and do not manifest behavioral abnormalities.

EEG shows biphasic high-voltage central temporal spikes followed by slow waves and a normal background activity. Genetic predisposition is frequent and there is some male predominance.

Prognosis is excellent and seizures always cease spontaneously by the age of 16. Genetic predisposition with an autosomal dominant trait and low penetrance has been suggested. Drug therapy is only necessary in about 30 percent of patients (Fejerman and Engel). Children who only have isolated nocturnal seizures do not require treatment. If therapy is indicated, the drugs of choice are carbamazepine, divalproex sodium, and gabapentin.

Another benign childhood epilepsy with partial features is the benign occipital epilepsy of childhood, which manifests with seizures that consist of visual symptoms (e.g., simple or complex visual hallucinations, hemianopsia) followed by nonvisual signs, such as altered level of consciousness, with automatisms, clonic ot tonic-clonic seizures, and postictal headache in some children. Prognosis is good and EEG shows occipital epileptiform activity observed on eye closure.

Benign childhood epilepsy with centrotemporal spike need to be differentiated from mesial temporal lobe epilepsy, but clinical history and EEG studies help pinpoint the correct diagnosis.

Status Epilepticus

Vignette

A 2-year-old boy with prior history of seizure disorder and mild mental retardation, after becoming febrile, experienced a generalized tonic-clonic convulsion upon awakening, which did not stop. In the ER his temperature was 103.5°F and he was noted to have increased tone in all extremities and abnormal eye movements.

Summary A 2-year-old boy with prior history of seizure disorder and mental retardation experiencing high temperature and continuous epileptic seizure activity.

Localization, Differential Diagnosis, and Diagnosis

This child is considered as experiencing status epilepticus.

The definition of status epilepticus is based on certain parameters that include the duration of a seizure activity longer than 30 minutes or recurrent seizures without full recovery of consciousness between them (Pellock and Meyer). Status epilepticus can represent the exacerbation of a preexisting seizure disorder or can indicate an acute insult that primarily or secondarily involves the central nervous system. In children, the most common factors that can precipitate status epilepticus are intercurrent infectious processes localized to the central nervous system or due to a systemic involvement, and change, withdrawal, or noncompliance with anticonvulsant medications.

Also drug toxicity can precipitate status epilepticus. Other etiological factors include fever, trauma, systemic and metabolic disorders, electrolyte imbalance, hypoxia, sleep deprivation, and various toxins.

Systemic complications of generalized convulsive status epilepticus include metabolic complications, such as hypoxemia, lactic acidemia, hypoglycemia, hyperkalemia, and so on; cardiorespiratory complications, such as hypertension, arrhythmia, airway obstruction, and hypercapnia; and renal complications, such as myoglobinuria and acute renal insufficiency. Neurological complications include increased intracranial pressure and cerebral edema.

Generalized convulsive status epilepticus always constitutes an emergency.

Treatment

The treatment goals for status epilepticus include prompt stabilization of cardiac and respiratory functions, rapid termination of both clinical and electrical seizures, identification and treatment of precipitating factors (infection, fever, hypoglycemia, electrolyte imbalance, etc.), and prevention of systemic complications (Pellock and Meyer).

The recommended treatment sequence for status epilepticus from the Children's Hospital in Boston, Massachusetts includes the following interventions (Riviello):

- Incipient, early, and late stages have been determined as well as a refractory stage. The incipient stage (0 to 5 minutes) includes the ABC with airway, breathing, and circulatory support. The early stage (0 to 30 minutes) consists of prompt pharmacological intervention with the use of benzodiazepines (lorazepam 0.1 mg/kg that can be administered again after 10 minutes if the seizures persist). Then fosphenytoin (20 mg/kg of phenytoin equivalents) and/or phenobarbital (20 mg/kg in neoneates, 15 mg/kg in all others) must be given.
- In the late stage (30 to 60 minutes), when still there is no effective control of the seizures, an additional fosphenytoin infusion can be administered and if this measure fails, valproic acid (10 to 20 mg/kg) should be utilized.
- The refractory stage consists of intractable seizures over 60 minutes and is associated with the use of phenobarbital infusion (2 to 10 mg/kg) followed by 0.5 to 1 mg/kg/hr) or midazolam (0.2 mg/kg followed by 0.5 to 1 mg/kg/hr) or general anesthesia (isoflurane).

References

Neonatal Seizures

Berg, B.O. Principles of Child Neurology. New York: McGraw-Hill, 223–284, 1996.

Bergman, I. et al. Neonatal seizures. Semin. Perinatol. 6:54–67, 1982.

Curtis, P.D. et al. Neonatal seizures: The Dublin Collaborative Study. Arch. Dis. Child. 63:1065–1068, 1988.

Dodson, W.E. and Pellock, J.M. (eds.). Pediatric Epilepsy: Diagnosis and Therapy. New York: Demos, 107–128, 1993.

Fenichel, G. Neonatal Neurology, ed. 3. New York: Churchill Livingstone, 17–34, 1990.

Holmes, G.L. Diagnosis and Management of Seizures in Children. Philadelphia: W.B. Saunders, 237–259, 1987.

Mizrahi, E.M. and Kellaway, P. Characterizations and classification of neonatal seizures. Neurology 37:1837–1844, 1987.

Mizrahi, E.M. and Kellaway, P. Diagnosis and Management of Neonatal Seizures. New York: Lippincott Raven, 1998.

O'Donohoe, N.V. Epilepsies of Childhood, ed. 3. Boston: Butterworth-Heinemann, 18–33, 1994.

Pellock, J.M. and Myer, E.C. Neurologic Emergencies in Infancy and Childhood, ed. 2. Boston: Butterworth-Heinemann, 24–41, 1993.

Scher, M.S. Seizures in the newborn infant: Diagnosis, treatment and outcome. Clin. Perinatol. 24:735–771, 1997.

Volpe, J.J. Neonatal seizures: Current concepts and revised classification. Pediatrics 84:422–428, 1989.

Infantile Spasms and Tuberous Sclerosis

Berg, B.O Neurocutaneous syndromes: Phakomatoses and allied conditions. In: Swaiman, K.F. (Ed.). Pediatric Neurology: Principles and Practice, Vol. II. St. Louis: Mosby, 795–817, 1989.

Brett, E.M. Pediatric Neurology. New York: Churchill Livingstone, 571–576, 1991.

Brodie, M.J. and Schachter, S.C. Epilepsy, ed. 2. Oxford: Health Press, 2001.

Dodson, W.E. and Pellock, J.M. Pediatric Epilepsy: Diagnosis and Therapy. New York: Demos, 135–145, 1993.

Dulac, O. et al. Infantile spasms and West syndrome. Philadelphia: W.B. Saunders, 1994.

Fenichel, G.M. Clinical Pediatric Neurology, ed. 3. Philadelphia: W.B. Saunders, 138–139, 1997.

Griesemer, D.A. Subependymoma. Neurology MedLink, Arbor, 1993–2001.

Holmes, G.L. Epilepsy and other seizure disorders. In: Berg B.O. (Ed.). Principles of Child Neurology. New York: McGraw-Hill, 247–248, 1996.

Menkes, J.H and Sarnat, H.B. Neurocutaneous syndromes. In: Child Neurology, ed. 6. Philadelphia: Lippincott Williams & Wilkins, 865–872, 2000.

Monaghan, H.P. et al. Tuberous sclerosis complex in children Am. J. Dis. Child. 135:912–917, 1981.

Osborne, J.P. Diagnosis of tuberous sclerosis. Arch. Dis. Child. 63:1423–1425, 1988.

Swaiman, K.F. Pediatric Neurology: Principles and Practice. St. Louis: Mosby 800–804, 1989.

Rodriguez Gomez, M. Tuberous Sclerosis Complex, ed. 3. New York: Oxford University Press, 1999.

Wiss, K. Neurocutaneous disorders: Tuberous sclerosis, incontinentia pigmenti and hypomelanosis of. Ito. Semin. Neurol. 12:364–373, 1992.

Absence Seizures

Dodson, W.D. and Pellock, J.M. (Eds.). Pediatric Epilepsy: Diagnosis and Therapy. New York: Demos, 157–169, 1993.

Engel, J. Jr. and Pedley, T.A. (Eds.). Epilepsy: A Comprehensive Textbook. Philadelphia: Lippincott Raven, 2327–2346, 1997.

Fenichel, G.M. Clinical Pediatric Neurology, ed. 3. Philadelphia: W.B. Saunders, 26–30, 1997.

Menkes, J.H. and Sarnat, H.B. Paroxysmal Disorders. In: Child Neurology, ed. 6. Philadelphia: Lippincott Williams & Wilkins, 919–1026, 2000.

Murphy, J.V. (Ed.). Handbook of Pediatric Epilepsy. New York: Marcel Dekker, 69–75, 1992.

Riela, A.R. Pediatric Epilepsy Update. American Academy of Neurology, 52nd Annual Meeting, San Diego, 2000.

Wyllie, E. The Treatment of Epilepsy: Principles and Practice. Philadelphia: Lea and Febiger, 401–410, 547–570, 1993.

Wyllie, E. EEG in Pediatric Epilepsy Syndromes. American Academy of Neurology, 52nd Annual Meeting, San Diego, 2000.

Febrile Seizures

Brett, E.M. Paediatric Neurology, ed. 2. New York: Churchill Livingstone, 330–337, 1991.

Dodson, W.E and Pellock, J.M. Pediatric Epilepsy: Diagnosis and Therapy. New York: Demos, 129–133, 1991.

Fenichel, G.M. Clinical Pediatric Neurology, ed. 3. Philadelphia: W.B. Saunders, 18–19, 1997.

Ferry, P.C. and Banner, W. Jr. Seizure Disorders in Children. Philadelphia: J.B. Lippincott, 143–152, 1986.

Menkes, J.H. Textbook of Child Neurology, ed. 4. Philadelphia: Lea and Febiger, 653–655, 1990.

Niedermeyer, E. and Lopes de Silva, F. Electroencephalography, ed. 2. Baltimore-Munich: Urban and Schwarzenberg, 439–440, 1987.

Wyllie, E. The Treatment of Epilepsy. Philadelphia: Lea and Febiger, 647–653, 1993.

Juvenile Myoclonic Seizures

Dodson, W.E. and Pellock, J.M. Pediatric Epilepsy: Diagnosis and Therapy. New York: Demos, 171–181, 1993.

Fenichel, G.M. Clinical Pediatric Neurology, ed. 3. Philadelphia: W.B. Saunders, 28–31, 1997.

Schmitz, B. and Sander, T. (Eds.). Juvenile Myoclonic Epilepsy: The Janz Syndrome. Wrightson Biomedical, 2000.

Wyllie, E. The Treatment of Epilepsy: Principles and Practice. Philadelphia: Lea and Febiger, 552–583, 1993.

Lennox-Gastaut Syndrome

De Vivo, D.C. Pediatric neurology. Continuum 6:94–113, 2000.

Dodson, W.E. and Pellock, J.M. Pediatric Epilepsy: Diagnosis and Therapy. New York: Demos, 171–181, 1993.

Livingston J.H. The Lennox-Gastaut Syndrome. Dev. Med. Child Neurol. 30:536–549, 1988.

Niedermeyer, E. and Lopes de Silva, F. Electroencephalography, ed. 2. Baltimore-Munich: Urban and Schwarzenberg, 441–445, 1987.

Roger, J. et al. The Lennox-Gastaut syndrome. Cleve. Clin. J. Med. 56:172–180, 1989.

Shields, W.D. Trends in the treatment of Lennox-Gastaut syndrome. Seizure Disorder and Epilepsy 1:3–5, 1998

Wheless, J.W. and Constantinou, J.E.C. Lennox-Gastaut syndrome. Pediatr. Neurol. 17:203–11, 1997.

Wyllie, E. The Treatment of Epilepsy. Philadelphia: Lea and Febiger, 604–613, 1993.

Benign Childhood Epilepsy

Dodson, W.E. and Pellock, J.M. Pediatric Epilepsy: Diagnosis and Therapy. New York: Demos, 183–195, 1993.

Fejerman, N. and Engel, J. Benign childhood epilepsy with centrotemporal spikes. Neurobase MedLink, Arbor, 1993–2000.

Glauser, T.A. Benign epilepsy with centro-temporal spikes. Epilepsy: Case based self-study for practicing neurologists, 1998.

Legarda, S. et al. Benign Rolandic epilepsy: High central and low central subgroups. Epilepsia 35:1125–1129, 1994.

Pellock, J.M. Seizures and epilepsy in infancy and childhood. Neurol. clin. 11:755–775, 1993.

Status Epilepticus

Dodson, W.R. and Pellock, J.M. Pediatric Epilepsy: Diagnosis and Therapy. New York: Demos, 197–206, 1993.

Pellock, J.M. and Meyer, E.C. Neurologic emergencies. In: Infancy and Childhood, ed. 2. Boston: Butterworth-Heinemann, 167–178, 1993.

Riviello, J.J. Status epilepticus in the pediatric patient: Advanced studies in medicine, Vol. 1, No. 4, 135–140, May 2001, The Johns Hopkins University School of Medicine office of continuing medical education.

Rothner, A.D. Status epilepticus in children: Case studies. In: Luders, H.O. Epilepsy: Comprehensive Review and Case Discussion. London: Martin Dunitz, 334–343, 2001.

Wyllie, E. The treatment of epilepsy: Principles and Practice. Philadelphia: Lea and Febiger, 678–685, 1993.

17
Pediatric Brain Tumors

Brainstem Glioma

Vignette

A 7-old-girl, for the preceding six weeks, seemed irritable, depressed, and less interested in her usual school activities and dance classes. The teacher noticed that she was unsteady, at times staggering and falling, and that her speech was garbled. She had a few episodes of unexplained vomiting. On examination, gaze to the right was limited with incomplete abduction of the right eye. She blinked poorly on the right side and had a mild right facial weakness. Gag was decreased and the uvula pulled slightly to the left. There was a left pronator drift and increased reflexes compared with the right. Gait was wide-based, unsteady.

Summary A 7-year-old girl with personality changes associated with focal neurological signs.

Localization

The involvement of multiple cranial nerves and a crossed motor paralysis (cranial nerves on one side and long tract signs on the opposite side) are indicative of a lesion intrinsic to the brainstem. In this particular case, the lesion localizes to the right brainstem, with involvement of fifth, sixth, seventh, and tenth cranial nerve nuclei, long tract pyramidal system, and cerebellum or its peduncles.

Differential Diagnosis

The differential diagnosis includes tumors, infections, and vascular malformations. Considering tumors first, diffuse instrinsic brainstem gliomas typically present with cranial nerve involvement, ataxia, and long tract signs, and should rank high in the differential diagnosis of this child. The location of the tumor is responsible for the clinical manifestations. Other posterior fossa tumors, including cerebellar astrocytoma, medulloblastoma, and ependymoma, are usually characterized by early signs of increased intracranial pressure that manifest with headache, vomiting, visual dysfunction, and altered consciousness. Vomiting is one of the most constant signs of increased intracranial pressure in children (Maria and Menkes). It represents a nonlocalizing sign and can also occur in isolation, particularly in the morning.

Contrary to adult patients with increased intracranial pressure, in whom headache represents a typical and steady sign, this is a less constant feature in children with brain tumors. Headache in children can be transitory, tend to manifest in the morning, and can be localized in the frontal or occipital areas. Occipital headache, neck stiffness, and head tilt may indicate a posterior fossa mass. Altered vision can be due to papilledema or unilateral or bilateral paresis of the lateral rectus muscle. Altered consciousness can cause drowsiness, stupor, or coma.

The association of long tract signs with ataxia and cranial nerve dysfunction is usually suggestive of brainstem pathology, whereas scanning speech, dysmetria, and ataxia are more often indicative of a cerebellar process (Duchatelier and Wolf in Keating et al.).

Infectious processes, such as brainstem encephalitis, enter the differential diagnosis because they can cause ataxia and cranial nerve dysfunction. Other symptoms are usually present and help the diagnosis, including fever, altered level of consciousness, hallucinations, meningeal signs, headache, photophobia, seizures, and so on. Chronic fungal or tubercular meningitides involving the base of the brain may cause multiple cranial neuropathies and ataxia, but other important signs, such as headache, fever, mental status changes, signs of meningeal irritation, and seizures, may predominate.

Cerebral abscesses localized to the brainstem usually are characterized by a more acute symptomatology and can present with low-grade fever, altered mentation, headache, persistent vomiting, and focal neurological findings.

Vascular malformations of the posterior fossa can occasionally simulate a neoplasm, manifesting with insidious and progressive brainstem and cerebellar signs but are relatively rare in children.

Clinical Features

Tumors intrinsic to the brainstem represent 10 to 25 percent of all pediatric brain tumors, with diffuse intrinsic brainstem gliomas accounting for 60 to 80 percent of brainstem tumors (Blum and Goodrich Tait in Keating). Packer separates brainstem gliomas based on the location into three groups that can be overlapping and include diffuse pontine gliomas, which carry the worst prognosis; tectal lesions, which have a benign histology and manifest a slow clinical progression; and cervical medullary junction tumors, which have a low grade of malignancy, manifest an indolent course and are amenable to surgical treatment with possibility of good recovery.

Diffuse intrinsic brainstem gliomas, which almost always shows involvement of the pons and can extend rostrally to the midbrain and caudally to the medulla, preferentially affect the first decade of life, particularly children between 6 and 10 years of age. Diffuse pontomedullary brainstem gliomas classically present with the combination of cranial nerve palsies, ataxia, and long tract signs. The neurological manifestations are based on the localization of the mass.

Cranial neuropathies commonly include abducens and facial nerve paralysis that can be the initial symptom of a growing brainstem tumor and reflect the pontine location of the mass. The involvement of the ninth and tenth nerves is not usually an initial feature.

Signs of corticospinal tract dysfunction manifest with spastic weakness, hyperreflexia, and Babinski's signs. Ataxia, which is due to involvement of the cerebellum and its peduncles, represents another clinical sign of diffuse brainstem glioma and is responsible, together with the spastic paresis, for the gait disturbance.

Mental changes include memory dysfunction, apathy, and crying alternating with irritability, etc. (Strange and Wohlert). The reason for such personality changes is unclear but could be attributed to the interruption of thalamic projections (Packer).

Signs of increased intracranial pressure are usually a late manifestation, but vomiting unaccompanied by headache can occur at the time of the initial presentation and is caused by direct infiltration of the medullary vomiting center.

Diffuse brainstem gliomas tend to have an insidious onset and carry a very poor prognosis with few children surviving after 18 months (according to Packer less than 10 percent are alive and free of progressive disease 18 months after the diagnosis). In contrast, focal brainstem tumors are circumscribed masses and manifest few neu-

rological signs and slow progression. Focal intrinsic tumors localized in the upper midbrain and lower medulla are demarcated from the surrounding tissue and often carry a favorable prognosis.

Diagnosis

MRI of the brain remains the study of choice for the diagnosis of brainstem tumors. Characteristic feature of the neoplasm should be identified, such as location, degree of infiltration, enlargement and distortion of the brainstem, and associated cystic, hemorrhagic, or necrotic components. Malignant gliomas tend to show hypointensity on T_1- and hyperintensity on T_2-weighted images with varying degrees of contrast enhancement. Other features that can be demonstrated are distortion of the pons with exophytic growth, edema, mass effect, and presence of necrosis and hemorrhages. The fourth ventricle can be displaced posteriorly or assume a slit-like shape. With the advent of the neuroimaging studies, patients are usually diagnosed within two months.

Treatment

Brainstem gliomas are very difficult to treat due to their resistance to radiotherapy and poor response to chemotherapy. Radiation therapy remains the only treatment that is beneficial, at least transiently, in order to arrest the disease progression. Tumors that carry a more favorable prognosis, such as those that arise in the cervicomedullary junction, can be treated surgically with total or partial resection followed by radiothearpy or chemotherapy.

References

Brett, E.M. Paediatric Neurology, ed. 2. New York: Churchill Livingstone, 1991.

Cogen, P.H. and Nolan C.P. Intracranial and intraspinal tumors of children. In: Berg, B.O. (Ed.). Principles of Child Neurology. New York: McGraw-Hill, 731–748, 1996.

Keating, R.F. et al. Tumors of the Pediatric Central Nervous System. New York: Thieme, 206–220, 2001.

Littman, P. et al. Pediatric Brain Stem Gliomas. Cancer 45:2787–2792, 1980.

Maria, B.L and Menkes, J.H. Tumors of the Nervous System. In: Menkes, J.H. and Sarnat, H.B. (Eds.). Child Neurology, ed. 6. Philadelphia: Lippincott Williams & Wilkins, 787–858, 2000.

Maria, B.L. et al. Brainstem and other malignant gliomas: II. Possible mechanisms of brain infiltration by tumor cells. J. Child. Neurol. 8:292–305, 1993.

Munsat, T.L. Primary brain tumors in children and adolescents. Continuum, Part A 1:48–52, 1994.

Packer, R.J. Brainstem gliomas in childhood. Neurobase MedLink; Arbor, 2000.

Strange, P. and Wohlert, L. Primary brainstem tumors. Acta Neurochirurg. 62:219–232, 1982.

18
Pediatric Neuromuscular Disorders

Hypotonic Infant

Vignette

A 6-month-old girl was brought to your attention because of poor motor development. She was never able to roll over and had a very poor head control in a sitting position. She was the full-term product of an uncomplicated pregnancy, labor, and delivery. Two weeks after birth, she started having breathing difficulty as well as feeding and swallowing problems. On examination, she appeared bright and alert, with appropriate language and social development, and normal facial expression without dysmorphic features. Extraocular movements were intact. There was poor head control with hand traction, and poor trunk and limb control in ventral suspension. In the legs, she had total immobility. Small amount of movement was confined to the feet and marked proximal muscle weakness was noted. Deep tendon reflexes were absent, and the breathing was mainly diaphragmatic.

Summary A 6-month-old infant presenting with hypotonia, weakness, and respiratory problems, without apparent dysmorphic features and with normal extraocular muscles, appearing bright and alert.

> **Key word:** floppy infant.

Localization

The first issue is to determine whether the patient is weak or hypotonic, or both, because if not all hypotonic infants are weak, all weak infants are hypotonic. The patient in the vignette has clear evidence of weakness and hypotonia.

In order to localize, we need to determine if the problem is central (cerebral hypotonia), or if it involves the spinal cord or the motor unit (peripheral hypotonia). If indeed it is a neuromuscular problem, it is important to assess which part of the motor unit is affected—the anterior horn cell, the peripheral nerves, the neuromuscular junction, or the muscles.

In the vignette both hypotonia and weakness are described. It is also indicated that the problem was discovered shortly after birth (two weeks after birth she started having breathing and feeding difficulties).

Cerebral hypotonia can easily be excluded in this infant. Babies with cerebral hypotonia manifest signs of nervous system involvement other than those reflecting muscle function, such as lethargy, altered level of consciousness, poor response to visual or auditory stimuli, seizures, and so on (Dubowitz). Other factors suggestive of central hypotonia are the presence of dysmorphic features, particularly involving the face and scalp, and malformations of other organ systems such as heart and limb defects (Miller et al.).

Spinal cord injury as a cause of hypotonia is also easily clinically excluded in this infant who was the full-term product of uncomplicated pregnancy, labor and delivery. An injury to the spinal cord due to traction can occur during vaginal delivery, particularly when the baby presents in a breech position (according to Fenichel, 75 percent with breech presentation and 25 percent with cephalic presentation). Clinically, spinal cord lesions manifest with weakness and hypotonia in association with sensory-level and sphincteric abnormalities. Altered level of consciousness can also occur. Again, the vignette indicated normal labor and delivery without complications.

In this case—a baby who is mentally bright and alert, interacting well socially, without any dysmorphism, but severely weak and areflexic—a disorder of the motor unit should rank high on the list (Fenichel). The degree and distribution of weakness and associated features can also help to localize within the different parts of the motor unit. Important points in the vignette are normal cognition, normal extraocular muscles, marked proximal leg weakness, areflexia, and diaphragmatic breathing. Disorders of different parts of the motor unit are considered in the differential diagnosis.

Differential Diagnosis

Disorders of the anterior horn cells, particularly infantile spinal muscular atrophy (SMA), ranks high in the differential diagnosis of this infant. Infantile SMA1 (infantile onset spinal muscular atrophy, Werdnig-Hoffman disease) manifests at birth or during the first few months of life with severe weakness, particularly involving the proximal muscles, hypotonia, and areflexia. Sensation is normal and there is no sphincteric abnormality. Infants are bright, alert, and expressive, with a very floppy body.

A disorder of the peripheral nerves to be considered as part of the differential diagnosis because it can present during the neonatal period is congenital dismyelinating neuropathy. Peripheral neuropathies, including acute inflammatory demyelinating polyneuropathy (Guillain-Barré syndrome), are very rare in newborn babies. Cases of GBS occurring during the first few months of life have been described in few cases with severe hypotonia, ascending paralysis, areflexia, and feeding, respiratory, and autonomic compromise. An exception is congenital hypomyelinating neuropathy, which can present in the neonatal period with progressive weakness, hypotonia, atrophy, and areflexia, and can simulate the picture of acute infantile spinal muscular atrophy. Extraocular muscles are intact and feeding and respiratory problems can be fatal. Sural nerve biopsy demonstrates almost total absence of myelin formation. CSF studies show elevated proteins.

Disorders of the neuromuscular junction to be considered in the differential diagnosis of a hypotonic infant include congenital myasthenic syndromes, transient neonatal myasthenia gravis, and infantile botulism. Congenital myasthenic syndromes are rare disorders of the neuromuscular junction manifesting in the newborn period with weakness, hypotonia, fatigue during sucking, fluctuating ptosis, and weak cry, in babies who are seronegative.

Transient neonatal myasthenia gravis occurs in approximately 10 percent of infants whose mothers have myasthenia gravis (Dumitru et al.) and varies in severity of manifestations, which can include generalized weakness, hypotonia, weak cry, feeding and respiratory difficulties, facial weakness, and ptosis. Acetylcholine receptor antibodies are discovered in babies who have a seropositive mother and the disorder is self-limited with most patients being symptom-free within six weeks.

Infantile botulism usually manifests between 6 weeks and 6 months of age with neurological and nonneurological symptoms, the most constant of the latter ones being constipation. Neurological signs include a descending paralysis sometimes associated with hyporeflexia, weak cry, hypotonia, ophthalmoplegia, facial paralysis, pupillary dilatation, and so on.

In summary, neuromuscular junction disorders with their clinical characteristics seem less likely as a possible diagnosis in the vignette presented.

Finally, consideration is given to disorders of the muscle. Myopathies that enter the differential diagnosis of a hypotonic infant are the congenital myopathies, the infantile form of myotonic dystrophy, congenital muscular dystrophies, and acid maltase deficiency. Congenital myopathies can present at birth with weakness and hypotonia.

In particular, nemaline myopathy has a severe infantile form manifesting at birth with marked hypotonia and generalized weakness, including the respiratory muscles that often require ventilatory support. Dysmorphic features can be noted with long narrow face and deformity of the palate. This form has a poor prognosis, with death caused by respiratory failure and pneumonia. Muscle biopsy demonstrates the accumulation of intranuclear rods.

Congenital myotonic dystrophy, which affects infants born to mothers who have myotonic dystrophy, is manifested at birth with severe hypotonia, prominent weakness of proximal muscles, facial diplegia, sucking and feeding difficulties, and respiratory failure that can be fatal.

Congenital muscular dystrophies also manifest at birth with hypotonia in combination with generalized weakness, including the face, and sucking and respiratory difficulties, with varying degrees of severity. Other anomalies, such as ocular and brain malformations, can also occur in some of the congenital muscular dystrophies, such as hypoplasia of the optic nerve, microophthalmia, corneal opacity, pachygyria, polymicrogyria, vermis hypoplasia, and so on. Muscle biopsy demonstrates dystrophic changes.

The infantile form of acid maltase deficiency, which represents a severe metabolic myopathy due to deficiency of alpha-glucosidase, manifests with progressive weakness and significant hypotonia, usually during the first trimester of life. The involvement of multiple organs with hepatomegaly, cardiomegaly, and macroglossia also occurs.

In conclusion, considering all the possible causes of hypotonia in infancy, the best diagnosis in the vignette is infantile spinal muscular atrophy.

Clinical Features

The spinal muscular atrophies are hereditary autosomal recessive disorders affecting the anterior horn cells and cranial nuclei and characterized by progressive weakness, diffuse denervation, and atrophy. Three forms of SMA have been decsribed, the most severe being the early infantile or type 1 (Werdnig-Hoffman disease). The other two are the late infantile form or type 2 (intermediate) and the juvenile or type 3 (Kugelberg-Welander disease).

Spinal Muscular Atrophy Type 1

SMA type 1, also called acute infantile paralysis or Werdnig-Hoffman disease, presents at birth or during the first few months of life with severe proximal weakness, preferentially affecting the lower extremities, and marked hypotonia. Weakness can be so profound that only movements in the hands and feet can be observed. Sometimes a subtle tremor of the fingers called polyminimyoclonus is noted. The baby tends to assume a frog-like position and breathing is mainly diaphragmatic due to intercostal muscle weakness, which can cause the bell-shaped deformity. Other characteristic features include fasciculations and atrophy of the tongue, areflexia, normal sensation, and normal sphincteric function. Extraocular and facial muscles are also spared. Affected infants are bright and alert.

The prognosis is poor due to severe respiratory compromise and most succumb before reaching 2 years of age.

Spinal Muscular Atrophy Type 2

SMA type 2, or intermediate form, is characterized by a later occurrence of the symptoms, usually after 6 months of age, proximal lower extremity weakness, hypotonia, hypo-reflexia, areflexia, tongue fasciculations, and normal intellectual function. Many patients are able to sit without support but only a limited number reach the ability to stand and walk with assistance.

The prognosis is more favorable than with type 1 and the survival longer, but joint contractures and kyphoscoliosis can occur and respiratory compromise represents the most serious complication.

Spinal Muscular Atrophy Type 3

SMA type 3, or Kugelberg-Welander disease, manifests after the age of 18 months with proximal muscle weakness, particularly in the lower limbs, that can be responsible for a waddling gait in ambulatory patients, often in association with lumbar lordosis and prominent abdomen. Deep tendon reflexes are decreased or absent and diffuse fasciculations are observed, particularly of the tongue. Extraocular muscles are always intact.

The course is slowly progressive with a survival that can reach the second decade of life.

Diagnosis

Genetic studies are important because all these disorders are due to mutations in the spinal motor neuron gene located on chromosome 5q13.

Serum measurements of creatine kinase may or may not show elevation, but are usually normal in SMA type 1 and 2.

Electrodiagnostic evaluation may demonstrate normal conduction velocities, decreased amplitude of the compound muscle action potential, and signs of denervation and reinnervation on needle EMG study.

Muscle biopsy shows evidence of neurogenic atrophy with atrophic round fibers and fiber type grouping.

Treatment

There is no available treatment and the management is based on preventing and treating complications, in particular respiratory compromise, joint and spinal deformities, and failure to thrive.

Muscular Dystrophies

The dystrophies are genetic, progressive myopathies caused by defects in structural proteins.

Duchenne's Muscular Dystrophy

Vignette

A 7-year-old boy was brought to your attention because of a gait disorder. He was a full-term product of uncomplicated pregnancy and delivery with no evidence of fetal distress. He started crawling at 8 months and walking at 15 months. At the age of 3 his mother noticed that he was falling more frequently than his playmates and seemed to have difficulties climbing stairs. He could never jump over his shoes or a toy on the floor. There was no double vision or speech difficulties. The mother had mild diabetes and a maternal uncle was wheelchair-bound since his teens and died of heart disease. On examination the boy appeared dull and distractible. Cranial nerve examination was unremarkable except for a large tongue. Lumbar lordosis and protuberance of the abdomen were noted as well as Achilles' tendon contractures and mild hyperthrophy of the gastrocnemius muscle. Strength in the arms was decreased, especially serratus anterior and pectorals, and prominent scapular winging was noted. Deep tendon reflexes were absent and Babinski's sign was negative. When walking, his heels did not strike the ground and his gait was waddling.

Summary A 7-year-old boy with progressive weakness.

Localization and Differential Diagnosis

The history and neurological examination help in localizing the lesion to a specific component of the motor unit. Progressive weakness can be due to disorders of the following:

- Anterior horn cells, such as spinal muscular atrophy or other motor neuron diseases.
- Peripheral nerves, such as hereditary, or acquired: (idiopathic, metabolic, infectious, and inflammatory neuropathies).
- Neuromuscular junction, such as myasthenia gravis.
- Muscle, such as muscular dystrophies; congenital; metabolic; or inflammatory myopathies.

The history and neurological examination help localize to a disorder of the muscles.

Gait abnormality can be caused by proximal or distal lower extremity weakness. In the vignette, there is clear indication of proximal muscle weakness. With proximal weakness, the pelvis is not stabilized and waddles from side to side as the child walks (Fenichel 1997). Lumbar lordosis and protuberance of the abdomen are due to weakness of the abdomen, back, and pelvic girdle muscles. Progressive proximal weakness of insidious onset in children is often an indication of an underlying myopathic process, in particular a muscular dystrophy (preferred diagnosis).

On the other hand, juvenile spinal muscular atrophy, which is a neurogenic process involving the anterior horn cells, also manifests with progressive proximal weakness predominantly affecting the lower extremities, lumbar lordosis, and a waddling gait. Juvenile SMA has other distinctive clinical features, including minipolymyoclonus that can be prominent, fasciculations of the tongue, signs of bulbar involvement, variable reflexes, and extensor plantar responses in some cases.

Neurogenic and myopathic processes can usually be differentiated by the clinical features and also by diagnostic studies, particularly needle EMG and muscle biopsy.

Disorders of the neuromuscular junction, such as juvenile myasthenia gravis, are easily clinically excluded by the case presented in the vignette because of the lack of typical characteristics of MG, such as fatigable weakness and ocular and bulbar involvement, and the description in the vignette of clinical findings not related to myothenia (muscle hypertrophy, contractures, absent deep tendon reflexes, and so on).

Therefore, the best initial diagnosis of the vignette remains a disorder of the muscle. Loss of tendon reflexes in myopathic processes occurs if the degree of weakness is severe.

Childhood myopathies can be distinguished into acquired and inherited disorders. Acquired disorders of muscle include

- Inflammatory myopathies, such as dermatomyositis and polymyositis.
- Infectious myopathies, such as viral myositis (HIV, coxsackievirus) or parasitic myositis (trichinosis, toxoplasmosis, and so on).
- Toxic myopathies due to alcohol or drugs, such as steroids, vincristine, cloroquine, and so on.
- Myopathies associated with endocrine or systemic dysfunction such as hypothyroidism or hyperthyroidism, Addison's disease, Cushing's syndrome, renal and electrolyte dysfunction, and so on.

Inflammatory myopathies, especially dermatomyositis, with the typical features of fever, rash, muscle pain, and weakness are not featured in the vignette. Polymyositis without evidence of other target organ involvement is uncommon before puberty (Fenichel). None of the acquired childhood myopathies secondary to endocrinopathy, toxic exposure, or infection are supported by the clinical findings in the vignette.

Many factors suggest that the boy described in the vignette has a hereditary myopathic disorder. These factors include the insidious onset and relentless progression of the symptoms and the positive family history significant for a maternal uncle wheelchair-bound since his teens and deceased for cardiac problems. This may point to a possible X-linked disorder of the muscles.

We can easily exclude many inherited muscle disorders. Congenital myopathies, for example, are muscle disorders that present at birth with hypotonia, weakness, and respiratory dysfunction. The distribution of weakness is diffuse and in some cases, such as nemaline myopathy, predominantly distal. Skeletal deformities and dysmorphic features also also present. The diagnosis is based on muscle biopsy.

Other hereditary disorders of the muscle such as myotonic dystrophy, myotonia congenita, and periodic paralysis can be easily excluded. Patients with myotonic dystrophy, which is an autosomic dominant disorder, have a typical facial appearance due to marked weakness of the facial muscles. Myotonia is characteristic and the distribution of weakness is mainly distal with slow progression to the proximal muscles. Myotonia congenita manifests with muscle stiffness and myotonia in patient with normal strength and reflexes. Periodic paralysis is characterized by episodic and not chronic weakness precipitated by heavy meals, emotional stress, or strenuous physical activity.

Metabolic myopathies are hereditary disorders characterized by exercise intolerance. Some cases, such as the juvenile form of type II glycogenosis, can sometimes simulate a dystrophynopathy due to the clinical features of proximal muscle weakness, delayed motor milestones, waddling gait, and lumbar lordosis, presenting during the first decade of life. Hypertrophy of the calf muscles has also been described. Respiratory compromise can be severe and fatal. As opposed to the muscular dystrophies, cardiomegaly, hepatomegaly, and cranial nerve dysfunction, although uncommon, can manifest in some cases.

Finally, a very important category of inherited muscle disorders needs to be considered: the muscular dystrophies. Duchenne's muscular dystrophy appears to be the most likely diagnosis of the child described in the vignette who has a history of progressive proximal weakness, hypertrophic muscles, areflexia, and a maternal relative who was wheelchair-bound since his early teens (which in this case suggests a possible X-linked disorder).

Clinical Features

Duchenne's muscular dystrophy (DMD) is an X-linked recessive disorder that affects only males and manifests with progressive muscular weakness that becomes apparent when the boy starts walking. It affects 1 in 3500 live male births (Berg). Approximately one third of cases appear to be due to new mutations (Amato and Dumitru). The abnormal gene product in both Duchenne's and Becker's muscular dystrophy is a reduced muscle content of the structural protein dystrophin (Fenichel). In Duchenne's muscular dystrophy the dystrophin content is 0 to 3 percent of normal, whereas in Becker's muscular dystrophy the dystrophin content is 3 to 20 percent of normal.

The clinical manifestations become evident at the time of walking, and most children appear normal at birth and are able to reach some motor milestones, such as sitting and standing. Gait is usually clumsy and waddling and the boys experience frequent falls, cannot run with their peers, and have great difficulty climbing stairs. Toe walking caused by Achilles' tendon contractures, calf hypertrophy, and difficulty arising from the floor are also noted. The distribution of muscle weakness is mainly proximal, particularly involving the lower extremities, pelvic and paraspinal muscles, and also the shoulder girdle muscles. Prominent lumbar lordosis and abdominal protuberance also occur. Gower's sign, which is not specific for the muscular dystrophies but can also be observed in other neuromuscular disorders with significant proximal weakness such as spinal muscular atrophies, manifests with certain maneuvers that allow the boy to arise from the floor, such as pushing himself upright after getting onto his hands and knees and then climbing up the legs.

This disorder shows a progressive, relentless course to the point that ambulation becomes an impossible task and the patients are relegated to a wheelchair around the age of 12. Joint contractures and hyposcoliosis also develop, and respiratory compromise may represent a serious complication. Cranial nerve musculature is not affected but the tongue can be enlarged.

The involvement of other organs is also a feature of DMD. Signs of cardiac dysfunction vary from asymptomatic cases to congestive heart failure and cardiac arrhythmia. Gastrointestinal dysfunction can manifest with acute gastric dilatation, also called intestinal pseudo-obstruction.

Intellectual functions can also be affected, and the average IQ of the child with DMD is one standard deviation below the normal mean.

Diagnosis

Creatine kinase is significantly increased from 50 to 100 times the normal values. Abnormally high levels can be detected at birth before the clinical manifestations become apparent.

Needle electromyography shows increased insertional activity with positive sharp waves and fibrillation potentials, and short- and long-duration motor unit action potentials that recruit early.

Muscle biopsy may demonstrate regenerating and necrotic muscle fibers, large hypercontracted fibers, excessive variation of muscle fiber diameter, increased endomysial fibrosis, and muscle fiber loss with fat accumulation.

Genetic tests may show detectable mutations on routine DNA testing. The distrophin gene, located at Xp21, is the largest known gene and is very susceptible to mutations and deletions.

Treatment

Some improvement in muscle strength and pulmonary function has been obtained with the use of prednisone and deflazacort (a synthetic derivative of prednisolone) in randomized double-blind controlled trials.

Supportive care is the mainstay of treatment with orthopedic and cardiorespiratory management. Gene therapy with myoblast transfer and vector-mediated gene transfer are other new approaches.

Prenatal diagnosis determined in males is possible by testing for the deletion in chorionic villus or amniocentesis fluid.

Other Muscular Dystrophies

Following are capsule summaries of four other muscular dystrophies:

Becker's muscular dystrophy
- Later onset of symptoms than DMD, often after 8 years of age
- X-linked recessive inheritance.
- Ability to walk maintained beyond age 16.
- Pattern of muscle weakness similar to DMD but less frequent contractures.
- Longer survival: patients can reach middle age and beyond.

Emery-Dreyfuss muscular dysytrophy
- X-linked recessive inheritance.

- Early onset of prominent joint contractures, particularly of the Achilles' tendons, elbows, and posterior cervical muscles.
- Progressive muscular weakness and atrophy in a humeroperoneal distribution.
- Frequent cardiomyopathy with conduction abnormalities.
- CK levels only moderately elevated.

Facioscapulohumeral muscular dystrophy (see also later vignette)
- Autosomal dominant transmission with strong penetrance.
- Weakness of the shoulder girdle and scapular fixation muscles is characteristic.
- Biceps and triceps are affected with deltoid muscles relatively spared.
- Facial weakness is also an important feature.

Limb-Girdle muscular dystrophy
- Autosomal recessive transmission.
- Slowly progressive, symmetrical, proximal weakness, with or without facial involvement.
- Onset in the second or third decade.
- Elevated serum CK, but less than DMD.

Dermatomyositis

Vignette

A 5-year-old girl was noted to be having trouble climbing stairs during the last six months. She refused to walk for more than two blocks or ride her bicycle, complaining that her legs hurt. She has also been very irritable with low-grade fever and poor appetite. A pediatrician who examined the girl noticed some erythematous areas over the knees and elbows. Blood tests including a CK level were normal. On examination she was alert and cooperative. There was mild weakness of neck flexor and moderate weakness of the pelvic girdle muscles. DTR were hypoactive. She had a tiptoe gait.

Summary A 5-year-old girl presenting with progressive proximal muscle weakness and hyporeflexia associated with myalgia, systemic symptoms, and a rash over the knees and elbows. The CPK level is reported as normal.

Localization and Differential Diagnosis

The localization is clearly the peripheral nervous system. There are no signs of central nervous system involvement.

Next, it is important to determine which part of the motor unit is involved: anterior horn cells, peripheral nerves, neuromuscular junction, or muscle. Another distinction is between hereditary and acquired disorders.

This child presents with progressive proximal muscle weakness without any disturbance of sensory or autonomic function. The weakness is bilateral, mainly proximal, and associated with pain. All these symptoms point toward a muscle disorder. The different categories of muscle disorders include

- Muscular dystrophies.
- Metabolic myopathies.
- Myopathies secondary to metabolic, endocrine, toxic, and systemic disorders.
- Inflammatory myopathies.

Considering the muscular dystrophies first, Duchenne's and Becker's muscular dystrophies can be easily ruled out because they are X-linked hereditary disorders that affect only boys. The characteristic symptoms of progressive, insidious proximal weakness in these muscular dystrophies become apparent when the child begins to walk, and always before five years of age.

Facioscapulohumeral muscular dystrophy is characterized by marked facial and shoulder-girdle muscle weakness. In the lower extremities, the tibialis anterior muscle is the first and most significantly involved, resulting in a frequent foot drop.

Limb-girdle dystrophy includes several groups of disorders characterized by mild and severe forms presenting with progressive muscular weakness of the upper and lower extremities, sometimes associated with calf pseudohypertrophy and usually an autosomal recessive inheritance.

The metabolic myopathies are a group of muscle disorders characterized by a specific metabolic abnormality. They include disorders of glycogen metabolism, disorder of nucleotide and lipid metabolism, and mitochondrial myopathies. These disorders have specific characteristics that can be easily ruled out in the vignette (see vignette in Chapter 19).

The inflammatory myopathies are disorders characterized by progressive proximal weakness, inflammatory changes of muscle on biopsy, increased levels of CK, and signs of muscle membrane instability and fiber loss on electrodiagnostic studies. They include polymyositis, dermatomyositis, and inclusion body myositis. Dermatomyositis in particular, with its characteristic features of progressive symmetrical weakness preferentially affecting the proximal muscles, myalgia, skin changes, and systemic manifestations, represent the best possible diagnosis of the child described in the vignette.

Dermatomyositis tends to manifest between 5 and 10 years of age. The insidious onset of proximal weakness may be preceded by systemic manifestations that include low-grade fever, fatigue, anorexia, muscle pain and discomfort, and artralgia. The onset of the disease can be subacute over a few weeks or acute over a few days and is often preceded by an infection.

Proximal muscles are preferentially involved and common complaints are difficulty climbing up stairs, getting up from a low seat, and combing or blow drying the hair. Distal muscles may also be involved and, in particular, the involvement of the calf muscles may be responsible for contractures and toe walking. Weakness of the flexor muscles of the neck is observed in approximately one half of children (Menkes). Bulbar dysfunction with dysphagia and dysarthria can also occur in more severe cases. Deep tendon reflexes can be preserved or diminished.

Cutaneous manifestations are an important feature of the disorder and include a purplish erythematous rash in the periorbital area that can extend into the cheeks and forehead. Knuckles, elbows, and knees can also became affected. The periungual region in the hands also can show erythematous changes.

Subcutaneous calcifications are more common in children than in adults, and according to Dumitru, can occur in 30 to 70 percent of children. They tend to appear over pressure points (buttocks, knees, elbows) and can be of varying size, from barely palpable to very large and disfiguring, particularly in children inadequately treated. Systemic complications include cardiac involvement, gastroparesis, and gastrointestinal tract perforation. Other complications include residual weakness with contractures, and subcutaneous calcifications.

Diagnosis

Laboratory studies demonstrate elevation of serum levels of muscle enzymes: CK, LDH, SGOT, and SGPT. Serum CK can be significantly elevated up to 50 times the upper limits of normal. However, serum levels can also be normal, particularly in the early stages, and therefore a normal laboratory level does not exclude the diagnosis of polymyositis or dermatomyositis.

Electrodiagnostic studies, particularly needle EMG, show signs of membrane instability represented by profuse fibrillations and positive sharp waves. Motor unit potentials are of short duration and polyphasic, and may show early recruitment.

Muscle biopsy demonstrates the typical finding of perifascicular atrophy.

Treatment

Corticosteroids are considered the treatment of choice. The initial dose of prednisone is 2 mg/kg/day, not to exceed 100 mg/day, followed after clinical improvement by an alternate-day regimen. If the patient does not respond to this regimen, then immunosuppressive agents such as methothrexate, azathioprine, or cyclosporine can be used. Plasmapheresis is another option.

Infantile Botulism

Vignette

A 4½-month-old baby boy was brought to the ER because of respiratory distress. The mother noticed that for the last few days he had stopped rolling over and lifting his head and had experienced severe constipation. There was no fever or vomiting. On examination the child was hypotonic and areflexic. He had limited extraocular movements, and gag reflex was absent. Prenatal and perinatal histories as well as past medical history were normal with typical developmental milestones.

Summary A 4½-month-old baby, who had a normal medical history up until few days ago, when he stopped rolling over and lifting his head, experiencing constipation and respiratory problems.

Localization and Differential Diagnosis

The vignette describes a case of acute respiratory distress due to a neuromuscular disorder (signs of hypotonia and areflexia indicate a disorder of the motor unit). The next step is to determine which level of the motor unit is affected: anterior horn cells, peripheral nerve, neuromuscular junction, or muscle.

Among the disorders of the anterior horn cells, infantile spinal muscular atrophy can manifest with respiratory compromise in the neonatal period. Extraocular muscles are typically spared and severe constipation is not a feature. Acute anterior horn cell disease due to polyomyelitis is uncommon since the advent of polio immunization except in immunodepressed patients and is characterized by fever, meningeal signs and an asymmetrical flaccid paralysis.

Acute disorders of the peripheral nerves, such as GBS, is rare in children younger than 2 years of age (Evans). GBS usually presents with progressive ascending motor weakness and sensory symptoms. Respiratory dysfunction can complicate the course of the disorder but is unlikely to be an initial manifestation.

Disorders of the neuromuscular junction, typically infantile botulism (preferred diagnosis) can present between 3 and 18 weeks of age with weakness, hypotonia, and hyporeflexia or areflexia. The neurological manifestations can be preceded by several days or few weeks of constipation and poor feeding. On examination the child may appear lethargic and hypotonic with diminished spontaneous movements. Ptosis, extraocular and facial muscle weakness, reduced or absent gag reflex, and poor suck can also be noted. Pupillary reaction to light may be impaired. Respiratory function can be compromised due to weakness of the respiratory and pharyngeal muscles and infants may require assisted mechanical ventilation.

Disorders of the muscle that can manifest with respiratory compromise in the neonatal period include the congenital myotonic dystrophy and the rare metabolic myopathies (acid maltase deficiency and myophosphorylase deficiency). These disorders can easily be clinically ruled out from the vignette. Congenital myotonic dystrophy that may cause complications, such as polyhydramnios or decreased fetal movements, during the prenatal period is characterized by severe hypotonia and respiratory distress that become manifest immediately after birth. Acid maltase deficiency manifests at birth or during the first weeks of life with severe hypotonia and respiratory failure but severe organomegaly is also present. Myophosphorylase deficiency can rarely present with a severe infantile form characterized by marked hypotonia and respiratory failure and usually manifests during the teenage years with exercise intolerance, cramps, and myoglobinuria.

In summary, infantile botulism represents the preferred diagnosis of the child in the vignette.

Diagnosis

The diagnosis is confirmed when the toxin is identified in the stool specimen. Both type A and type B spores of *Clostridium botulinum* have been implicated.

Electrophysiological findings in botulism are indicative of a presynaptic defect of the neuromuscular junction and show a moderate increment of the compound muscle action potential present in the affected muscles after rapid repetitive stimulation.

Treatment

Treatment of infantile botulism is based on supportive measures including respiratory support and nasogastric feeding.

Neonatal Transient Myasthenia Gravis

Vignette

A 2-day-old baby boy was transferred to the ICU because of poor feeding, poor cry, generalized weakness, diminished activity, apathy, respiratory distress, and severe hypotonia. The infant was born four weeks premature through an emergency C-section after spontaneous rupture of the membranes. The initial examination was normal. The mother had a history of myasthenia gravis since the age of 21 and has had several miscarriages. The father of this child was unknown. One sibling had several bone deformities plus juvenile diabetes.

Summary A 2-day-old baby with severe hypotonia, generalized weakness, respiratory distress, apathy, and a weak cry.

Localization and Differential Diagnosis

Again, the distinction between cerebral versus motor-unit hypotonia should be made in this infant. There is no mention in the vignette of any decreased level of consciousness, seizures, dysmorphic features, or other organ malformation that may indicate a cerebral localization. If the symptoms are localized to the motor unit and the family history (myasthenic mother) is considered, transitory neonatal myasthenia ranks high on the list of the possibilities.

Transient neonatal autoimmune myasthenia gravis occurs in 10 percent of children born to mothers with myasthenia gravis (Dumitru et al.). The disorder is caused by the passive transfer through the placenta of circulating antiacetylcholine receptors antibodies from the myasthenic mother to the fetus. The onset of the symptoms is usually during the first three day of life with generalized weakness, hypotonia, respiratory distress, a weak cry, poor feeding due to suck problems, facial muscle weakness, and ptosis.

Diagnosis

The disorder is self-limited with a mean duration of symptoms of 18 to 20 days. Diagnostic approach includes the demonstration of high serum concentration of Ach-binding antibodies in the newborn and transient improvement of weakness by the subcutaneous or intravenous injection of edrophonium chloride 0.15 mg/kg.

Treatment

The treatment includes anticholinesterase medications, plasma exchange if the weakness is severe, and mechanical ventilation.

Charcot-Marie-Tooth Disease

Vignette

A 16-year-old boy started having difficulty running at the age of 6, which steadily progressed. By the age of 12, he had mild weakness and wasting of the thenar and interossei muscles and a bilateral foot drop. He was previously diagnosed as having a learning disability. There was no other medical history. The boy was adopted and the family history was not available. On examination there was distal limb atrophy. Hand grip, wrist and foot dorsiflexion and eversion were weak. DTR were absent except for trace in the biceps and triceps. Vibration was decreased at the ankles.

Summary A 16-year-old boy with a history of chronic progressive distal weakness atrophy and sensory disturbances.

Localization and Differential Diagnosis

Considering the different parts of the motor unit, there is no doubt that the vignette indicates involvement of the peripheral nerves. Next, it is important to determine if the disorder is hereditary or acquired.

After excluding a toxic or metabolic etiology, the most likely categories of chronic neuropathies to be considered are the hereditary neuropathies and chronic inflammatory demyelinating polyneuropathy (CIDP) (Ouvrier et al.). Hereditary neuropathies are considered the most common type of chronic neuropathies in children. Of the hereditary group, 40 percent had peroneal muscular atrophy (Covanis in Pantepiadis). When considering the hereditary neuropathies, it is important to determine if the neuropathy occurs as a sole manifestation of a peripheral nerve disorder or if it is associated with other symptoms suggestive of a more widespread involvement of the nervous system or other organs. The patient in the vignette had experienced a distal sensorimotor neuropathy without other clinical manifestations. This type of picture can represent Charcot-Marie-Tooth (CMT) disease, which is the most common of the inherited polyneuropathies.

Clinical manifestations of CMT are characterized by symmetrical weakness and atrophy, preferentially involving the lower extremities distally and to a lesser extent the upper extremities without any signs of a more widespread involvement. Charcot-Marie-Tooth disease is a heterogenous group of hereditary disorders. CMT type I is the most common variety and is characterized by an autosomal dominant inheritance and clinically by distal weakness, atrophy, sensory loss, and foot deformity, particularly pes cavus and hammer toe. Nerve biopsy shows evidence of extensive demyelination with onion bulb formation. CMT type II usually manifests later than type I with similar features but less prominent weakness and deformity and without enlargement of the peripheral nerves.

A third variety of inherited polyneuropathy, Dejerine-Sottas disease, or hereditary motor and sensory neuropathy (HMSN) type III, is an autosomal recessive disorder characterized by presentation in infancy or early childhood with generalized weakness, preferentially distal; hypotonia; deformities of hands, feet, and spine and enlarged peripheral nerves.

Other hereditary and metabolic neuropathies can be distinguished based on their clinical characteristics and more widespread central nervous system or other system involvement. Neuropathies associated with spinocerebellar degeneration include Friedreich's ataxia, which is an autosomal recessive disorder characterized by involvement of the peripheral nerves with distal weakness, wasting, sensory loss, and areflexia, and other characteristic symptoms, such as dysarthria, ataxia, titubation of the head, nystagmus, bilateral Babinski's sign, and so on.

Hereditary neuropathies associated with specific metabolic defects include disorders that can easily be excluded from the vignette. Refsum disease, associated with a defect of phytanic acid metabolism, has distinctive clinical features in addition to peripheral nerve dysfunction, such as retinitis pigmentosa presenting with night blindness, hypoacusis ataxia, and other cerebellar signs, such as tremor, nystagmus, and elevated protein level in the CSF.

Fabry disease, which is due to deficiency of the lysosomal enzyme alpha-galactosidase, is an X-linked disorder manifesting with painful distal paresthesias due to small fiber neuropathy and angiokeratoma, particularly over the trunk, buttocks, and scrotum.

Metachromatic leukodystrophy, caused by deficiency of the lysosomal enzyme arylsulfatase A, presents with gait dysfunction, hyporeflexia, and hypotonia, often preceding the signs of CNS, involvement in the late infantile form. In the juvenile form, the presentation is often with behavior dysfunction and cognitive impairment.

Globoid cell leukodystrophy, due to deficiency of galactosylceramidase can have signs of peripheral nerve involvement but the classic manifestations are represented by severe mental and motor impairment, seizures, optic atrophy, and so on.

Tangier disease and abetalipoproteinemia are mentioned here for completion. The former, due to deficiency of high-density lipoproteins, has typical features of neuropathy and enlarged yellow-orange tonsil, a pseudosyringomyelic picture of dissociated sensory loss combined with weakness and atrophy of the upper extremities or multifocal mononeuropathies. Abetalipoproteinemia, due to absence of apolipoprotein B, is characterized by progressive peripheral neuropathy associated with retinitis pigmentosa, and severe fat malabsorption.

Chronic acquired neuropathies of children, particularly CIDP, also need some consideration in the differential diagnosis of the child described in the vignette. CIDP is more common in adults than in children and is characterized by progressive or relapsing weakness that affects the upper and lower extremities proximally and distally. The proximal weakness can be pronounced but the atrophy is rarely significant.

Toxic and metabolic causes of neuropathies also need to be mentioned for completion. These can be drug induced (e.g., isoniazid, nitrofurantoin, vincristine, etc.) or secondary, for example, to diabetes or uremia.

In general, during childhood and adolescence, chronic peripheral neuropathies are usually caused by a hereditary metabolic or a familial degenerative disorder.

Finally, as part of the differential diagnosis, motor neuron diseases, such as hereditary spinal muscular atrophy, particularly types 2 and 3, may simulate CMT types I and II in some aspects but the weakness mainly affects the proximal muscles and sensation is completely normal. The hereditary distal myopathies and myotonic dystrophy have their typical characteristics that help the distinction.

Clinical Features and Diagnosis

The most common cause of peroneal muscular atrophy in children is a hereditary motor and sensory neuropathy, usually CMT. There are two main entities within the CMT phenotype:

- CMT-I (HMSN I): The hypertrophied or demyelinating form characterized by severe reduction in nerve conduction velocities and nerve biopsy findings consistent with demyelination and onion bulb formation.
- CMT-II (HMSN-II): The neuronal form with normal or near normal conduction velocity and nerve biopsy findings of axonal loss without significant demyelination.

CMT Type I

CMT type I is the most frequent form and is characterized by an autosomal dominant inheritance and onset during the first or second decade of life. Some cases can be secondary to spontaneous mutations. There are three genetic variants of this condition:

- CMT-IA is due to segmental duplication of 1.5 megabase of DNA at the region 17p 11.2–12, or to a mutation of the peripheral myelin protein 22.
- CMT-IB is caused by mutations in the myelin protein PO, which is located on chromosome 1q22–23.
- CMT-IC is not linked to any chromosome.

The clinical features manifest with gait impairment due to weakness and atrophy of the intrinsic foot and peroneal and anterior tibial muscles. Foot drop and steppage gait may result. Absent ankle jerk is a very common finding and the rest of the reflexes can be decreased or absent. Patients may also show the appearance of inverted champagne bottle legs due to severe atrophy below the knees. Sensory complains are usually rare but the examination may show decreased joint position sense and vibration in the distal extremities. Foot deformities are common, particularly pes cavum, equinovarus, and hammer toe.

Distal weakness and atrophy of the upper extremities can also gradually occur. Peripheral nerves are clinically enlarged in 25 percent of children with CMT type I (Dumitru et al.). The disorder has a slow course of progression.

Electrophysiological studies demonstrate significantly decreased conduction velocity on nerve conduction studies. The hereditary demyelinating neuropathies typically show a uniform and symmetrical slowing without conduction block or temporal dispersion. Nerve biopsy demonstrates extensive demyelination and onion bulb formation.

CMT Type II

This type is the neuronal form of peroneal muscular atrophy and is characterized by an autosomal dominant transmission and by similar clinical features to type I except for later onset, less severe weakness and deformities, and less common involvement of the upper extremities.

Peripheral nerves are not enlarged and electrophysiological findings demonstrate normal or minimally abnormal conduction velocities and features of axonal loss on needle EMG. Nerve biopsy demonstrates axonal atrophy and wallerian degeneration. The only major difference between this disease and CMT-I is in the electrophysiological and pathological findings.

Facioscapulohumeral Muscular Dystrophy

Vignette: Serratus Anterior

A 15-year-old girl started noticing difficulty running, climbing rope, and blow-drying her hair about eight months ago. Her medical history was unremarkable except for feeling tired when raising her arms for some time during the last year. When examined she stated that she has never been able to drink through a straw or whistle. She had a mild facial weakness, scapular winging, and mild weakness and atrophy of latissimus dorsi, trapezius, rhomboids, serratus, and anterior biceps and triceps muscles. Deltoids were of normal strength. She had a bilateral foot drop. Reflexes and sensation were normal. Family history was unremarkable except the father had scapular winging and could never whistle or do pull-ups.

Summary A 15-year-old girl with history of progressive weakness involving face, shoulder muscles, and distal legs, and scapular winging. The father has scapular winging and could never whistle or do pull-ups (this indicates weakness of the face, shoulders, and proximal upper extremities in the father).

Localization and Differential Diagnosis

Weakness associated with normal reflexes and intact sensation suggest a disorder of the muscles. Childhood myopathies can be inherited or acquired. The child described in the vignette had a father who manifested some common clinical features, such as scapular winging and inability to whistle, suggesting an inherited dominant disorder.

The pattern of weakness involving the facial, scapular, stabilizer, and proximal upper extremities muscles and anterior tibialis muscles with resultant foot drop, is typical of facioscapulohumeral muscular dystrophy (FSH). Patients cannot purse their lips, use a straw, or whistle. Weakness and atrophy mainly involves the humeral muscle groups sparing the forearm musculature and deltoid muscle but greatly affecting biceps and triceps. Scapular winging can be prominent and the anterior compartment muscles of the distal legs can also be affected.

Other muscular dystrophies can be easily distinguished by their clinical characteristics. Limb-girdle dystrophies are a heterogeneous group of autosomal recessive and autosomal dominant disorders that manifest with progressive weakness of the pelvic girdle and shoulder musculature of varying severity. Calf hypertrophy and scapular winging can occur. Facial weakness, which is typical of FSH, is not a feature.

Emery-Dreifuss muscular dystrophy is an X-linked recessive disorder affecting only males and characterized by progressive weakness and atrophy particularly of biceps, triceps, and peroneal muscles, early prominent contractures of the elbows and Achilles' tendon, and cardiomyopathy. Facial weakness is not a feature.

Duchenne's and Becker's muscular dystrophies can be easily excluded for obvious reasons (course of disease, distribution of weakness, progression, severity, X-linked inheritance affecting only males).

Myotonic dystrophy with its characteristics of myotonia, facial appearance, and distal limb weakness, can be easily distinguished and ruled out by the vignette.

Congenital myopathies that can be associated with an FSH dystrophy-like phenotype, such as nemaline myopathy and centronuclear myopathy, are commonly accompanied by dysmorphic features and skeletal abnormalities such as narrow facies and high arched palate, micrognathia, prognathism pectus escavatum; hyposcoliosis; pescavus or club feet. Deep tendon reflexes are reduced or absent.

Acquired myopathies, such as inflammatory or secondary to endocrine, toxic, or infectious processes, may have an insidious onset and always need to be ruled out when considering weakness in children because they can be treated.

Clinical Features and Diagnosis

FSH is an autosomal dominant disorder linked to the telomeric region of chromosome 4q35 (Dumitru et al.). The clinical features include weakness of the facial, shoulder girdle, and proximal upper extremity muscles with sparing of the deltoid muscles. The involvement of the biceps and triceps muscles with almost normal forearm muscles has suggested the definition of Popeye arms. Winging of the scapula occurs and can be prominent. In the lower extremities, the anterior tibialis muscle is usually affected with the result of foot drop and frequent falling.

Laboratory findings include a mild to moderate increase of the CK level and electrophysiological findings of short duration, small amplitude polyphasic potentials with early recruitment. Muscle biopsy shows variation in fiber size with rounded or angulated atrophic fibers. Mononuclear inflammatory cells may be demonstrated.

Myotonic Dystrophy

Vignette

An 8-year-old boy was referred to the school counselor because of inattentiveness, poor school performance, and hyperactivity. On examination he was mildly retarded and showed facial weakness with a tented upper lip. His mother was divorced and could not keep a steady job because she was always falling asleep at work during the day. She had cataracts removed at the age of 25 and showed facial weakness and bilateral foot drop.

Summary An 8-year-old boy with mental retardation and facial weakness. His mother has facial weakness and distal limb weakness and a history of cataracts removed at a young age. In addition she has daytime sleepiness that interferes with her job performance.

Localization and Differential Diagnosis

The history points to a hereditary disorder presenting with facial weakness and mental retardation. The mother had facial and distal leg weakness as well as a history of cataracts and hypersomnolence. Several inherited disorders, particularly muscular dystrophies can manifest with significant facial weakness.

Facioscapulohumeral dystrophy can present during infancy with marked facial weakness but other features important for the diagnosis observed in the patients and family members are shoulder girdle weakness and atrophy, and winging of the scapulae. Only rarely can mental retardation be observed.

In this vignette, the clinical features shown by the mother and the child do not indicate a case of FSH.

Myotonic dystrophy, particularly congenital myotonic dystrophy, can clearly represent the case described in the vignette. Facial muscle weakness is an important clinical manifestation. Children may show an expressionless face and triangular mouth with a tented upper lip or inverted V-shape appearance. Mild or moderate mental retardation is another significant feature. The vignette does not give information about the prenatal and perinatal history of this child. In congenital myotonic dystrophy, infants may present at birth with hypotonia, and feeding and respiratory difficulties. Decreased fetal movements can also be observed by the mother before the baby is born. Clinical myotonia cannot be present in infants but is usually demonstrated in older children after the age of 5 years. Congenital myotonic dystrophy is nearly always transmitted by a mother affected with myotonic dystrophy, even though in some cases she may not be aware of having the disorder.

Classic myotonic dystrophy manifests with facial and distal limb weakness. Myotonia, a disturbance of muscle relaxation after contraction, can be demonstrated by action or percussion particularly in the hands but also in the eyelids or tongue. Other features include behavioral and cognitive dysfunction with personality disorders and impairment of memory and spatial orientation. Posterior subscapular cataracts can be present. Signs of cardiac involvement with arrhythmias and sleep disorders, such as sleep apnea and daytime hypersomnolence, are other features.

Diagnosis

The diagnosis is based on the clinical characteristics and family history. CK can be mildly elevated. The needle EMG study may demonstrate the typical myotonic discharges with characteristic waxing and waning of both amplitude and frequency. DNA test for the expanded CTG (cytosine, thymine, guanine) repeat on chromosome 19 may show an unstable expansion of a CTG trinucleotide repeat sequence.

Treatment

No treatment is effective in improving muscle strength.

Periodic Paralysis

Vignette

A 14-year-old boy woke up in the middle of the night unable to move his limbs. He was able to talk and did not complain of double vision. The day of this event he was at a friend's birthday party, but he denied using alcohol or illicit drugs. He was alert and oriented. Cranial nerves examination showed normal extraocular movements, pupillary function, palatal movements, and gag reflex. There was a flaccid limb paralysis with areflexia. Sensory exam was intact to all modalities.

Summary A 14-year-old boy with acute motor weakness and areflexia. Other details provided by the history are: normal cranial nerves and normal sensory examination.

Localization and Differential Diagnosis

The symptoms are clearly associated with a disorder of the motor unit. Next is to determine the component involved: peripheral nerve, neuromuscular junction muscle, or anterior horn cell.

Disorders of peripheral nerve causing acute weakness include Guillain-Barré syndrome (GBS) as well as neuropathies secondary to infectious, metabolic, and toxic causes. In GBS there is progressive weakness over several days and rarely is the evolution rapid, in less than 24 hours. Cranial nerve involvement, autonomic dysfunction, sensory deficits, and paresthesias are common, and respiratory compromise can occur.

Infectious causes of neuropathies, such as diphtheria, have distinguishing characteristics, such as systemic symptoms and palatal paralysis. Metabolic disorders, such as acute intermittent porphyria, can present with an acute paralysis but abdominal symptoms such as pain, nausea, and vomiting, are often prominent, and autonomic and sensory symptoms are common. Seizures are another important finding. Toxic neuropathies due to drugs or toxins are associated with a recognizable offending agent. Most of the toxic neuropathies have a subacute or chronic evolution.

Disorders of the neuromuscular junction to be considered in the differential diagnosis of acute weakness are myasthenia gravis and botulism. In myasthenia gravis, symptoms are often related to involvement of ocular, facial, and bulbar muscles and reflexes are usually normal. The fatigable weakness is an important clinical sign. Botulism can be responsible for acute weakness, but cranial nerve involvement and large, poorly reactive pupils represent some typical findings.

Disorders of the anterior horn cell such as amyotrophic lateral sclerosis, spinal muscular atrophy, and polio, can be easily excluded from the vignette for the lack of characteristic signs and symptoms.

Considering muscle dysfunction as the origin of the acute weakness, the periodic paralysis needs great consideration because they can present with attacks of acute, severe limb weakness. Primary hyperkalemic periodic paralysis, also called potassium-sensitive periodic paralysis, is an autosomal dominant disorder with onset during childhood caused by mutations in the muscle membrane sodium channel. Clinically, it manifests with attacks of acute weakness usually lasting less than a few hours and triggered by rest following strenuous exercise. Serum potassium level is normal between attacks but can be increased during the acute paralysis.

Hypokalemic periodic paralysis, which represents the most common type of periodic paralysis, is an autosomal dominant hereditary disorder due to mutations in calcium channel of skeletal muscles. Symptoms appear during the first two decades, with episodes of acute paralysis that tend to occur during the night or early in the morning and are precipitated by meals rich in carbohydrates and sodium, stress, or sleep following heavy exercise. The weakness tends to involve the upper and lower extremity muscles sparing the facial and extraocular muscles and only rarely causing respiratory compromise. Sensation is normal and reflexes are diminished or absent. The paralysis lasts several hours with gradual return to normality over a few days. The episodes of weakness are associated with low potassium levels with normal potassium between attacks. The treatment is based on potassium administration and prophylactic measures.

Fabry's Disease

Vignette

A 13-year-old boy started complaining of a burning pain in his toes and fingers after playing soccer with his friends during the summer. His medical history revealed some prior attacks of diarrhea and abdominal pain diagnosed as food intolerance. The clinical examination revealed a reddish purple rash around the scrotum and umbilical area. Corneal opacity was noted on slit lamp examination. The neurological examination showed no objective signs of sensory impairment, reflex loss, or weakness. In the family history, a maternal uncle suffered multiple strokes and had heart disease and hypertension.

Summary A 13-year-old boy complaining of painful distal paresthesias precipitated by exercise. Neurological examination is apparently normal. Other symptoms and signs are: diarrhea, abdominal pain, skin lesions, and eye involvement with corneal opacity.

Localization and Differential Diagnosis

The vignette suggests a hereditary disorder with an X-linked transmission by mentioning in the family history that a maternal uncle had cardiac problems and hypertension and suffered multiple strokes. This is a metabolic hereditary multisystem disorder in which one of the clinical signs is intermittent painful paresthesias.

The categories of disorders to be considered are the juvenile metabolic polyneuropathies, in particular Fabry's disease, which is an X-linked disorder characterized by burning, lancinating pain in the extremities aggravated by hyperthermia. The neurological examination may not re-

veal objective findings. The involvement of other systems helps in the diagnosis of this syndrome, which is caused by a deficiency of the lysosomal enzyme alpha-galactosidase.

Other familial juvenile polyneuropathies have distinctive clinical characteristics. Refsum disease is an autosomal recessive disorder of lipid metabolism characterized by retinitis pigmentosa that presents as night blindness, cerebellar dysfunction, deafness, and peripheral neuropathy.

Acute intermittent porphyria is characterized by a predominantly motor neuropathy with weakness of the upper and lower extremities and facial and bulbar muscles accompanied by abdominal symptoms, seizures and psychiatric disturbances.

Tangier disease, which is caused by a deficiency of high-density lipoproteins, manifests with an asymmetrical or symmetrical peripheral neuropathy or with a syringomyelic presentation. A typical feature is the yellowish-orange colored tonsils.

Methachromatic leukodystrophy is characterized by progressive cerebral dysfunction with ataxia, spasticity, speech and intellectual deterioration, and optic atrophy and associated signs of peripheral nerve involvemnt.

The hereditary motor and sensory neuropathies (CMT-I and -II) are autosomal dominant disorders manifesting with distal weakness and atrophy and foot deformities. The hereditary motor and sensory neuropathy type III (Dejerine-Sottas) manifests with progressive weakness, atrophy, and sensory ataxia.

Clinical Features

Fabry's disease (angiokeratoma corporis diffusum) is an X-linked disorder due to deficiency of the lysosomal enzyme alpha-galactosidase. Clinical symptoms include characteristic episodic painful paresthesias, described as burning and lancinating pain, involving the distal extremities and triggered by hyperthermia due to strenuous exercise, infection, or other causes. The neurological examination shows no objective signs of sensory abnormality, reflex loss, or weakness. Motor and sensory nerve conduction studies and EMG are normal because Fabry's disease causes involvement of the small myelinated and unmyelinated nerve fibers.

Autonomic dysfunction manifests with episodic diarrhea, nausea, vomiting, and hypohydrosis. Dermatologic signs manifest with angiokeratoma, which is characterized by a dark red maculopapular rash involving the periumbilical area and the scrotum, inguinal area, and perineum. The ophthalmologic involvement is mainly characterized by corneal opacity.

Serious complications are represented by signs of vascular dysfunction with multiple strokes, hypertension, myocardial ischemia, premature atherosclerosis, and so on. Fatal complications are also due to renal failure.

Diagnosis

Laboratory investigations show a decreased level of alpha-galactosidase A activity. The disorder is linked on a mutation of the alpha-galactosidase gene located on chromosome Xq21–22.

Treatment

Treatment is symptomatic.

Metabolic Myopathies

McArdle's Disease

Vignette

A 13-year-old boy had experienced stiffness, muscle pain, and cramps while in the school gym lifting weights. This became a problem during a recent school-sponsored walk when he was forced to stop after two miles and at frequent intervals afterward. A few days later, while lifting weights again, he developed stiffness, cramps, and severe pain in his arms and shoulders. He was otherwise in good health and there was no history of weakness, numbness, incoordination, or difficulty walking. In the family, a paternal uncle had a history of muscle pain on exercise and renal disease.

Summary A 13-year-old boy with history of stiffness, pain, and cramps on exercise and normal neurological examination. A paternal uncle suffered from muscle pain and renal disease.

Localization and Differential Diagnosis

The vignette describes a case of exercise intolerance characterized by episodes of muscle pain, cramps, and stiffness triggered by exercise. This is a typical feature of metabolic muscle disease. The metabolic myopathies include disorders of glycogen, lipid, or mitochondrial metabolism. The only disorder of nucleotide metabolism involving muscle is myoadenilate deaminase deficiency. Typical symptoms of metabolic myopathies are exercise intolerance, muscle pain, stiffness, cramps, fatigue, myoglobinuria, and, in some cases, weakness of proximal or distal muscles.

In the patient described, the occurrence of symptoms following brief episodes of strenuous exercise (weight lifting) or prolonged low-intensity exercise (long walk) is typical of McArdle's disease (myophosphorylase deficiency). This disorder, whose hallmark is exercise intolerance during childhood, can be clinically similar to the other disorders of glycogen metabolism, and laboratory investigations need to point to the correct diagnosis.

The examination is usually normal between attacks but one third of patients with McArdle's disease may develop fixed, mild proximal weakness due to the recurrent attacks of rhabdomyolysis (Dumitru et al.).

Disorders of fatty acid metabolism that enter the differential diagnosis mainly include carnitine palmitoyl-transferase deficiency (CPTD). This disorder usually manifests with muscular pain, cramps, and fatigue after intense or prolonged exercise or hyperthermia. Recurrent myoglobinuria is precipitated by prolonged exercise or fasting and renal failure can occur. Patients do not experience the second-wind phenomenon as with McArdle disease and the examination is normal between the episodes. In myophosphorylase deficiency some patients may develop fixed proximal weakness due to rhabdomyolisis. In CPT deficiency, serum concentration of creatine kinase and EMG are normal between attacks. The forearm ischemic exercise is normal.

In the differential diagnosis of exercise intolerance, myoadenylate deaminase deficiency is another disorder to be considered. The onset of symptoms is late adolescence to middle age, with muscle pain of varying severity, fatigue, and myoglobinuria after exercise. The second-wind phenomenon does not occur. The forearm ischemic exercise test shows normal increase of serum lactate without a rise of ammonia level.

Mitochondrial myopathies can be excluded by the vignette, but they enter the differential diagnosis of exercise intolerance. Symptoms are heterogeneous and include hypotonia in infancy, myalgia, exercise intolerance, myoglobinuria, proximal weakness, and so on. A variety of neurological syndromes with a multiplicity of symptoms are also part of the mitochondrial disorders and include psychomotor retardation, seizures, dementia, movement disorders, migraine-type headache, stroke-like episodes, dysmorphic features, short stature, deafness, and multiple organ involvement.

Clinical Features

McArdle's disease (myophosphorylase deficiency) is an autosomal recessive disorder affecting preferably males and characterized by exercise intolerance with symptoms of myalgia, fatigue, stiffness, cramps, and weakness, typically precipitated by brief strenuous activity, such as lifting weights, or prolonged low-impact exercise, such as long walks or swimming.

The second-wind phenomenon is described as the ability to slow down and rest as soon as patients experience muscle pain to avoid an attack and continue exercising with better durability. Patients can reduce the intensity effort so that they can maintain the activity for a longer period of time.

The physical examination between attacks can be normal or show some degree of proximal weakness. Myoglobinuria and renal insufficiency may complicate the picture, usually in later stages.

Diagnosis

The serum CK level is usually elevated. The needle EMG is normal but myopathic features can also be found. The exercise forearm test demonstrates a rise in ammonia level, but not in the level of lactic acid. Muscle biopsy demonstrates abnormal glycogen accumulation in the subsarcolemmic and intermyofibrillar areas. McArdle's disease is due to a mutation in the gene encoding for myophosphorylase on chromosome 11q13.

Treatment

No therapy is available, although gene therapy is a possible consideration.

Acid Maltase Deficiency

Vignette

A 6-month-old boy had a history of severe hypotonia and feeding and respiratory difficulties, since the age of 3 months. On examination he was very floppy and weak and rested limply, with his tongue protruded. There was no evidence of atrophy or fasciculations. The pediatrician noted that he was tachypneic and had an enlarged liver and heart. Family history and perinatal history were unremarkable.

Summary A 6-month-old boy with hypotonia, weakness, feeding and respiratory problems, and organomegaly with hepatomegaly and cardiomegaly.

Localization and Differential Diagnosis

The first goal is to categorize the hypotonia as of central or peripheral origin.

Cerebral hypotonia is characterized by decreased level of alertness and the presence of dysmorphic features. Peripheral hypotonia is suggested when the infant is bright and alert but severely weak and areflexic. Another important consideration is the localization of the motor unit disorder at one of his different levels: the motor neuron, peripheral nerve, neuromuscular junction, or muscle. Sometimes there can be a combination of cerebral and motor unit hypotonia.

The presence of organomegaly, hepatomegaly, and cardiomegaly suggests a metabolic disorder, particularly a metabolic myopathy. Pompe's disease or glycogenosis type II (acid maltase deficiency, AMD), characterized by severe weakness, hypotonia, and feeding and respiratory compromise in association with organomegaly, can be clearly represented by the child described. The infantile form of AMD must be distinguished from other muscle disorders presenting with organomegaly. These include the infantile cytochrome C oxidase deficiency, debranching enzyme deficiency, and so on.

Cytochrome C oxidase deficiency, which can manifest with severe hypotonia, weakness, poor feeding, and respiratory difficulty in the newborn, can also be associated with cardiac dysfunction but rarely cardiomegaly.

Debranching enzyme deficiency or type III glycogenosis is not characterized by severe weakness and hypotonia, as is AMD, and typically can manifest with seizures related to hypoglycemia.

Infantile acid maltase deficiency needs to be differentiated from spinal muscular atrophy type I (Wernig-Hoffman disease) affecting the anterior horn cells, but the organomegaly, in particular cardiomegaly, is characteristic of AMD.

Clinical Features

Acid maltase deficiency, which has an autosomal recessive inheritance is caused by a deficiency of the lysosomal enzyme alpha-glucosidase due to mutations on the gene encoding for acid maltase, which is located on chromosome 17q 21–23. Three forms have been described: the severe infantile form, the childhood-onset type, and the adult-onset variant.

The infantile form is characterized by severe weakness and hypotonia, respiratory and feeding problems, in addition to organomegaly that includes hepatomegaly, cardiomegaly, and macroglossia. Onset is usually during the first three months and the disease is rapidly progressive and carries a poor prognosis.

The juvenile type manifests during the first decade of life with proximal muscle weakness and respiratory compromise. Organomegaly is rare.

The adult-onset form, which manifests in the third or fourth decade, is characterized by weakness, mainly involving the proximal muscles, simulating a limb-girdle muscular dystrophy.

Diagnosis

Laboratory studies show significant deficiency of alpha-glucosidase activity in the infantile form. The CK level in the serum is usually moderately elevated.

Electrophysiological tests demonstrate normal sensory and motor nerve conduction studies (except in advanced cases were the amplitude of the CMAP may drop). Needle EMG shows abnormal spontaneous activity, including myotonic discharges, fibrillation, positive waves, and complex repetitive discharges, particularly in the paraspinal muscles.

Muscle biopsy may demonstrate abnormal glycogen accumulation between and within the myofibrils and beneath the sarcolemma.

Treatment

Treatment is supportive and gene therapy needs some consideration.

References

Hypotonic Infant

Berg, B.O. Principles of Child Neurology. New York: McGraw-Hill, 1451–1458, 1966.

Berg, B.O. Child Neurology: A Clinical Manual, ed. 2. Philadelphia: J.B. Lippincott, 279–286, 1994.

Brown, R.H. Jr. Inherited motor neuron diseases: Recent progress. Semin. Neurol. 14:365–373, 1993.

Dubowitz, V. The floppy infant. Clinics in developmental medicine, No. 76, ed. 2. Spastics International Medical publications, 1980.

Dubowitz, V. Evaluation and differential diagnosis of the hypotonic infant. Pediatr. Rev. 6:237–243, 1985.

Dumitru, D. et al. Electrodiagnostic Medicine. Philadelphia: Hanley and Belfus, 2002.

Evans, O.B. Manual of Child Neurology. New York: Churchill Livingstone, 255–265, 1987.

Fenichel, G.M. Hypotonia, arthrogryposis, and rigidity. In: Neonatal Neurology, ed. 3. New York: Churchill Livingstone, 35–68, 1990.

Fenichel, G.M. Clinical Pediatric Neurology: A Sign and Symptoms Approach, ed. 3. New York: Churchill Livingstone, 153–175, 1997.

Jannaccone, S.T. Spinal muscular atrophy. Semin. Neurol. 18:19–26, 1998.

Leshner, R.T. and Trasley, J.E. Pediatric neuromuscular emergencies. In Pellock, J.M. and Myer, E.C. (Eds.). Neurologic Emergencies in Infancy and Childhood. Boston: Butterworth-Heinemann, 242–261. 1993.

Miller, V.S. et al. Neonatal hypotonia. Semin. Neurol. 13:73–83, 1993.

Rumack, C.M. Diagnostic value of ultrasonic and computed tomographic imaging in infants with hypotonia. Pediatr. Rev. 6:282–286, 1985.

Russman, B.S. and Spiro, A.J. Case studies in pediatric neurology: The hypotonic infant. Motor unit disorders. American Academy of Neurology, 50th Annual Meeting, Minneapolis, 1998.

Duchenne Muscular Dystrophy

Aicarai, J. Diseases of the Nervous System in Childhood. Oxford: Blackwell, 1172, 1992.

Brett, E.M. Paediatric neurology. Pediatr. Rev. 6:195–200, 1985.

Berg, B.O. Principles of Child Neurology. New York: McGraw-Hill, 1665–1702, 1996.

Carroll, J. Diagnosis and management of Duchenne muscular dystrophy. Pediatr. Rev. 6:195–200, 1985.

Dubowitz, V. Color Atlas of Muscle Disorders in Childhood. New York: Yearbook Medical, 8–25, 1989.

Dumitru, D. et al. Electrodiagnostic Medicine. Philadelphia: Hanley and Belfus, 2002.

Fenichel, G.M. Clinical Pediatric Neurology: A Sign and Symptoms Approach, ed. 3. Philadelphia: W.B. Saunders, 176–201, 1997.

Griggs, R.C. et al. Evaluation and Treatment of Myopathies. Philadelphia: F.A. Davis, 93, 1995.

Mancall, E.L. Neuromuscular disease. Continuum, Part A. 8–15, 1993.

Menkes, J.H. and Sarnat, H.B. Child Neurology, ed. 6. Philadelphia: Lippincott Williams & Wilkins, 1046–1092, 2000.

Panteliadis, C.P. and Darras B.T. Pediatric Neurology: Theory and Praxis. Thessaloniki, 617–632, 1995.

Tawil, R. Outlook for therapy in the muscular dystrophies. Semin. Neurol. 19:81–85, 1999.

Tsao, C-Y. and Mendell, J.R. The childhood muscular dystrophies: Making order out of chaos. Semin. Neurol. 19:9–23, 1999.

Dermatomyositis

Brett, E.H. Paediatric Neurology, ed. 2. New York: Churchill Livingstone, 53–115, 1991.

Dubowitz, V. Color Atlas of Muscle Disorders in Childhood. New York: Yearbook Medical, 158–180, 1989.

Dumitru, D. et al. Electrodiagnostic Medicine. Philadelphia: Hanley and Belfus, 2002.

Engel, A.G. and Franzini-Armstrong, C. Myology, ed. 2. New York: McGraw-Hill, 1336–1337, 1994.

Fenichel, G.M. Clinical Pediatric Neurology, ed. 3. Philadelphia: W.B. Saunders, 176–204, 1997.

Menkes, J.H. Textbook of Child Neurology, ed. 4. Philadelphia: Lea and Febiger, 1990.

Spiro, A.J. Childhood Dermatomyositis and Polymyositis Pediatr. Rev. 6:163–172, 1984.

Infantile Botulism

Brett, E.M. Pediatric Neurology, ed. 2. New York: Churchill Livingstone, 649–651, 1991.

Dubowitz, V.R. Evaluation and Differential Diagnosis of the Hypotonic Infant. Pediatr. Rev. 6:237–243, 1985.

Evans, O.B. Guillain-Barré Syndrome in Children. Pediatr. Rev. 8:69–74, 1986.

Fenichel, G.M. Clinical Pediatric Neurology, ed. 3. Philadelphia: W.B. Saunders, 153–175, 1997.

Pellock, J.M. and Myer, E.C. Neurologic Emergencies in Infancy and Childhood, ed. 2. Boston: Butterworth-Heinemann, 242–261, 1993.

Rodder, A.H. Guillian-Barré syndrome. Philadelphia: F.A. Davis, 1991.

Russman, B.S. Case Studies in Pediatric Neurology. Education Program Syllabus, 50th Annual Meeting, Minneapolis, 1998.

Neonatal Transient Myasthenia Gravis

Dumitru, D. et al. Electrodiagnostic Medicine. Philadelphia: Hanley and Belfus, 2002.

Engel, A.C. and Amstrong, C.F. Myology, ed. 2, Vol. 2. New York: McGraw-Hill, 1772–1773, 1996.

Fenichel, G.M. Clinical Pediatric Neurology, ed. 3. Philadelphia: W.B. Saunders, 107, 1997.

Harper, C.M. Pediatric Disorders of the Neuromuscular Junction. American Academy of Neurology, 52nd Annual Meeting, San Diego, 2000.

Menkes, J.H. and Sarnat H.B. Child Neurology, ed. 6. Philadelphia: Lippincott Williams & Wilkins, 1040–1046, 2000.

Charcot-Marie-Tooth Disease

Berg, B.O. Child Neurology: A Clinical Manual, ed. 2. New York: J.B. Lippincott, 95–137, 1994.

Lyon, G. et al. Neurology of Hereditary Metabolic Diseases of Children, ed. 2. New York: McGraw-Hill, 177–272, 1996.

Mendell, J.R. Charcot-Marie-Tooth neuropathies and related disorders. Semin. Neurol. 18:41–47, 1998.

Ouvrier, R.A. et al. Peripheral Neuropathy in Childhood, ed. 2. London: MacKeith, 67–135, 1999.

Panteliadis, C.P. Pediatric Neurology: Theory and Praxis. Thessaloniki, 423–446, 1995.

Facioscapulohumeral Muscular Dystrophy

Engel, A.G. and Franzini-Armstrong, C. Myology, ed. 2. New York: McGraw-Hill, 1220–1232, 1994.

Fenichel, G.M. Clinical Pediatric Neurology, ed. 3. Philadelphia: W.B. Saunders, 177–204, 1997.

Kissel, J.T. Facioscapulohumeral Dystrophy. Semin. Neurol. 19:35–43, 1999.

Myotonic Dystrophy

Kaye, E.M. Fabry's Disease. Neurobase MedLink, Arbor, 1993–2000.

Lyon G. et al. Neurology of Hereditary Metabolic Diseases of Children. New York: Mc Graw Hill, 177–272, 1996.

Schaumburg H.H. et al. Disorders of Peripheral Nerves. Philadelphia: F. A. Davis, 89–98, 1983.

McArdle's Disease/Acid Maltase Deficiency

DiMauro, S. and Tsujino, S. Acid maltase deficiency. Neurobase MedLink, Arbor, 1993–2000.

Dumitru, D. et al. Electrodiagnostic Medicine. Philadelphia: Hanley and Belfus, 2002.

Dubowitz, V. Color Atlas of Muscle Disorders in Childhood. New York: Yearbook Medical, 125–132, 1989.

Engel, A.G. and Franzini Armstrong, C. Myology, ed. 2. New York: McGraw-Hill, 1533–1576, 1994.

Griggs, R.C. et al. Evaluation and Treatment of Myopathies. Philadelphia: F.A. Davis, 247–293, 1995.

Lyon, G. et al. Neurology of Hereditary Metabolic Diseases of Children. New York: McGraw-Hill, 64–66, 1996.

Menkes, J.H. and Sarnet, H.B. Child Neurology, ed. 6. New York: Lippincott Williams & Wilkins, 74–79, 2000.

Muscle disease. Continuum, Part A. Vol. 6, No. 2. April 2000.

19
Mitochondrial Disorders

Mitochondrial Encephalomyopathy

Vignette

In the last six months a 5-year-old girl started experiencing clumsiness during walking with great difficulty climbing stairs, headaches, unexplained episodes of vomiting, and seizures, following an upper respiratry tract infection. After one generalized tonic-clonic seizure, she complained of visual loss for several hours. The ER resident noticed that her pupils were normal with good reaction and funduscopic examination was intact. She also experienced several episodes of inability to find the right word that also resolved. During her hospitalization, a neurologist noted a left visual field defect, mild left sided weakness, and bilateral sensorineural hearing loss. During an early examination she was noted to have mild proximal muscle weakness with a positive Gower's sign. She was the full-term product of an uncomplicated pregnancy and delivery with a normal early developmental history. She had short stature and was easily fatigued by physical exercise. Her mother and maternal uncle had hearing loss. Her 6-year-old brother had seizures, mental retardation, and hearing loss.

Summary   This is a complicated vignette. At its core, the features of the case are the following:

- Seizures.
- Transitory blindness and transitory episodes of word-finding difficulty.
- Left visual field defect and hemiparesis.
- Hearing loss.
- Proximal muscle weakness with a positive Gower's sign.

- Family history significant for multiple abnormalities including seizures, hearing loss, and mental retardation.

Localization and Differential Diagnosis

The localization is multifocal and this seems to be a progressive disorder involving multiple systems. Some of the neurological symptoms such as seizures, aphasia, cortical blindness (as indicated by the normal pupils and intact funduscopic examination) suggest a cortical localization. The focal neurological deficits can be attributed to a demyelinating process or to a vascular ischemic mechanism. Another consideration is an aura phenomenon of migraine.

Proximal weakness with a positive Gower's sign is nonspecific and may indicate a disorder of muscles. This is also suggested by the easy fatigability after exercise (characteristic of metabolic myopathies).

Several characteristic features point to an underlying metabolic hereditary disorder such as:

- The occurrence of a neurological problem in siblings or relatives. (The child described in the vignette had the mother and a maternal uncle with hearing loss and an older brother with seizures, mental retardation and hearing loss.)
- Intermittent vomiting, and progressive cerebral dysfunction.

Several hereditary and metabolic disorders, such as homocytinuria, are associated with stroke and stroke-like episodes in children.

In the vignette presented, the neurological signs and symptoms and the multisystem involvement suggest the possibility of a juvenile mitochondrial encephalopathy. Some of the features of mitochondrial disorders include:

- Progressive disorder characterized by peripheral neuropathy, gastrointestinal dysfunction with pseudo-obstruction, ophthalmoplegia, and ptosis.

- Multiple stroke-like episodes, such as hemiparesis, aphasia, cortical blindness, and migraine-like headache with nausea and vomiting, precipitated by infections or hyperthermia.
- Progressive external ophthalmoplegia associated with retinitis pigmentosa with or without weakness and cardiac defects.
- Myoclonus, seizures, ataxia, weakness, and sensory neural hearing loss.
- Exercise intolerance, weakness, and other neurological findings.
- Short stature and progressive hearing loss, which are some common features of many mitochondrial disorders.

Syndromes such as mitochondrial myopathy, encephalopathy, lactic acidosis, and stroke (MELAS) seem to clinically fit the case described in the vignette.

Diagnosis

The mitochondrial encephalomyopathies are an heterogenous group of disorders affecting multiple systems, in particular the central and peripheral nervous system and in the latter the muscles seem typically susceptible to mitochondrial dysfunction. Other organs commonly affected are the heart, eyes, and ears.

Progressive external ophthalmoplegia, retinitis pigmentosa, and sensorineural hearing loss are some typical findings. Recurrent focal neurological deficits, hemiparesis, cortical blindness, speech difficulties, and seizures can occur. Exercise intolerance is another important sign of mitochondrial disorders. Cardiac dysfunction, endocrinopathies, and short stature can also be encountered in these disorders.

The diagnosis can be suggested by findings of elevated lactate level in the serum and CSF, and the demonstration of ragged red fibers on muscle biopsy due to subsarcolemmic accumulation of abnormal mitochondria.

Mitochondrial Encephalomyopathy with Lactic Acidosis and Stroke-like Episodes (MELAS)

MELAS is a mitochondrial disorder that usually presents in the first or second decade of life with stroke-like episodes, encephalopathy, focal and generalized seizures, dementia, and mitochondrial myopathy with lactic acidosis or ragged red fibers, or both. The episodes of focal neurological deficits that simulate stroke consist of aphasia, hemiparesis, visual field defects, cortical blindness, and so on. Exercise intolerance and proximal muscle weakness are also present. Many patients present with short stature and hearing loss. Recurrent unexplained vomiting and migraine-type headache are other features.

Some authors have attributed the intermittent episodes to intermittent vasospasm, caused by the abnormal smooth muscle cells of the vasculature.

Diagnosis

CT scan and MRI may demonstrate cortical hypointense lesions and basal ganglia calcifications. Lactate and pyruvate levels are increased at rest and may demonstrate a dramatic elevation after moderate exercise. Skeletal muscle biopsy shows ragged red fibers on modified Gomori's trichrome stain. In MELAS (as well as in myoclonic epilepsy and ragged red fibers and Kearns-Sayre syndromes) mitochondrial DNA mutations can be demonstrated.

Sleep Disorders: Kleine-Levin Syndrome

Vignette

A 14-year-old boy was brought to the emergency room by his concerned parents because of abnormal behavior. During the last two weeks he was sleeping most of the time, waking up only to eat voraciously, particularly sweets, and was seen to masturbate frequently. A similar episode occurred six months prior and resolved completely. In the emergency room he was asleep and when aroused, he became very irritable and uncooperative. His medical history was otherwise unremarkable.

Summary A 14-year-old boy with hypersomnolence, hyperphagia, and hypersexuality.

Localization and Differential Diagnosis

Several categories of disorders need to be considered, such as sleep disorders, psychiatric disorders, and processes involving the central nervous system (tumors, infections, trauma, vascular disorders).

Considering sleep disorders first, Kleine-Levin syndrome typically manifests in adolescent boys with episodes of marked hypersomnolence, hyperphagia, and hypersexuality lasting days to weeks and alternating with periods of normality. Idiopathic recurrent stupor presents with periods of altered level of consciousness that may further lead to stupor or coma lasting 2 to 72 hours.

Psychiatric disorders such as major depression and bipolar affective disorder can have symptoms of hypersomnolence, hyperphagia, and abnormal libido.

Tumors of the third ventricle can manifest with symptoms of diabetes insipidus, hypothermia or hyperthermia, and hypersomnolence of several weeks' duration.

Hypersomnolence can also be caused by infections such as encephalitis, traumatic head injury, or cerebrovascular pathology that involves the area of the mesencephalon or diencephalon.

Diagnosis

The Kleine-Levin syndrome manifests with episodes of hypersomnia lasting days to weeks and affects adolescent boys. Increased food intake usually occurs in most cases and other features such as hypersexuality with frequent masturbation can also be part of this disorder. Other behavioral abnormalities such as social withdrawal, memory dysfunction, irritability, incoherence, and inattentiveness can occur.

Kleine-Levine syndrome is a rare disease and the diagnosis is mainly clinical. EEG studies may be normal or demonstrate generalized slowing background activity during the episodes of hypersomnolence. Neuroimaging studies are normal.

Prognosis is favorable and this disorder is self-limited and tends to resolve during adulthood.

Congenital Defects: Mobius' Syndrome

Vignette

A 2-week-old baby girl was brought to you by her concerned mother because of sucking difficulties and because she did not seem to sleep with the eyes closed. She was the product of a full-term, uncomplicated pregnancy and vaginal delivery. On examination she appeared to lack facial expression and movement when crying. Additionally, a palsy of both external recti and mild atrophy of the left side of the tongue were noted. No other abnormalities were observed.

Summary A 2-week-old baby girl with multiple cranial nerve dysfunction. Facial nerve weakness is indicated by the sucking difficulties, inability to close the eyes during sleep, lack of facial expression, and absence of movement when crying. Other findings described are abducens nerve paralysis (bilateral external recti palsy) and hypoglossal nerve involvement with tongue atrophy.

Localization and Differential Diagnosis

Facial weakness can suggest different localizations and can be caused by a supranuclear palsy (pseudobulbar palsy), brainstem disorders, or motor unit dysfunctions (which include disorders of the facial nerve, neuromuscular juction, or facial muscles).

In the newborn, facial paralysis can be attributed to a developmental disorder or can have a traumatic etiology. Developmental abnormalities tend to preferentially involve the upper part of the face and be unnoticed at birth. The mother may first realize that the baby has difficulty sucking and does not completely close the eyelids during sleep. Other congenital defects can be present and suggest a congenital disorder.

Mobius' syndrome is the best known congenital aplasia of facial nerve nuclei and facial muscles (Fenichel). There is also usually involvement of the abducens and hypoglossal nerves.

When the etiology is traumatic, the facial paralysis occurs in isolation and usually involves one side of the face, particularly in children born vaginally after a prolonged and difficult labor. It is attributed to compression of the infant's mastoid area from the maternal sacral prominence (Fenichel).

Other neuromuscular disorders presenting with facial paralysis in a newborn are myotonic dystrophy, facioscapulohumeral muscular dystrophy, myasthenia gravis, and other myopathies.

Congenital myotonic dystrophy, which usually affects infants born to mothers with MD, may present with facial diplegia in the newborn but other symptoms are severe weakness, hypotonia, and respiratory distress. Abducens and hypoglossal nerves are not involved.

Facioscapulohumeral muscular dystrophy, characterized by facial diplegia, can simulate congenital aplasia of facial muscles. Abducens palsy and tongue atrophy are not features.

Transient neonatal myasthenia gravis can present in the newborn with ophthalmoplegia and facial weakness but tends to resolve within 20 days and affects children born to mothers with MG.

Congenital myasthenic syndromes may present with poor sucking, poor cry, and ophthalmoplegia but the weakness is fatigable and intermittent ptosis and respiratory weakness are important symptoms.

Considering the case presented in the vignette, Mobius' syndrome emerges as the preferred diagnosis.

Clinical Features

Mobius' syndrome consists of facial diplegia associated with paralysis of lateral gaze due to abducens paralysis. Poor sucking and decreased facial expression during crying are usually noticed first. The paralysis of the face is often bilateral and associated with paralysis of the abducens and hypoglossal nerves.

Other features include limb and craniofacial abnormalities such as tongue hemiatrophy, external ear anomalies, micrognatia, hypoplasia of digits, clubfoot deformity, and so on.

The disorder can be complicated by feeding difficulty that may lead to aspiration, speech problems, and corneal ulceration due to poor eyelid closure.

References

Mitochondrial Encephalomyopathy

Case records of the Massachussetts General Hospital. Case. N. Engl. J. Med. 39:914–23, 1998.

Hirano, M. Mitochondrial encephalomyopathy, lactic acidosis and stroke-like episodes syndrome. Neurobase MedLink, Arbor, 1993–2000.

Lyon, G. et al. Childhood and adolescent hereditary metabolic disorders. In: Neurology of Hereditary and Metabolic Diseases of Children, ed. 2. New York: McGraw-Hill, 254–257, 1996.

Roach, E.S. and Riela, A.R. Genetic causes of cerebrovascular disease. In: Pediatric Cerebrovascular Disorders, ed. 2. New York: Futura, 1995.

Kleine-Levin Syndrome

Adams, R.D. and Victor, M. Principles of Neurology, ed. 5. New York: McGraw-Hill, 343, 1993.

Aldrich, M. Idiopathic recurring stupor. Neurology MedLink, Arbor, 1993–2001.

Mobius' Syndrome

Fenichel, G.M. Clinical Pediatric Neurology, ed. 3. Philadelphia: W.B. Saunders, 344–353, 1997.

Glaser, J.S. Neuroophthalmology, ed. 2. Philadelphia: J.B. Lippincott, 424–425, 1990.

Menkes, J.H. and Sarnat, H.B. Child Neurology, ed. 6. Philadelphia: Lippincott Williams & Wilkins, 380–381, 2000.

Raymond, G. Mobius syndrome. Neurology MedLink, Arbor, 1993–2000.

20
Pediatric Ataxia

Ataxia-Telangiectasia

Vignette

A 3-year-old boy started having some problems walking at the age of 20 months, with clumsiness, irregular steps, lateral veering, and wide-based awkward motions. For the past three months he had developed slow, sinuous, involuntary movements with his right hand. Perinatal developmental and family histories were normal. His medical history was unremarkable except for frequent ear infections and several episodes of unexplained fever. He was bright, alert and cooperative. The resident noted some dilated venules on his ear lobes. His right upper extremity showed some choreoathetoid movements. He had mild dysarthria and unsteady wide-based gait. Deep tendon reflexes were diminished and plantar responses were equivocal.

Summary A 3-year-old boy with progressive ataxia. Other neurological findings include choreoathetoid movements, dysarthria, and hyporeflexia. Systemic symptoms characterized by recurrent otitis and unexplained fever are described as well as cutaneous findings, such as dilated venules on the ear lobes.

Localization and Differential Diagnosis

The localizations typically point to two structures: cerebellum and basal ganglia.

In the evaluation of ataxia it must first be determined if the process is static or progressive, and acute or chronic. The vignette illustrates a case of chronic progressive ataxia.

Tumors of the posterior fossa are important causes of progressive ataxia and should always be ruled out particularly because they are more common than supraten-torial tumors between the ages of 1 and 8 years (Fenichel). They usually manifest with signs of cerebellar involvement, such as unsteady gait, incoordination, and nystagmus, and signs of increased intracranial pressure due to obstruction of the fourth ventricle. Vomiting and headache are commonly an initial complaint. Papilledema, sixth and other cranial nerve palsies can also occur. These signs are not illustrated in the vignette.

Supratentorial brain tumors can also cause chronic ataxia (Fenichel) and manifest with gait abnormalities and cerebellar signs.

Progressive or intermittent cerebellar ataxia can also be a prominent sign of hereditary metabolic disorders where it can occur in isolation or be accompanied by other signs and symptoms that indicate a more widespread involvement of the central or peripheral nervous system. In addition to ataxia, neurological findings may include spasticity, hyperreflexia, optic nerve atrophy, extrapyramidal signs, seizures, myoclonus, dementia, psychomotor retardation, peripheral neuropathy, and so on.

Among the progressive hereditary degenerative encephalopathies, ataxia-telangiectasia best explains the findings described in the vignette. Ataxia-telangiectasia is characterized by progressive ataxia, dysarthria, choreoathetosis, typical cutaneous telangiectasias and recurrent infections.

Other hereditary disorders with ataxia that manifest in late infancy or early childhood include, for example, GM$_2$ gangliosidosis characterized by ataxia but also dysarthria, optic atrophy, and progressive cognitive decline. Ataxia is also a manifestation of the late infantile form of neuronal ceroid lipofuscinosis but typical features are myoclonic or other type of seizures that can be the presenting symptom. In addition, clinical findings include retinal degeneration, developmental regression, progressive dementia, and so on. Metachromatic leukodystrophy can manifest with a gait disturbance in the late infantile form but other important features are tremor, spasticity, progressive intellectual decline, optic atrophy, and so on.

Another progressive disorder causing ataxia is Friedreich's ataxia, characterized by significant cerebellar dysfunction, but other features such as spasticity, areflexia, and sensory disturbances help pinpoint the correct diagnosis.

Wilson's disease, abetalipoproteinemia, Refsum's syndrome, mitochondrial disorders, and early-onset cerebellar ataxia with retained tendon reflexes are also hereditary disorders manifesting with ataxia in childhood but the clinical findings help in formulating the diagnosis.

Other causes of chronic or progressive ataxias are congenital malformations, such as Arnold-Chiari malformation, that manifest with ataxia but prominent symptoms are usually occipital with neck pain, head tilt, cranial nerve abnormalities, hyperreflexia, and so on.

In summary, based on the information in the vignette, ataxia-telangiectasia is the preferred diagnosis.

Clinical Features

Ataxia-telangiectasia is a hereditary neurocutaneous disorder transmitted by autosomal recessive inheritance and characterized by a multitude of manifestations involving different systems. The gene's mutations are localized on chromosome 11q22.23.

Neurological symptoms include progressive truncal ataxia that is noted when the child starts walking, and dysarthria. Dystonia, choreoathetosis, and signs of extrapyramidal dysfunction may occur as well as symptoms of peripheral nerve involvement with decreased or absent deep tendon reflexes. Oculomotor abnormalities are other important signs, particularly oculomotor apraxia, which manifests with an inability to initiate lateral movements voluntarily or on command despite integrity of the anatomical pathway subserving motor function. Cognitive impairment with mild mental retardation may became apparent after a few years.

Extraneurological signs represent an important part of the disease. Telangiectasias are venous plexuses that are first noted when the child is 3 to 5 years of age, particularly on the bulbar conjunctiva, ear lobes, nose, flexor surfaces of the extremities, upper chest, and so on. They tend to prefer the areas exposed to the sun or to friction.

Abnormalities of both cell-mediated and antibody immunity increase the risk of recurrent infections, in particular recurrent sinopulmonary and middle ear infections. There is also an increased susceptibility to neoplasms, particularly Hodgkin's and non-Hodgkin's lymphomas and acute T cell leukemias.

Endocrine abnormalities are also reported, such as insulin-resistant diabetes, gonadal dysfunction, and so on.

Diagnosis

The clinical combination of progressive ataxia, oculomotor apraxia, cutaneous telangiectasias, and recurrent infections strongly suggest the diagnosis. The levels of serum alpha-fetoprotein and carcinoembryonic antigen are usually elevated. Immunological deficiencies can also be demonstrated.

Treatment

The treatment of infections should be very aggressive because sinopulmonary infections are considered the most common cause of death (Lechtenberg). Radiation exposure should be minimized due to patient's great sensitivity to radiation that may produce cellular and chromosomal abnormalities.

Prognosis is poor and the causes of death are recurrent complicated infections and neoplasms.

Friedreich's Ataxia

Vignette

An 8-year-old girl was noted by her gym teacher as being particularly clumsy. The pediatrician only found some mild scoliosis. By the age of 10, she was showing speech problems, gait difficulties, and bilateral hand tremor. On neurological examination, bilateral horizontal nystagmus and mild disc pallor were noted. Speech was dysarthric. She was unable to stand on one leg. Plantar responses were both extensor, and DTR could not be elicited in the legs. Gait was wide based and unsteady. Romberg's sign was markedly positive. Past history and family history were unremarkable except for a great-aunt with diabetes and clumsiness.

Summary A 10-year-old girl presenting with progressive ataxia with associated dysarthria and bilateral hand tremor. The neurological examination reveals bilateral nystagmus, disc pallor, dysarthria, positive Romberg's sign, gait ataxia, leg areflexia, and bilateral upgoing toes. Past history includes two years of progressively increasing symptoms. Family history includes a great-aunt with diabetes and clumsiness.

Localization and Differential Diagnosis

This clinical case describes a chronic progressive disorder, characterized by ataxia in association with other neurological abnormalities.

Signs of midline cerebellar syndrome (McDonald in Berg) are nystagmus and gait ataxia. Sensory ataxia that results from loss of proprioceptive function manifests with a positive Romberg's sign, wide-base unsteady gait, and reflex loss (McDonald).

Several disorders can cause chronic progressive ataxia in children as we mentioned in the prior vignette. They include hereditary metabolic or neurodegenerative disorders or acquired disorders, in particular brain tumors, which always need to be ruled out in cases of progressive ataxia and no prior apparent neurological problems. Congenital malformations such as Chiari's malformation and platybasia can present with progressive ataxia but important features are occipital pain, head tilt, lower cranial nerve dysfunction, and hyperreflexia. Subacute viral infections may also cause progressive ataxia, particularly in immunodepressed children. Demyeliniated disorders, such as multiple sclerosis, also enter the differential diagnosis of ataxia, either intermittent or progressive, but reflex loss is not a feature.

The vignette presented suggests a possible hereditary disorder with an autosomal recessive pattern of inheritance by indicating in the family history of the child a great-aunt with clumsiness and diabetes. Therefore the inherited ataxias should be considered in the differential diagnosis.

The inherited ataxias manifest with progressive gait abnormality, limb ataxia, and other signs of cerebellar dysfunction associated with neurological findings that may consist of oculomotor abnormalities, extrapyramidal and pyramidal signs, visual loss, cognitive impairment, and signs of peripheral nerve dysfunction. Acquired disorders, particularly cerebellar tumors, congenital malformations, and multiple sclerosis need to be excluded.

Among the progressive inherited ataxias, Friedreich's ataxia, which combines sensory and cerebellar ataxia and is characterized by progressive ataxia, dysarthria, proprioceptive loss, areflexia, and extensor plantar responses, should be considered first and should rank high on the list of the differential diagnostic possibilities.

Sensory and cerebellar ataxia are also features of abetalipoproteinemia, which manifests with progressive cerebellar and limb ataxia, dysarthria, sensory loss, and areflexia, but also retinitis pigmentosa and acanthocytosis.

Ataxia with vitamin E deficiency can simulate Friedreich's ataxia and may create a diagnostic challenge manifesting with progressive ataxia, sensory loss, areflexia, and sometimes cardiac and skeletal abnormalities.

Juvenile GM_2 gangliosidosis can have similarities with Friedreich's ataxia. Additional findings in juvenile GM_2 gangliosidosis are spasticity, optic atrophy, dementia, and so on.

Myoclonic epilepsy and ragged red fibers (MERRF) may also show features resembling those of Friedreich's ataxia but important typical findings are myoclonus, seizures, and the mytochondrial myopathy.

Wilson's disease can manifest with signs of cerebellar dysfunction but other features such as the Kaiser-Fleischer ring point to the correct diagnosis.

Clinical Features

Friedreich's ataxia is the most common form of hereditary ataxia and is characterized by an autosomal recessive inheritance and onset of manifestations in the first decade of life. The mutation in the gene is localized on chromosome 9q13.

Typical symptoms include insidious progressive gait and limb ataxia, associated with dysarthria and areflexia. Extensor plantar responses can also be demonstrated in the majority of patients in combination with areflexia. Nystagmus is common, usually horizontal, and optic atrophy can also be found.

Disturbance of proprioception is manifested by absence or decreased joint position sense and vibration in the lower extremities but the upper extremities can also be involved. Skeletal deformities include high-arched foot (pes cavus) with hammer toes and hyposcoliosis. Cardiac manifestations are represented by a cardiomyopathy. Diabetes can also occur.

Summary of the clinical characteristics:

- Neurological features
  - Progressive ataxia.
  - Dysarthria.
  - Dysmetria.
  - Nystagmus.
  - Proprioceptive loss.
  - Areflexia.
  - Bilateral Babinski's sign.
  - Optic atrophy.
- Skeletal features
  - Pes cavus.
  - Hammer toes.
  - Scoliosis.
- Cardiac and other features
  - Cardiomyopathy.
  - Nonspecific ST and T wave changes.
  - Diabetes mellitus.

Diagnosis

MRI study may demonstrate cerebellar atrophy and is important in ruling out cerebellar tumors and malformations. Nerve conduction studies typically show absent or very reduced sensory nerve action potentials. Serum vitamin E levels should always be measured.

Treatment

Treatment is supportive and symptomatic.

Posterior Fossa Tumor as Cause of Chronic Ataxia

Vignette

A previously healthy 7-year-old boy, after returning from a school trip, started complaining of early morning headache and vomiting for a few days that resolved and were treated as a stomach virus by the pediatrician. Two weeks later he again complained of headache and vomiting and developed a squint. In school, the gym teacher noted that he was clumsy, irritable, easily knocked over, and had an akward gait. Finally the pediatrician referred him to a neurologist who found bilateral abduction defect and gross nystagmus on lateral gaze. Funduscopic examination revealed blurry margins. DTRs were hyperactive and the gait wide based and unsteady.

Summary A 7-year-old boy who developed headache, vomiting, a squint, and unsteady gait. Neurological examination shows bilateral paralysis of abduction, nystagmus, papilledema, hyperactive reflexes, and ataxia.

Localization and Differential Diagnosis

The vignette suggests the following:

- Nonlocalizing signs suggestive of increased intracranial pressure: headache, vomiting, papilledema, bilateral VI (false localizing sign).
- Localizing signs, such as ataxia, that indicate involvement of the midline cerebellar structures.

Brain tumor needs always to be excluded in a previously healthy child who presents with progressive ataxia accompanied by early headache and vomiting. Vomiting is an important sign of increased intracranial pressure and also the most common presenting sign of cerebellar tumors (Menkes). Cranial nerve dysfunction, particularly sixth nerve paralysis (pseudosixth), commonly accompanies increased intracranial pressure. Cerebellar tumors include, in particular, medulloblastoma, cerebellar astrocytoma, and ependymoma.

Medulloblastomas are highly malignant and rapidly growing tumors that originate from the velum of the fourth ventricle. The most common symptoms are due to hydrocephalus and increased intracranial pressure and include headache, nausea, and vomiting that typically occur early in the morning. Vomiting usually represents the most common presenting sign and can be due to the increased intracranial pressure or to an effect on the vomiting center. Papilledema and sixth nerve paralysis are other important signs. Gait abnormality with progressive ataxia is also common. Seeding of the tumor to the subarachnoid space and spinal region can also occur. The MRI study demonstrates an isointense or hypointense mass on T_1 involving the vermis and fourth ventricle with hyperintensity on T_2. The mass is highly enhancing after Gd-DPTA. Medulloblastomas have a poor prognosis, particularly in younger children or when there is significant postoperative residual mass or leptomeningeal seeding.

Cerebellar astrocytomas are well-circumscribed, slowly growing tumors that can originate in the cerebellar hemispheres or in the vermis and tend to cause unsteady gait, incoordination, and symptoms of increased intracranial pressure.

Ependymomas originate from the roof and floor of the fourth ventricle and are characterized by a slower course of presentation than medulloblastomas and marked signs of increased intracranial pressure with symptoms that are usually progressive but sometimes intermittent. Ataxia and cranial nerve dysfunction also occur.

Acute Ataxia

Vignette

A previously healthy 2-year-old girl woke up unable to stand or walk. Ten days earlier, she had experienced several bouts of diarrhea that resolved in a few days. On examination, she was alert and cooperative. Bilateral horizontal nystagmus and head titubation were noted. Walking was very awkward and accompanied by a great deal of staggering, holding on to furniture, and occasional falling. There was no history of headache.

Summary Acute ataxia in a 2-year-old girl.

Localization and Differential Diagnosis

Acute ataxia can be due to cerebellar dysfunction or to loss of proprioceptive function due to a disorder of the posterior columnae or the peripheral nerves.

Ataxia due to cerebellar dysfunction manifests with a staggering, unsteady wide-based gait. Other signs include dysarthria with scanned speech, dysmetria, head titubation, nystagmus, and so on. Sensory ataxia manifests with a cautious broad-based gait that relies on visual guidance to maintain the balance and typically worsens with the eye closed (positive Romberg's sign). Deep tendon reflexes are absent or diminished and abnormal joint position sense and vibration are noted in the lower extremities.

The child in the vignette shows signs of cerebellar dysfunction with marked ataxia, horizontal nystagmus, and head titubation. The history reveals that 10 days prior to the event she suffered several bouts of diarrhea, which could imply a gastrointestinal infection. Acute ataxia in children is usually caused by an infectious process or by ingestion of drugs. Postinfectious, acute cerebellar ataxia is common.

Viral infections, particularly respiratory or gastrointestinal, may precede the onset of ataxia. Varicella in particular can frequently be associated with acute cerebellar ataxia in children. The symptoms occur acutely with mild unsteady gait or total inability to stand and walk in an otherwise alert child. Nystagmus and dysarthria can also be observed. Ataxia has the maximum intensity at onset and is self-limited, slowly decreasing with a complete recovery that varies from days to several months. Treatment is symptomatic.

Brainstem encephalitis can manifest with acute cerebellar ataxia, but most children have other neurological abnormalities, such as signs of cranial nerve and brainstem dysfunction, headache, fever, vomiting, altered level of consciousness, seizures, and so on. These features are not present in the vignette.

Miller Fisher syndrome manifests with acute ataxia following a viral illness but ophthalmoplegia and reflex loss are additional features.

Acute or subacute ataxia can be part of the opsoclonus-myoclonus-ataxia syndrome that is accompanied by chaotic eye movements, myoclonic jerks, personality changes, and may precede the discovery of an occult neuroblastoma.

Drug intoxication, especially accidental drug ingestion, is another important cause of acute ataxia in children particularly between 1 and 4 years of age (Fenichel). Agents such as alcohol, thallium, anticonvulsant drugs, and antihistamines can be responsible and a toxic screen is always a priority in the diagnosis of a child presenting with acute ataxia.

MRI of the brain is also important because brain tumors always need to be excluded. Posterior fossa tumors generally present with insidious chronic ataxia but an acute picture can be due to complications such as hemorrhage into the tumor or hydrocephalus.

Vascular disorders, such as cerebellar hemorrhage, infarct, vasculitis, coagulopathy, and homocystinuria, may cause acute ataxia often accompanied by other acute neurological symptoms.

Trauma and migraine, particularly basilar migraine, can manifest with acute ataxia, usually in association with other signs of vertebrobasilar dysfunction.

Acute vestibular neuronitis presenting with episodes of severe vertigo and inability to stand and walk may sometimes cause some diagnostic difficulty.

Finally, multiple sclerosis can present with acute ataxia following a febrile illness but the diagnosis requires the evidence of multiple attacks of neurological dysfunction separated in time and space.

References

Ataxia-Telangiectasia

Berg, B.O. Child Neurology: A Clinical Manual, ed. 2. Philadelphia: J.B. Lippincott, 287–305, 1994.

Brett, E.M. (Ed.) Paediatric Neurology, ed. 2. New York: Churchill Livingstone, 232–523, 1991.

Fenichel, G.M. Clinical Pediatric Neurology: A Sign and Symptoms Approach, ed. 3. Philadelphia: W.B. Saunders, 231–252, 1997.

Leghtenberg R. (Ed.) Handbook of Cerebellar Diseases. New York: Marcel Dekker, 477–490, 1993.

Lyon, G. et al. Neurology of Hereditary Metabolic Diseases of Children, ed. 2. New York: McGraw-Hill, 124–176, 1996.

Subramony, S.H. and Nance, M. Diagnosis and Management of the Inherited Ataxias. Neurologist 4:327–338, 1998.

Friedreich's Ataxia

Berg, B.O. Child Neurology: A Clinical Manual, ed. 2. Philadelphia: J.B. Lippincott, 287–305, 1994

Brett, E.M. Paediatric Neurology, ed. 2. New York: Churchill Livingstone, 223–228, 1991.

De Jong, J.M.B.V. (Ed.). Friedreich's disease. In: Handbook of Clinical Neurology. Vol. 16: Hereditary neuropathies and spinocerebellar atrophies. New York: Elsevier, 299–330, 1991.

DeMichele, G. et al. Childhood onset of Friedreich ataxia: A clinical and genetic study of 36 cases. Neuropediatrics 27: 3–7, 1996.

Durr, A. et al. Clinical and genetic abnormalities in patients with Friedreich's ataxia. N. Engl. J. Med. 335:1169–75, 1996.

Fenichel, G.M. Clinical Pediatric Neurology, ed. 3. Philadelphia: W.B. Saunders, 230–252, 1997.

Ouvrier, R.A. et al. Peripheral Neuropathy in Childhood, ed. 2. London: MacKeith, 1999.

Subramony, S.H. and Nance, M. Diagnosis and management of the inherited ataxias. Neurologist 4:327–338, 1998.

Posterior Fossa Tumor

Brett, E.M. Paediatric Neurology, ed. 2. New York: Churchill Livingstone, 511–544, 1991.

Fenichel, G.M. Clinical Pediatric Neurology, ed. 3. Philadelphia: W.B. Saunders, 230–252, 1997.

Lee, M.S. et al. Sixth nerve palsies in children. Pediatr. Neurol. 20:49–52, 1999.

Menkes, J.H. Textbook of Child Neurology, ed. 4. Philadelphia: Lea and Febiger, 526–582, 1990.

Mollman J.E. Neuro-oncology. Continuum, Vol. 1, No. 2, 48–62, Dec. 1994.

Packer, R.J. Brain and spinal cord tumors. American Academy of Neurology, 52nd Annual Meeting, San Diego, 2000.

Acute Ataxias

Chutorian, A.M. and Pavlakis S.G. Acute ataxia. In: Pellock, J.M. and Myer, E.C. (Eds.). Neurologic Emergencies in Infancy and Childhood, ed. 2. Boston: Butterworth-Heinemann, 208–219, 1993.

Fenichel, G.M. Clinical Pediatric Neurology, ed. 3. Philadelphia: W.B. Saunders, 230–252, 1997.

Stumpf, D.A. Acute ataxia. Pediatr. Rev. 8:303–306, 1987.

21
Pediatric Cerebrovascular Disorders

Paradoxical Emboli

Vignette

A 10-year-old, healthy boy, while listening to his favorite music, suddenly sneezed several times. He then noticed some frontal and retroorbital headache accompanied by a complete inability to move his left arm. In the emergency room there was marked weakness of the left face and arm with minimal weakness of his leg and some decreased sensation to pinprick. Visual fields and extraocular movements were intact. There was no prior history of headache and a drug screen was reported as negative. The family history was unremarkable.

Summary A 10-year-old boy with acute onset of left hemiparesis and hypoesthesia after sneezing associated with frontal and retroorbital headache.

Localization and Differential Diagnosis

The vignette describes an acute neurological event characterized by headache, and focal signs involving predominantly the left face and upper extremity and to a lesser extent the left lower extremity.

The differential diagnosis includes several possibilities:

- Acute vascular event (stroke): ischemic (embolic or thrombotic) or hemorrhagic due to various etiologies.
- Space-occupying lesion, such as tumor, complicated by acute hemorrhage.
- Inflammatory disorders causing vasculitis.
- Intracerebral abscess causing edema and localized compression.
- Complications of migraine (hemiplegic or migrainous stroke).
- Trauma.

- Seizures with postictal paralysis.
- Metabolic abnormalities such as hypoglycemia or diabetes.

All these mechanisms can cause an acute focal event.

The child described experienced sudden onset of headache and focal weakness after sneezing several times. This sequence may bring into consideration a mechanism involving an increased intrathoracic pressure and right heart pressure during Valsalva's maneuver that can accompany excessive sneezing, coughing, or stool straining. This mechanism may be responsible for the occurrence of paradoxical emboli originating from thrombi located in the pelvic area or lower extremities in children, for example, with septal defects or patent foramen ovale.

Cerebral embolism manifests with an acute neurological deficit that is maximal at onset. The occlusion of a superficial branch of the right middle cerebral artery may explain weakness more severe in the face and upper extremity with relative sparing of the lower extremity. Therefore, in the differential diagnosis of an acute vascular event occurring in a child, cerebral embolism is considered first but it is also important to rule out thrombotic or hemorrhagic disorders causing hemiplegia. Cerebral embolism is the most common nontraumatic cerebrovascular disorder in children (Roach and Riela).

Ischemic Strokes

Ischemic strokes account for approximately 45 percent of all pediatric cases of strokes (Mendoza and Conway). Three possible mechanisms are responsible for the cerebral ischemia: embolism, thrombosis, and hypoperfusion. The most common category of disease that leads to cerebral infarction in children is congenital or acquired heart disease (Riela). Cardiac disease is a common predisposing factor for cerebral emboli that originate from clots within the cardiac chambers or from vegetations on the valvular leaflets. Table 21.1 presents common etiology of brain ischemia due to embolism and thrombosis in pediatric patients.

Embolic Stroke

Cerebral embolism is characterized by a sudden neurological deficit that is maximal at onset and may show a partial or total improvement due to lysis and reinstatement of the perfusion. Emboli in children usually originate from the heart when congenital or acquired structural abnormalities are present. Sources of cerebral emboli in children include

Cardiac sources
- Congenital heart defects.
  - Cyanotic congenital heart disease.
  - Atrial and ventricular septal defect.
  - Coarctation of the aorta.
  - Transposition of great vessels.
- Acquired heart disease.
  - Rheumatic heart disease.
  - Bacterial and nonbacterial endocarditis.
  - Cardiomyopathy.
  - Atrial myxoma.
  - Mitral valve prolapse.
  - Arrhythmias: Atrial fibrillation occurs in children with rheumatic heart disease, Ebstein's anomaly, atrial septal defect, and total anomalous pulmonary venous return (Riela).

Arterial sources
- Vasculopathies: Moya-moya, fibromuscular dysplasia.
- Catheterization and other procedures.
- Arteritis and arterial aneurysms.
- Trauma.

Other sources
- Air/fat embolism.
- Paradoxical emboli.

Paradoxical Emboli and Differential Diagnosis of an Acute Focal Event

Paradoxical embolization occurs when a cardiac defect allows direct entrance of embolic formations into the systemic circulation. The source of embolization derives from thrombi that form in the lower extremities or pelvic veins but also from pulmonary fistulas. Congenital heart defects, such as atrial or ventricular septal defects, patent foramen ovale with significant shunt, truncus arteriosus, and so on, or large pulmonary arteriovenous fistulas that can be found in children with hereditary hemorrhagic telangiectasias, can result in the occurrence of paradoxical embolism.

In the differential diagnosis of the vignette, an acute vascular event is first considered but other causes of acute focal weakness need to be presented.

Space-occupying lesions, such as neoplasms, usually manifest with progressive hemiparesis but if a hemor-

TABLE 21.1 Common embolic and thrombotic causes of pediatric brain ischemia.

Category	Condition
Heart disease	Congenital cardiac defects
	Cyanotic congenital heart disease
	Atrial and ventricular septal defects
	Patent ductus arteriosus
	Aortic and mitral stenosis
	Mitral valve prolapse
	Coarctation
	Acquired heart disease
	Rheumatic fever
	Endocarditis
	Myocarditis
	Cardiomyopathies
	Cardiac arrhythmia
	Atrial myxoma
Hematological abnormalities	Sickle cell anemia
	Disorders causing a hypercoagulable state:
	—Antithrombin III deficiency
	—Protein C/S deficiency
	—Lupus anticoagulant
	Leukemia
	Polycytemia
	Trombocytosis
	Liver disorders
Vasculitis/vasculopathy	Moya-moya disease
	Fibromuscular dysplasia
	Infectious and autoimmune vasculitides
	Primary cerebral angiitis
	Venous thrombosis
Metabolic and genetic disorders	Homocystinuria
	Fabry's disease
	Mitochondrial disorders (MELAS)
	Methylmalonic aciduria
	Neurofibromatosis
Migraine	Migrainous stroke
	Drug ingestion, toxins causing vasospasm and stroke
	Cocaine or amphetamines use
	Glue sniffing
	Oral contraceptives
Systemic disorders	Hypertension
	Diabetes
	Systemic hypotension
	Hypernatremia
Genetic disorders	Mitochondrial disorders
	Homocystinuria
	Fabry's disease
	Pseudoxanthoma elasticum

rhage acutely occurs into the tumor, this will result in an acute focal deficit in addition to headache and decreased level of consciousness.

Complicated migraines can manifest with transitory neurological deficits, particularly hemiplegia and less commonly ophthalmoplegia, that can occur prior to or after the headache and also in the absence of headache. This is not always an easy diagnosis, particularly if the characteristic migraine symptoms are not present. Other etiologies that need to be excluded are antiphospholipid antibodies and other disorders that can cause a hypercoagulable state.

Trauma and infections can also cause acute hemiplegia but can easily be excluded from the vignette. Bacterial and viral infections can be responsible for an acute focal neurological deficit because of various mechanisms, including vascular inflammation, cerebral infarction, sinus occlusion, and parenchymal necrosis. Additional symptoms are usually present, such as fever, nausea, vomiting, altered sensorium, and seizures.

Focal seizures, particularly if prolonged, can be followed by hemiplegia and may suggest an underlying vascular lesion, such as a cerebral malformation or an infarction.

Metabolic disorders, particularly hypoglycemia, diabetes mellitus, or homocystinuria need to be mentioned as causes of acute hemiplegia that enter into the differential diagnosis of this vignette.

Diagnosis

- Physical and neurological evaluation.
- Laboratory studies.
  - Blood count PT and PTT.
  - Special studies, in selected cases.
    - Hemoglobin electrophoresis.
    - Protein C/S.
    - Antithrombin III.
    - Antiphospholipid antibodies.
    - Lupus anticoagulant.
    - Lactate pyruvate (for mitochondrial dysfunction).
    - HIV, VDRL.
- Neuroimaging studies.
  - CT.
  - MRI.
  - MRA and angiography in selected cases.
- Cardiac studies.
  - EKG.
  - Transesophageal echocardiogram in cases of congenital cardiac defects or to demonstrate an intracardiac thrombus or valvular vegetations.

Treatment

Roach and Riela recommend the short-term use of heparin for patients at risk for recurrent, nonseptic cerebral embolism and with minimal risk of secondary hemorrhage. The long-term use of anticoagulation with warfarin is based on situations that carry a high risk of stroke, such as in children with congenital and acquired heart disease, venous sinus thrombosis, coagulopathies and hypercoagulable states, arterial dissection, and so on.

The use of antiplatelet agents in children is controversial, particularly regarding the efficacy and effective dose of aspirin, which has been used in low daily doses.

Bacterial endocarditis and septic embolism are treated with intravenous antibiotics for at least six to eight weeks.

Homocystinuria

Vignette

A 10-year-old boy, mildly retarderd and with history of cataract, underwent an emergency appendectomy. The postoperative period was complicated by right hemiplegia and aphasia. There was no history of heart disease, TIA, seizures, trauma, or infections. He never experienced migraine and his family history was unremarkable. He was tall and slender. The pediatric resident noted that he had pes cavus, hyposcoliosis, highly arched palate, and multiple erythematous spots over his cheeks but did not detect any organomegaly. Neurological examination showed expressive aphasia and dense right hemiplegia, more severe in the face and upper extremities with relative sparing of the lower extremities.

Summary A 10-year-old boy experiencing an acute vascular event after surgery. Involvement of several other systems is indicated:

- Ocular system: Cataract.
- Skeletal system: Pes cavus, hyposcoliosis, highly arched palate.
- Skin: Multiple erythematous spots over the cheeks.
- CNS: Mental retardation, acute hemiplegia, and aphasia.

Localization and Differential Diagnosis

The expressive aphasia with right hemiplegia more severe in the face and upper extremity, with relative sparing of the lower extremity, localized to a lesion involving the upper trunk of the left middle cerebral artery. The involvement of multiple systems, including skeletal, eye, skin, and central nervous system, points to a neurometabolic disorder where stroke is a significant part of the clinical manifestations.

Four neurometabolic genetic disorders—homocystinuria, Fabry's disease, MELAS, and methylenetetrafolate reductase deficiency—are responsible for strokes in children and young adults due to vasculopathies and venous or arterial occlusion.

Homocystinuria is the most common genetic disorder that affects the brain vasculature and leads to premature atherosclerosis and stroke (Caplan). The clinical symptomatology involves multiple systems with skeletal deformities such as pes cavus and hyposcoliosis, dermatological features such as malar flush, ocular abnormalities with lens dislocation, cataract, and so on, and neurological abnormalities with mental retardation and multiple cerebrovascular accidents. The clinical vignette clearly describes a case of homocystinuria.

MELAS (mitochondrial encephalomyopathy with lactic acidosis and stroke-like episodes) is a mitochondrial disorder characterized by multiple manifestations that include stroke-like episodes, migraine-type headache, recurrent vomiting, epileptic seizures, proximal muscle weakness, short stature, and exercise intolerance. Lactic acid levels are increased in blood and CSF and muscle biopsy demonstrates ragged red fibers.

Fabry's disease is a sex-linked lysosomal storage disease due to deficiency of alpha-galactosidase A. The clinical manifestations include signs of peripheral neuropathy manifesting with painful paresthesias, cutaneous lesions presenting with a red-purple maculopapular rash, and cerebrovascular complications, in particular hemiplegia and aphasia due to premature atherosclerosis.

Methylenetetrafolate reductase deficiency can manifest with cerebrovascular complications due to thrombotic occlusion, but also vomiting, seizures, mental deterioration, and so on, in the absence of any ocular or skeletal abnormalities.

Clinical Features

Homocystinuria is a disorder of methionine metabolism, due to a defect of cystathionine B-synthase, which catalyzes the conversion of homocystine and serine to cystathionine. This abnormality results in homocystinuria and increased plasma and CSF levels of homocystine and methionine. The transmission is autosomal recessive.

Homocystinuria is responsible for a multitude of manifestations due to involvement of ocular, skeletal, cutaneous, vascular, and CNS systems. Ocular manifestations are represented by ectopia lentis, glaucoma, retinal detachment, and cataracts. Skeletal abnormalities include pes cavus, hyposcoliosis, high-arched palate, arachnodactyly, and so on. Children and adolescents are tall and slender and have features that simulate Marfan's syndrome. Skin anomalies manifest with livedo reticularis and multiple erythematous spots over the maxillary area and cheeks.

Mental retardation may occur and cognitive impairment can also be attributed to multiple infarcts. Focal and generalized seizures have been described, even in the absence of strokes.

Vascular complications that can occur particularly following surgery, even if minor, or intravenous injection, are responsible for a multitude of manifestations that include myocardial infarction, deep venous thrombosis

with pulmonary embolism, renal artery and vein thrombosis, and cerebral thromboembolic events.

Diagnosis

The diagnosis of homocystinuria can be demonstrated by the increased urinary excretion of homocystine, elevated plasma levels of methionine and homocystine, and a positive urinary cyanide-nitroprusside reaction.

It is important to reach the diagnosis as promptly as possible because early therapeutic intervention may prevent some of the complications.

Treatment

Pyridoxine or betaine therapy and dietary manipulation with restriction of methionine and cystine supplementation have shown efficacy in some patients.

Intracranial Hemorrhage

Vignette

An 8-year-old girl was playing basketball with her teammates when she suddenly screamed, complained of headache, and vomited. Her mother could not keep her awake. There was no previous history of trauma or seizure disorder. In the emergency room she was drowsy and her neck was rigid. Preretinal hemorrhages were present on the left eye. During the next several hours she experienced two generalized tonic-clonic seizures.

Summary A previously healthy 8-year-old girl experiencing sudden onset of headache, vomiting, decreased level of consciousness, stiff neck, and seizures.

Localization

A sudden onset of headache, vomiting, and decreased level of consciousness accompanied by signs of meningeal irritation and increased intracranial pressure in the absence of focal neurological deficits is highly suggestive of subarachnoid hemorrhage (SAH).

Infants and young children may have a less typical presentation with low-grade fever, hypersensitivity, irritability, seizures, and vomiting.

Focal and generalized convulsions can occur and focal neurological deficits are not noted unless there is extension into the brain parenchyma or if vasospasm causes brain infarcts. Signs of increased intracranial pressure manifest with headache, vomiting, and papilledema. Cranial nerve dysfunction mainly affects the sixth and third nerve, the latter in particular can be an indication of a posterior communicating artery aneurysm.

Subarachnoid hemorrhage in children is attributed primarily to trauma.

Nontraumatic causes of SAH include sickle cell disease and coagulopathies, aneurysmal rupture, arteriovenous malformations, and so on.

Table 21.2 presents the etiology of intracranial (subarachnoid and intraparenchymal) hemorrhage in children.

Acute Hemiplegia

Vignette

A previously healthy, 20-month-old girl started experiencing attacks of head shaking and eye rolling several days after a febrile upper respiratory infection. She then developed acute left-sided weakness. On examination, left hemiparesis, hyperreflexia and a left Babinski's sign were noted. Cranial nerves were normal. She was drowsy and uncooperative during the rest of the examination.

Summary A previously healthy, 20-month-old girl experiencing episodes that could represent seizures (head shaking and eye rolling) after a respiratory infection with subsequent acute left hemiplegia.

Differential Diagnosis

The differential diagnosis of acute hemiplegia in children includes several categories of disorders, and among them, stroke is the most common cause of weakness.

Acute hemiplegia can be due to a vascular disorder, can follow an epileptic seizure, or can be a migraine component (hemiplegic migraine). Other possibilities include metabolic abnormalities, infectious processes, trauma, or a neoplastic lesion (Griesemer). Etiological factors predisposing to an acute vascular event such as congenital or acquired heart disease, sickle cell anemia, coagulopathies, vasculitis, or vasculopathies can be recognized in many but not all cases of strokes in children.

Cerebrovascular disorders have been divided based on the pathophysiology into ischemic (embolic and thrombotic) and hemorrhagic.

Cardiac abnormalities, congenital or acquired, are usually the source of emboli in children. They include disorders such as septal defects, aortic and mitral valve insufficiency, complex cardiac abnormalities, rheumatic valvular disease, myocarditis, cardiomyopathy, atrial myxoma, and so on.

Vasculitis of the intracranial vessels, which is usually attributed to infections or autoimmune disorders, may

TABLE 21.2 Etiology of pediatric subarachnoid and intraparenchymal hemorrhage.

Category	Condition
Trauma	The most common cause of intracranial hemorrhage in children. In infants SAH should always bring into consideration the possibility of child abuse.
Prematurity	Germinal matrix hemorrhage.
Structural vascular malformations	Cerebral aneurysm. Symptomatic intracranial aneurysms are uncommon in the pediatric group. Children tend to have more aneurysms in the posterior circulation and carotid bifurcation and tend to have larger aneurysm. Males are more affected than females. Subarachnoid hemorrhage is usually the initial presentation of an intracranial aneurysm in both children and adults.
	Arteriovenous malformations. Characterized by direct communication of arteries with veins. The symptoms of AVMs are influenced by size, location, and age at presentation. Vein of Galen malformations manifest in the neonatal period with congestive heart failure and in infants with macrocephaly, hydrocephalus and so on. In older children or adolescents, AVM typically manifests with headache, seizures and intraparenchymal or subarachnoid hemorrhage.
	Cavernous malformations. Characterized by well-circumscribed, dilated vessels, sometimes multiple, and manifesting with headache, recurrent seizures, intracranial hemorrhage, etc.
Coagulopathies	Hereditary Hemophilia A, B, and other factor deficiency. Thrombocytopenia. Acquired Vitamin K deficiency. Liver dysfunction with coagulation defects.
Hemoglobinopathies	Sickle cell anemia.
Vasculitis	
Sinovenous thrombosis	
Hemorrhagic infarction	
Hemorrhagic encephalopathy due to hypernatremia	
Tumor, infections	

manifest with arterial thrombosis, intraparenchymal or subarachnoid hemorrhage, or sinovenous occlusion. Infections may predispose to cerebrovascular occlusive disease, and often an upper respiratory infection may precede the onset of the stroke. Bacterial meningitis can be complicated by cerebral vasculitis and strokes in children due to acute inflammation of the vessel's wall and occlusion.

Other causes of intracranial arteritis include tuberculous meningitis, HIV, varicella infection, and so on. Among the autoimmune vasculitides, systemic lupus erythematosus can manifest with cerebral infarction due to arterial thrombosis, but also with hemorrhage and venous occlusion.

Hematological disorders may be characterized by arterial or venous occlusion or hemorrhage. Sickle cell disease in particular can predispose to stroke, especially ischemic infarction, often during the time of a crisis when the child is febrile or dehydrated following an infection. Venous occlusion and subarachnoid hemorrhage are also complications of sickle cell disease. Other hematological disorders, such as trombocytopenia, polycytemia, and disorders of coagulation such as hemophilia A (X-linked factor VIII deficiency) may be responsible for stroke and acute hemiplegia.

Metabolic disease (homocystinuria, Fabry's disease, MELAS) can produce arterial and venous occlusions.

Among the vasculopathies, moya-moya syndrome can present with acute hemiplegia. Clinical symptoms vary from transitory ischemic attacks to strokes, seizures, and cognitive decline. The Japanese word *moyamoya* meaning "like a puff of smoke" best describes the angiographic picture of abnormal vascular network at the base of the brain.

Trauma can cause carotid occlusion in children, for example, after a fall when the child is carrying some object in the mouth such as a lollipop or a pencil, and can be responsible for acute hemiparesis.

In the differential diagnosis of acute hemiplegia in children, other categories aside from stroke (most common form of weakness) need to be considered, such as epilepsy, encephalitis, cerebral abscess, tumor, trauma, migraine, metabolic disorders, etc.

Hemiplegia can follow a jacksonian seizure (Todd's paralysis), usually lasting a few hours, but can also be an expression of prolonged focal seizures such as seen with Rasmussen's encephalitis, herpes encephalitis, or as a manifestation of an underlyng vascular malformation (Griesemer).

Brain neoplasm complicated by acute hemorrhage can present with acute hemiplegia or focal seizures followed by postictal hemiparesis.

Acute focal deficit can also be associated with metabolic abnormalities such as hypoglycemia or diabetes mellitus.

Transient neurological deficits, particularly hemiplegia, accompany complicated migraine in children. In alternating hemiplegia, which has been described as a form of complicated migraine, there are recurrent episodes of unexplained hemiplegia often associated with head pain prior to or following the attack and accompanied by other neurological symptoms and developmental abnormalities.

Finally, multiple sclerosis can present with acute hemiplegia but the clinical diagnosis requires the presence of neurological deficits disseminated in time and space.

Diagnosis

An accurate history and physical and neurological examination are very important in the formulation of the diagnosis, particularly considering the possibilities of trauma, convulsions, developmental status, cognitive impairment, family history, and so on. The examination of the cardiovascular system should cautiously consider murmurs, abnormal heart sounds, abnormal rhythms, hypertension, and bruits. The funduscopic examination may reveal retinal pigmentation, hemorrhages, or exudates, and also inspection of the skin may show abnormalities such as rash, hyper-/hypopigmentation, and so on.

The diagnostic workup should include laboratory tests such as complete blood count to rule out infection, sickle cell anemia, polycythemia, leukemia, or thrombocytopenia. Hemoglobin electrophoresis is important if hemoglobinopathies are considered in the differential diagnosis. Also, sedimentation rate, prothrombin time, and partial prothrombin time are obtained. Serum chemistries will rule out the possibility of hyperglycemia and hypoglycemia.

Neuroimaging (CT/MRI of the brain) and cardiac studies are essential in the evaluation of a child with acute hemiplegia. Lumbar puncture is important if there is no cerebral mass effect and there is suspicion that the hemiplegia is due to a brain infection.

Angiography may be reserved for selected cases of arterial dissection, moya-moya disease, cerebral vasculitis, and so on.

Treatment

The treatment of acute hemiplegia, medical or surgical, is based on the underlying etiology.

Subdural Hematoma

Vignette

A 6-month-old boy, previously in good health, was found unresponsive in his crib by his babysitter. He then experienced a generalized seizure and in the emergency room was comatose. Pupils were poorly reactive to light and bilateral retinal hemorrhages were noted. He was afebrile and normotensive. A chest x-ray indicated possible healing fractures of the posterior rib cage.

Summary A 6-month-old boy suddenly became comatose. Poorly reactive pupils and bilateral retinal hemorrhages were noted, as well as possible healing fractures on chest x-ray.

Localization and Differential Diagnosis

In the differential diagnosis of a comatose child, several causes are considered, including trauma, vascular disorders, infections, tumors, toxic, metabolic, and systemic disorders (Table 21.3). In this particular case, a traumatic etiology is highly suspicious particularly because of healing fracture of the posterior rib cage.

Child abuse is an important consideration in the etiology of intracranial vascular lesions. Cranial trauma due to direct punch to the head with or without a skull fracture, can be responsible for subdural, subarachnoid, or intraparenchymal bleeding, swelling, and herniation. Shaken baby syndrome may be responsible for a comatose baby due to posttraumatic subarachnoid hemorrhage or subdural hematoma even in the absence of signs of external injury. The ophthalmoscopic examination may demonstrate retinal hemorrhages, which are commonly seen in child abuse after inflicted trauma, particularly when there are no other signs of external injuries.

Subdural hematoma is common in battered babies and can be bilateral, particularly in infants.

TABLE 21.3 Causes of coma in children.

Category	Condition
Traumatic injuries	Hemorrhage
	Epidural
	Subdural
	Subarachnoid
	Malignant brain edema
Vascular disorders	Intracranial
	Nontraumatic
	Hemorrhagic
	Vasculitis
	Venous thrombosis
	Cerebral infarction
Infectious/parainfectious disorders	Meningitis
	Encephalitis
	Encephalomyelitis
	Cerebral abscess
Metabolic and systemic disorders	Hyper/hypoglycemia
	Hyper/hyponatremia
	Hepatic coma
	Uremic coma
	Hypophosphatemia
Toxic disorders	
Brain tumors	
Hydrocephalus	

Clinical Features

Infantile subdural hematoma can be acute or chronic, and when presenting acutely, manifests with altered level of consciousness, generalized seizures, vomiting, and bulging fontanelle. Retinal or subhyoid hemorrhages are frequently encountered. A skull fracture can also be demonstrated in almost half the patients. Acute subdural hematoma usually is due to tearing of cerebral veins bridging to the sagittal sinus, with blood accumulating beneath the dura against the brain parenchyma.

Diagnosis

The CT scan in acute subdural hematoma may show a high-density, crescent-shaped extracerebral fluid collection or signs of cerebral mass effect and swollen brain. MRI can give further details.

Treatment

The treatment is based on surgical intervention with evacuation of large hematoma with mass effect.

Headache

Basilar Migraine

Vignette

While playing basketball in school, a 14-year-old boy complained of sudden visual loss and fainted. When he regained consciousness, he had a throbbing headache and was vomiting. In the emergency room, pupillary testing and an ophthalmoscopic examination were unremarkable.

Summary A 14-year-old boy with bilateral visual loss, syncope, and headache.

Localization and Differential Diagnosis

The character of the visual loss reflects its posterior visual pathway origin and localizes to the occipital cortical area. All the possible causes of bilateral visual loss of cortical origin should be considered. Even if more benign conditions, such as basilar artery migraine, are suspected, alternative diagnoses need also to be ruled out.

Vascular disorders involving the posterior circulation, characterized by infarction of the posterior cerebral arteries bilaterally due to embolization with occlusion of the distal basilar artery, may present with cortical blindness and headache, although this event is not common in children. Subacute bacterial endocarditis and a prolapsing mitral valve are the most common sources of such emboli (Pellock).

Consideration needs to be given also to other disorders such as vertebral artery dissection, cerebral vasculitis, moya-moya disease, and vasospasm following subarachnoid hemorrhage. Hematological disorders creating a hypercoagulable state and sickle cell disease may also cause occipital lobe dysfunction. Hemorrhage, such as those due to arteriovenous malformations, also needs to be considered.

Tumors of the posterior fossa usually manifest with progressive symptoms, mostly dominated by signs of increased intracranial pressure, cranial nerve dysfunction, ataxia, and so on. Traumatic injuries to the occipital lobe can be responsible for cortical visual loss. The head injuries are usually mild, frequently involving blows to the frontal or occipital region. Commonly, loss of vision is complete or almost complete (Pellock). The association of migraine or seizure disorder increases susceptibility to posttraumatic transient cerebral blindness (Albert). Blindness can also follow severe generalized convulsions in infants or toddlers. It can be easily excluded in this vignette.

Other causes of acquired cerebral visual impairment during childhood that need to be mentioned, even if easily excluded from this vignette, are CNS infections such as meningitis and encephalitis (SSP, CJD, and so on) and hypoxic-ischemic encephalopathies due to asphyxia, cardiac arrest or hypotension during surgical procedure.

Visual loss of psychogenic origin in absence of organicity can manifest in preadolescent and adolescent children and needs to be carefully evaluated in the above vignette.

Finally, hereditary metabolic disorders such as MELAS may also present with occipital blindness in addition to a multitude of symptoms.

Basilar artery migraine is an important consideration in the differential diagnosis but because the history is limited and there is no evidence in this child of other features common to migraine, a more cautious and aggressive approach should be mantained by obtaining MRI of the brain to exclude structural lesions and even MRA or angiography to rule out aneurysmal formations, vasculitis, and so on.

Basilar migraine is the most common type of complicated migraine variant in children and manifests with aura symptoms indicative of dysfunction of the brainstem or both occipital lobes. The headache classification committee of the International Headache Society has designed diagnostic criteria for basilar migraine that, in addition to the criteria of migraine with aura, should include two or more of the following: visual symptoms in the temporal and nasal field of both eyes, dysartria, vertigo, tinnitus, hearing loss, diplopia, ataxia, bilateral paresthesias, paraparesis, and altered level of consciousness.

Clinical Features

The clinical presentation includes different symptoms, in particular visual abnormalities characterized by blurred vision, bilateral visual loss, tunnel vision, scintillating scotoma, and positive or negative hallucinations. The visual disturbances during an attack indicate a posterior visual pathway involvement with normal pupillary responses and funduscopic examinations. Ataxia and vertigo with or without tinnitus also commonly occur as well as dysartria.

Altered level of consciousness is also common and can manifest with syncope, or drop attacks accompanied by loss of consciousness and amnesia.

The aura generally lasts 10 to 60 minutes.

Diagnosis

Even if the history is suggestive, a cautious approach should always be maintained in order to rule out alternative diagnoses.

MRI and MRA should be included in the diagnostic studies as well as hematological tests such as cell count, hemoglobin, anticardiolipin antibodies, VDRL, and so on.

Treatment

The treatment is symptomatic and preventive for reoccurrences.

Ophthalmoplegic Migraine

Vignette

A 3-year-old girl started experiencing severe right retroorbital pain, irritability, vomiting, drowsiness, and abdominal pain for two days. On the third day, her right pupil dilated and she developed right ptosis and outward deviation of the eye. On examination, she was alert, comfortable, afebrile, and had no physical or neurological abnormalities except complete right ptosis, pupillary dilatation, and the inability to move the right eye in any direction except laterally. She was a full-term product of a normal pregnancy and vaginal delivery. Her neonatal period was uneventful and she had developed normally from all points of view. She is the only child of healthy parents.

Summary A 3-year-old girl developed a right, third nerve palsy after two days of systemic symptoms: irritability, drowsiness, vomiting, abdominal pain, and right retroorbital pain.

Localization and Differential Diagnosis

The differential diagnosis of a child presenting with acute onset of third nerve palsy includes several possibilities.

Trauma is an important and the most common cause of an acquired third nerve palsy in the pediatric population (Liu). Other disorders include neoplastic processes, infectious and inflammatory disorders, and ophthalmoplegic migraine. Severe head injuries accompanied by an orbital or base of skull fracture or midbrain hemorrhage may be responsible for cranial neuropathies (Liu). The vignette does not mention or imply any previous traumatic event, so this cause can be easily ruled out.

Intracranial tumors must always be considered in a child presenting with ophthalmoplegia. Brainstem gliomas may be characterized by ophthalmoplegia, usually in combination with progressive ataxia and other cranial nerve abnormalities and long tract signs. When tumor-related third nerve palsies occur, lesions affecting the orbit, orbital apex, and leptomeninges may also be involved and other signs and symptoms can be present, such as abducens paresis and proptosis with orbital lesions.

Infectious and inflammatory processes are other important causes of third nerve palsies. Chronic sinusitis with a mucocele of the sphenoid sinus may be associated with recurrent headache and third nerve palsies (Hockaday). Patients usually have a history of chronic sinus infection. Meningitis due to pneumococci and *H. influenzae,* as well as tuberculous meningitis, may present with third nerve palsy, usually in association with headache and systemic symptoms.

Tolosa-Hunt syndrome, characterized by nonspecific granulomatous inflammation of the cavernous sinus and superior orbital fissure, is rare in children and is characterized by painful ophthalmoplegia with partial or total involvement of extraocular muscles innervated by nerves III, IV, or VI in any combination; various pupillary dysfunctions, and sensory abnormalities in the area of the ophthalmic-trigeminal nerve. Tolosa-Hunt syndrome can sometimes simulate ophthalmoplegic migraine but the course is prolonged and headache and ophthalmoplegia occur at the same time.

Isolated third nerve palsies due to posterior communicating aneurysms are very uncommon in the pediatric population and usually occur in combination with hydrocephalus and signs of SAH.

Cranial neuropathies due to diabetes are exceptionally rare in children.

Myasthenia gravis can be easily excluded because it is usually characterized by bilateral signs that fluctuate and do not involve the pupils.

Finally, we need to consider ophthalmoplegic migraine as the appropriate diagnosis after excluding other, more severe causes. Ophthalmoplegic migraine is a rare variant of complicated migraine that usually causes an isolated third nerve paresis. The onset of symptoms is usually in the first decade of life. The diagnostic workup in this child should include

- Careful history and neurological evaluation.
- MRI and MRA in order to exclude orbital or cavernous sinus pathology or aneurysm.
- Lumbar puncture if the neuroimaging studies are negative and an infectious process is suspected.
- Cerebral angiogram in a patient 10 years old or older to exclude aneurysm.

Clinical Features

Ophthalmoplegic migraine is characterized by one or recurrent episodes of ophthalmoplegia associated with severe headache that usually precede the ocular paresis.

The third nerve is affected in the majority of the cases with involvement of the pupil but the sixth nerve can also be involved, and rarely the fourth nerve. The pain is commonly ipsilateral, localized in the orbital, retroorbital, and temporal area and associated with nausea and vomiting. With the onset of ophthalmoplegia, the headache often subsides.

The episodes of ophthalmoplegic migraine, which usually involve the same eye, vary in frequency of attacks, and the duration of the ophthalmoplegia is also variable from a few hours up to several months.

The International Headache Society has defined diagnostic criteria for ophthalmoplegic migraine that include at least two attacks characterized by headache associated with paresis of one or more of the cranial nerves III, IV, and VI in the absence of parasellar lesion excluded by the appropriate investigations.

Diagnosis

The diagnostic workup in an infant or young child should include magnetic resonance imaging (MRI) and magnetic resonance angiography. If the patient is over 12 years of age, angiography to rule out posterior communicating aneurysm is indicated.

Treatment

Full recovery is the rule, but after repeated severe attacks residual deficits can be noted. Prevention of repeated episodes and residual abnormalities by the use of prophylactic drugs is important.

References

Paradoxical Emboli

Caplan, L. Stroke: A Clinical Approach, ed. 2. Boston: Butterworth-Heinemann, 1993.

Fenichel, G. Clinical Pediatric Neurology, ed. 3. Philadelphia: W.B. Saunders, 1997.

Griesemer, D.A. Acute hemiplegia in childhood. Neurobase MedLink, Arbor, 1993–2000.

Jones, H.R. Jr. et al. Cerebral emboli of paradoxical origin. Ann. Neurol. 13:314–319, 1983.

Loscalzo, J. Paradoxical embolism: Clinical presentation, diagnostic strategies, and therapeutic options. Am. Heart J. 112:141–149, 1986.

Mendoza, P. and Conway, E.E. Jr. Cerebrovascular events in pediatric patients. Pediatr. Ann. 27:665–674, 1998.

Nagaraja, D. et al. Cerebrovascular disease in children. ACTA Neurol. Scand. 90:251–255, 1994.

Nicolaides, P. and Appleton, R.E. Stroke in children. Dev. Med. Child Neurol. 38:172–180, 1996.

Rivkin, M.J. and Volpe, J.J. Strokes in children. Pediatr. Rev. 17:265, 1996.

Roach, E.S. and Riela, A.R. Pediatric Cerebrovascular Disorders, ed. 2. New York: Futura, 1995.

Homocystinuria

Brett, E.M. Paediatric Neurology, ed. 2. New York: Churchill Livingstone, 1991.

Lyon, G. et al. Neurology of Hereditary and Metabolic Diseases of Children, ed. 2. New York: McGraw-Hill, 264–268, 1996.

Menkes, J.M. and Sarnat, H.B. Cererebrovascular Disorders in Child Neurology, ed. 6. Philadelphia: Lippincott Williams & Wilkins, 885–917, 2000.

Roach, E.S. and Riela, A.R. Pediatric Cerebrovascular Disorders, ed. 2. New York: Futura, 1995.

Intracranial Hemorrage/Acute Hemiplegia

Berg, B.O. Principles of Child Neurology. New York: McGraw-Hill, 1996.

Biller, J. et al. Strokes in children and young adults. Boston: Butterworth-Heinemann, 1994.

Griesemer, D.A. Acute hemiplegia in childhood. Neurobase MedLink Arbor, 1993–2000.

Mendoza, P.L. and Conway, E.E. Jr. Cerebrovascular events in pediatric patients. Pediatr. Ann. 27:665–674, 1998.

Pellock, J.M. and Myer, E.C. Neurologic Emergencies in Infancy and Childhood, ed. 2. Boston: Butterworth-Heinemann, 1993.

Riela, A.R. and Roach, E.S. Etiology of stroke in children. J. Child Neurol. 8:201–220, 1993.

Rivkin, M.J. and Volpe, J.J. Strokes in children. Pediatr. Rev. 17:265, 1996.

Roach, E.S. et al. Cerebrovascular disease in children and adolescents. American Academy of Neurology, 52nd Annual Meeting, San Diego, 2000.

Subdural Hematoma

Berg, B.O. Principles of Child Neurology. New York: McGraw-Hill, 937–952, 1996.

Fenichel, G.M. Clinical Pediatric Neurology: A Sign and Symptom Approach. Philadelphia: W.B. Saunders, 71–75, 1997.

Pellock, J.M. and Myer, E.C. Neurologic Emergencies in Infancy and Childhood. Boston: Butterworth-Heinemann, 91–102, 1993.

Roach, E.S. and Riela, A.R. Pediatric Cerebrovascular Disorders, ed. 2. New York: Futura, 291–312, 1995.

Basilar Migraine

Albert, D.M. et al. Principle and Practice of Ophthalmology. Philadelphia: W.B. Saunders, 2634–2639, 1994.

Davidoff, R.A. Migraine: Manifestations, Pathogenesis and Management. Philadelphia: F.A. Davis, 1995.

Hockaday, J.M. Migraine in Childhood and Other Nonepileptic Paroxysmal Disorders. Boston: Butterworths, 1988.

Hockaday, J.M. Migraine in childhood. In: Berg, B.O. (Ed.). Principles of Child Neurology. New York: McGraw-Hill, 693–706, 1996.

Molofski, W.J. Headaches in children. Pediatr. Ann. 27:614–621, 1998.

Pellock, J.M. and Myer, E.C. Neurologic Emergencies in Infancy and Childhood, ed. 2. Boston: Butterworth-Heinemann, 268–269, 1993.

Rothner, A.D. The migraine syndrome in children and adolescents. Pediatr. Neurol. 2:121–126, 1986.

Singer, H.S. Migraine headaches in children. Pediatr. Rev. 15:94–101, 1994.

Welch, K.M.A. Basilar Migraine. Neurobase MedLink, Arbor, 1993–2000.

Wright, K.W. Pediatric Ophthalmology and Strabismus. St. Louis: Mosby, 801–805, 1995.

Ophthalmoplegic Migraine

Davidoff, R.A. Migraine: Manifestations, Pathogenesis, and Management. Philadelphia: F.A. Davis, 1995.

Glaser, J. S. and Bachynski, B. Infranuclear disorders of eye movement. In: Glaser, J.S. Neuroophthalmology, ed 2. Philadelphia: J.B. Lippincott, 361–419, 1990.

Hockaday, J.M. Migraine in childhood. Boston: Butterworths, 1988.

Lee, A.G. and Brazis, P. Ophthalmoplegic migraine. Neurobase MedLink Arbor, 1993–2000.

Liu, G.T. Pediatric 3rd, 4th and 5th nerve palsy. American Academy of Neurology, 51st Annual Meeting, Toronto, 1999.

22
Pediatric Neurocutaneous Disorders

Neurofibromatosis

Vignette

A 15-year-old boy from Santo Domingo has complained of bifrontal headache and intermittent vomiting for one month. His past medical history is significant for generalized seizures since the age of 12 months. His developmental history is normal. On examination, several hyperpigmented spots, skinfold axillary freckling, and subcutaneous nodules are noted. He is alert and cooperative. Funduscopic examination shows absent venous pulsations. Bilateral horizontal nystagmus, left dysmetria, and wide-based gait are also noted.

Summary A 15-year-old boy with headache and intermittent vomiting for one month. Past medical history is significant for generalized seizures since 12 months of age. The neurological examination shows absent venous pulsation on funduscopic examination, left dysmetria, and gait ataxia. Also, neurocutaneous findings, hyperpigmented spots, axillary freckling, and subcutaneous nodules are described.

Localization and Differential Diagnosis

The clinical findings indicate signs of increased intracranial pressure as well as signs of left cerebellar dysfunction. There is also a long-standing history of generalized convulsions, which point to a cortical irritative process. An important finding in the vignette is the description of the cutaneous lesions, which are represented by hyperpigmented macules, skinfold freckling, and subcutaneous nodules. All these features point to a neurocutaneous disorder.

Neurocutaneous syndromes include disorders characterized by cutaneous and neurological manifestations. The major neurocutaneous syndromes include

- Neurofibromatosis (Von Recklinghausen's disease).
- Tuberous sclerosis.
- Sturge-Weber syndrome.
- Von Hippel-Lindau syndrome.
- Ataxia-telangiectasia.

In this vignette, the clinical findings described suggest the diagnosis of neurofibromatosis (NF). The cutaneous manifestations are characteristic and the signs of cerebellar dysfunction may indicate the possibility of an intracranial tumor. Hyperpigmented macules ("café au lait spots") are an important cutaneous feature of neurofibromatosis type 1, which is the most common type, but are nonspecific and can be observed in other neurocutaneous syndromes and less frequently in neurofibromatosis type 2. Skinfold freckling is usually seen in the axillary and inguinal area. Subcutaneous neurofibromas as well as plexiform neurofibromas are also common manifestations of NF type 1.

Intracranial, spinal, and peripheral nerve tumors can complicate NF type 1 but are more common in the type 2. Unilateral or bilateral optic nerve glioma is considered the most commonly observed in NF type 1.

Clinical Features

There are two distinct types of neurofibromatosis: type 1 and type 2. Neurofibromatosis type 1 (NF1), or Von Recklinghausen disease, is the most common form affecting 1 in 4000 to 5000 individuals (Menkes and Maria) and resulting from a spontaneous mutation in almost 50 percent of the cases. The cutaneous manifestations characteristic of NF1 include café au lait spots, skinfold freckling, and neurofibromas. Café au lait spots are characterized by hyperpigmented macules widely distributed over the body, manifesting at birth and clearly obvious during the first year of life. According to the diagnostic criteria, at least six or more café au lait spots greater than 5 mm in diameter need to be present in prepubertal children and greater than 15 mm in postpubertal patients (Robertson).

Skinfold freckling consists of small pigmented lesions, usually noted in the areas not exposed to the sun, such as the axillary, inguinal area, inferior part of the chin, and so on.

Neurofibromas, which can be dermal or subcutaneous, are benign tumors that originate from peripheral nerves and tend to increase after puberty. They vary in size and number and can cause nerve compression with pain and loss of function. Plexiform neurofibromas can affect the trunk, face, and neck and cause significant deformity.

Lisch nodules are pigmented hamartomas of the iris and are usually asymptomatic.

The neurological manifestations of NF1 include the possible occurrence of tumors, particularly involving the brain, spinal cord, and peripheral nerves. Among the central nervous system tumors, optic nerve glioma is the most commonly found in NF1 and may manifest with progressive visual loss and optic atrophy.

Meningiomas, ependymomas and astrocytomas can also be discovered in NF1. Skeletal abnormalities include bone dysplasia of the sphenoid wing of the temporal bone and pseudoarthrosis of the tibia.

Diagnosis

Neurofibromatosis is a hereditary disorder transmitted with an autosomal dominant trait. The gene for NF1 is linked on the long arm of chromosome 17 (17g11.2) that of NF2 is on the long arm of chromosome 22 (22g11.2). Several criteria have been established in order to fulfill the diagnosis of NF1. They include

- Six or more "café au lait spots" greater than 5 mm in diameter in prepubertal children and greater than 15 mm in postpubertal patients.
- Two or more neurofibromas of any type or one plexiform neurofibroma.
- Axillary or inguinal freckling.
- Two or more iris hamartomas (Lisch nodules).
- Optic glioma.
- Typical osseous lesions, such as sphenoid dysplasia or tibial pseudoarthrosis.
- One or more first-degree relatives with NF1.

For NF2, any of the following:

- Bilateral vestibular schwannomas seen with imaging techniques.
- Unilateral vestibular schwannoma in association with any two of the following: meningioma, neurofibroma, schwannoma, and juvenile posterior subcapsular lenticular opacity.
- Unilateral eighth nerve tumor or other spinal or brain tumor in first-degree relative.

Neurofibromatosis type 2, which is less common than type 1, is characterized by less consistent cutaneous manifestations than type 1 and the typical occurrence of bilateral vestibular schwannomas. Symptoms include hearing loss, tinnitus, headache, and vertigo. Meningiomas of the brain and spine can also occur.

References

Aicardi, J. Diseases of the nervous system in childhood. McKeith Press. 1992. 203–11.

Berg, B.D. Child neurology: a clinical manual. Second ed. Philadelphia: J.B. Lippincott Co. 1994. Ch. 9: 185–95.

Brett, E.M. Paediatric neurology. Second ed. New York: Churchill Livingstone. 1991.

Conneally, M., Bird, T.D. et al. Neurocutaneous syndromes in Neurogenetics Continuum Part A program of the American Academy of Neurology Vol. 6, No. 6, Dec. 2000. 35–58.

Gutman, D.H. The diagnosis and management of neurofibromatosis 1. The neurologist. Nov. 1998; Vol. 4: 313–38.

Mackool, B.T. and Fitzpatrick, T.B. Diagnosis of neurofibromatosis by cutaneous examination. Semin. Neurol. 1992; Vol. 12: 358–63.

Menkes, J.H. and Maria, B.L. Neurocutaneous syndromes in child neurology. Menkes, J.H. and Sarnat, H.B. Sixth ed., Philadelphia: Lippincott Williams & Wilkins 2000. Ch 11: 859–884.

Roach, E.S. Diagnosis and management of neurocutaneous syndromes. Semin. Neurol. 1988; Vol. 8: 83–96.

Robertson P. Neurofibromatosis type 1; Neurofibromatosis type 2, Medlink Arbor-Publishing Corp. 1993–2001.

23
Pediatric Movement Disorders

Huntington's Disease

Vignette

An 8-year-old girl became irritable, apathetic, distractible, and lost interest in her schoolwork and dance classes. She was noted to have sudden jerking movements in her arms and started experiencing generalized tonic-clonic seizures. A year later she was more withdrawn, not following questions or commands, sometimes remaining in a catatonic posture. On examination, there was rigidity with loss of facial expression. Her prior developmental history was unremarkable. She had no siblings. Her father had involuntary movements and grimacing and was demented.

Summary An 8-year-old girl with progressive cognitive impairment associated with seizures and parkinsonian features (rigidity, loss of facial expression). In the family history, her father has dementia, facial grimacing, and involuntary movements.

Localization and Differential Diagnosis

The vignette describes an extrapyramidal disorder that occurs during childhood and is associated with progressive dementia and seizures.

The family history with a father affected by dementia and involuntary movements suggests a hereditary dominant disorder. Among the hereditary, predominantly extrapyramidal, syndromes occurring during late childhood and adolescence the following should be considered first:

- Childhood and juvenile forms of Huntington's disease.
- Wilson's disease.

- Hallervorden-Spatz disease.

Huntington's disease is a progressive degenerative disorder with an autosomal dominant pattern of transmission. The clinical manifestations in children are dominated by cognitive and behavior abnormalities, rigidity, loss of facial expression, decreased voluntary movements, and seizures. In the majority of childhood-onset cases there is an affected father.

Wilson's disease, which always needs to be ruled out in a child presenting with signs of extrapyramidal system dysfunction is an autosomal recessive disorder characterized by the accumulation of copper in the liver, basal ganglia, and cornea. Younger children usually present with signs and symptoms of significant liver dysfunction rather than neurological involvement. Neurological manifestations, with only minimal symptoms of liver disease, are more likely when the onset of symptoms is in the second decade (Fenichel). Speech abnormalities with dysarthria as well as tremor dystonia and gait disturbances are often the presenting neurological symptoms. Emotional lability and psychosis can also be the initial feature, but seizures and marked dementia are not usually a significant characteristic of the disease except in few cases.

Hallervorden-Spatz disease is a familial disorder that manifests with signs of involvement of the extrapyramidal system such as rigidity, dysarthria, choreoathetosis, and gait dysfunction, in association with signs of pyramidal involvement such as spasticity and hyperreflexia. Behavioral abnormalities and cognitive impairment can occur and visual abnormalities such as retinitis pigmentosa and optic atrophy can also be present. Seizures are not common. Typical pathological findings include hyperpigmentation of the pallidum and substantia nigra.

Other extrapyramidal disorders such as idiopathic torsion dystonia, familial calcification of the basal ganglia, juvenile paralysis agitans, chorea-acanthocytosis, and so on are easily differentiated by their clinical features.

Considering the information presented in the vignette, Huntington's disease is the preferred diagnosis.

Clinical Features

Huntington's disease (HD) in the pediatric population usually presents in the first decade of life (between 5 and 12 years of age) with symptoms characterized by behavioral and cognitive deterioration, rigidity, dystonia, and seizures.

Seizures, which are usually not observed in adult patients with HD, can be a prominent initial manifestation and may affect about 50 percent of children with HD (Menkes). Epileptic seizures can be represented by tonic-clonic convulsions, absence, and myoclonic seizures. Tonic-clonic or myoclonic status can also occur.

Rigidity causing gait disturbances is common, and dystonia, loss of facial expression and associated movements, and decreased voluntary movements are significant features in the majority of pediatric patients. Choreoathetosis and hyperkinesia are not common in the pediatric age group with HD.

Mental deterioration with progressive dementia is an important characteristic feature. Behavior abnormalities manifest with irritability, distractibility, emotional lability, negativism, and even catatonia. Most of childhood-onset cases have inherited the gene from an affected father. The HD gene has been localized to the short arm of chromosome 4 and contains an abnormal repeat of the trinucleotide CAG (cytidine-adenine-guanidine).

Diagnosis

The diagnosis is based on the clinical features and family history. Neuroimaging studies demonstrate caudate atrophy and PET studies reveal significant reduction in caudate glucose metabolism. DNA analysis detects the abnormal gene.

Treatment

The treatment is symptomatic and is based on the use of anti-parkinsonian medications to control rigidity and dystonia. Behavioral abnormalities may respond to neuroleptics. The use of baclofen (GABA agonist) and diltiazem (calcium-channel blocker that might block the action of glutamate on calcium channels) is controversial.

Sydenham's Chorea

Vignette

A 10-year-old Mexican immigrant was reported by her teacher as being restless, inattentive, over-emotional, and fidgety. Irregular jerking movements of her distal upper extremities and face were noted, and she seemed particularly troubled when eating, drinking from a cup, or writing. Her family and developmental histories were normal. Six months earlier, while still in Mexico, she had experienced knee pain and swelling accompanied with fever. Her family reported no other medical history.

Summary A 10-year-old girl with onset of involuntary movements and prior history of knee pain, swelling, and fever.

Localization and Differential Diagnosis

The involuntary, irregular jerking movements that interfere with activities such as writing or feeding in this patient, plus the fidgety, restless, and overemotional behavior observed by her teacher most likely are indications of a choreic disorder. Childhood chorea can be attributed to various etiologies:

- Infectious disorders, such as Sydenham's chorea, diphtheria, viral encephalitis, and so on.
- Immunological disorders, such as systemic lupus erythematosus, periarteritis nodosa, and sarcoidosis.
- Drug-induced causes, such as related to the use of neuroleptics, anticonvulsants, and so on.
- Toxic causes, such as due to manganese, carbon monoxide, toluene, and alcohol.
- Metabolic and endocrine disorders, such as hypoglycemia, hyperglycemia, hypocalcemia, hyperthyroidism, and Addison's disease.
- Structural disorders, such as tumors and arteriovenous malformations.
- Bilateral cerebral dysfunction, such as postanoxia.
- Genetic and hereditary degenerative disorders, such as childood Huntington's disease, Hallervorden-Spatz disease, Lesch-Nyhan syndrome, and so on.

Sydenham's chorea (St. Vitus' dance) is a well-known choreic sequelae of infection with group A streptococcus. It affects children between 5 and 15 years of age, particularly females. A beta-hemolitic streptococcal infection of the pharynx may occur 1 to 7 months prior to the onset of the neurological manifestations in most patients. The movements are typically choreoathetoid and preferentially involve the face and upper extremities, unilaterally or bilaterally. Sydenham's chorea, polyarthritis, and carditis are important features of rheumatic fever, the result of an antecedent group A streptococcal pharyngeal infection. A prior history of pharyngitis is not always given by the patient and families. The duration of the chorea varies from three months to two years.

Other infectious processes that can be responsible for

the occurrence of chorea include bacterial, such as sub-acute bacterial endocarditis, neurosyphilis, diphtheria, tuberculosis, Lyme disease, and viral infections, such as viral encephalitis, mononucleosis, HIV, Epstein-Barr, varicella, pertussis, and so on.

Immunological causes of chorea include, in particular, systemic lupus erythematosus, Behçet's disease, Schonlein-Henoch purpura, antiphospholipid antibodies syndrome, and so on. Systemic lupus erythematosus in children can manifest with psychosis, seizures, cranial neuropathy, and rarely with chorea as the only presentation. The presence of systemic symptoms such as fever, rash, lymphadenopathy, hematuria, albuminuria, and so on, and laboratory studies, particularly antibodies against DNA, help confirm the diagnosis.

Drug-induced causes are now considered the most common cause of chorea in children (Robertson et al.). Among the drugs, neuroleptics, anticonvulsants, antiemetic, noradrenergic stimulants, and so on, can be included. Tardive dyskinesia indicates a condition associated with the use of neuroleptics and characterized by abnormal involuntary movements such as choreic movements involving the face and limbs. Withdrawal emergent syndrome (Robertson et al.) refers to the first appearance of involuntary movements and chorea after interruption of neuroleptic treatment.

Toxic agents that may induce chorea include carbon monoxide, thallium, toluene (glue sniffing), and so on. Metabolic and endocrine disturbances can also cause secondary chorea. Electrolyte disturbances such as hypoglycemia, hyperglycemia, hypocalcemia, hypomanganesemia, and hepatic and renal failure can be responsible for secondary chorea. The endocrine disorders primarily include hyperthyroidism, but also hypoparathyroidism, Addison's disease, and so on. Some vitamin deficiencies such as vitamin B_{12}, beriberi, and pellagra can present with chorea.

Chorea can also be secondary to diffuse cerebral dysfunction due to perinatal anoxia or decreased cerebral perfusion due to postcardiopulmonary bypass. Structural cerebral lesions like tumor, arteriovenous malformations or cerebrovascular accidents can also present with chorea. Trauma has also been involved in some cases.

Hereditary degenerative disorders manifesting with chorea include the following:

- Juvenile Huntington's disease, as previously described, is an autosomal dominant disorder usually transmitted by the affected father and characterized by progressive cognitive impairment, rigidity, seizures, and choreoathetosis.
- Wilson's disease is an autosomal recessive disorder of copper metabolism characterized by hepatic failure and neurological features particularly involving the extrapyramidal system with tremor, rigidity, dystonia, dysarthria, choreoathetosis, and so on.

- Hallervorden-Spatz disease is a rare autosomal recessive disorder of iron metabolism, manifesting with choreic movements, athetosis, dystonia, rigidity, cognitive impairment, retinitis pigmentosa, seizures, and so on.
- Pelizaeus-Merzbacher disease is an X-linked recessive disorder of myelin formation characterized by involuntary movements with chorea or athetosis, cerebellar ataxia, pendular nystagmus, developmental regression, spasticity, optic atrophy, and so on.
- Fahr's disease, or familial calcification of the basal ganglia, manifests with choreoathetosis, mental impairment, microcephaly, and seizures. There is progressive calcification of the basal ganglia.
- Neuroacanthocytosis is characterized by chorea in association with seizures, orolingual dystonia, and acanthocytosis (acanthocytes are abnormal erythrocytes that have thorny projections from the cell surface).
- Ataxia-telangiectasia is a hereditary autosomal recessive disorder clinically characterized by progressive ataxia, telangiectasias, and recurrent sinopulmonary infections. Choreoathetosis can also be observed, particularly in infants.
- Benign familial hereditary chorea is an autosomal dominant hereditary disorder manifesting with chorea, dysarthria, and normal cognitive function.
- Genetic metabolic disorders such as GM_1 and GM_2 gangliosidosis, Leigh syndrome, lipofuscinoses, and so on, can also include chorea in their symptomatology.

Hereditary paroxysmal choreas need also to be mentioned:

- Paroxysmal dystonic choreoathetosis is an autosomal dominant hereditary disorder that manifests with episodes of choreic movements and dystonia of various duration from minutes to hours.
- Familial paroxysmal kinesiogenic choreoathetosis is a hereditary disorder characterized by brief, recurrent episodes of unilateral choreoathetosis precipitated by a sudden movement (Robertson).

Clinical Features

Sydenham's chorea represents a late sequelae of group A streptococcal pharyngitis. The neurological manifestations usually tend to present one to six months after the streptococcal infection. Affected children range from 5 to 15 years of age and are preferentially girls. The disorder manifests insidiously or acutely with involuntary movements that involve the face and distal part of the upper extremities. The involuntary movements disappear during sleep or sedation. The child is first noted to be restless, clumsy, and fidgety. The speech becames dysarthric, and hypotonia may create abnormal postures. The hand grip waxes and wanes when the child is asked to squeeze the examiner's hand, a phenomenon called "milkmaid sign." Seizures rarely occur. Behavioral dysfunction, includes, in particular, tics and obsessive-compulsive disorder.

Diagnosis

MRI of the brain, which is important in order to rule out structural lesions, is usually normal but may show high signal on T_2-weighted images in the head of the caudate and in the putamen.

Some laboratory tests should be considered including

- Blood count and differential.
- Blood chemistry.
- Thyroid function tests, erythrocyte sedimentation rate.
- Antinuclear antibodies titer.
- Anticardiolipid antibodies.
- Antistreptolisin O titer.

In selected cases, other laboratory studies include

- Blood smear for acantocytes.
- Ceruloplasmin, serum copper.
- VDRL.
- HIV.
- Heavy metal screen.
- Lysosomal enzymes.

Treatment

Streptococcal infection should be aggressively treated with penicillin. Treatment of chorea is based on the use of dopamine antagonists, benzodiazepines, or valproate. Neuroleptics with more specific D_2 receptor antagonism (such as haloperidol) are effective for the more intense chorea, but carry a risk of tardive dyskinesia (O'Brien).

Dystonia Musculorum Deformans

Vignette

A 10-year-old boy started having difficulty walking at the age of 6 because of intermittent abnormal posture of his left foot with plantar flexion and inversion as it approached the ground. The symptoms slowly progressed and, at age 9, the boy was unable to walk because both feet were constantly flexed. Eventually, involuntary flexion appeared at the left wrist as well as torticollis and facial grimacing. His medical and developmental history were normal. The patient was the product of a full-term, uncomplicated pregnancy. A paternal uncle in the family history had difficulty with handwriting. Upon examination the boy had normal intelligence. Cranial nerves, motor strength, reflexes, and sensation were intact.

Summary A 10-year-old boy with involuntary movements of his lower extremities consisting of abnormal plantar flexion and inversion of his ankles that progressed from age 6. In addition, left wrist flexion torticollis and facial grimacing are described. Birth and developmental history are normal. Mental status, cranial nerves, motor strength, sensation, and reflexes are normal. In the family history, one uncle has trouble with handwriting.

Localization

The disorder affecting this child may be localized to pathology involving the extrapyramidal system. The vignette describes a case of dystonia, which by definition is characterized by sustained muscle contraction of agonist and antagonist muscles, frequently causing repetitive abnormal movements and posture.

Diagnosis and Differential Diagnosis

The vignette indicates a normal perinatal and developmental history and no past history of exposure to drugs or toxins. The neurological examination shows a child with normal cognitive function and normal strength, sensation, and reflexes. This helps in narrowing the diagnostic possibilities.

A family history consistent with an uncle with "handwriting problems" points to a hereditary disorder. Torsion dystonia can clearly explain all the symptoms expressed in the vignette. It is a hereditary disorder characterized by involuntary, sustained muscular contractions commonly involving the foot, with movements of plantar flexion and inversion, which initially occur intermittently and then became constant.

The most important consideration in the differential diagnosis is Wilson's disease since it is a treatable condition and needs to be excluded in all patients developing movement disorders. In Wilson's disease, signs of hepatic dysfunction may predominate in children. Neurological symptoms include rigidity, tremor, bradykinesia, and dysarthria in addition to dystonia. Kaiser-Fleisher rings are characteristic and the serum ceruloplasmin is generally decreased.

Hereditary neurodegenerative disorders, such as Huntington's disease, Hallervorden-Spatz syndrome, Fahr's disease, ceroid lipofuscinosis, ataxia-telangiectasia, neuroacanthocytosis, and so on, may manifest with dystonia but usually they are also characterized by other neurological and multifocal abnormalities, such as mental deterioration, seizures, retinitis pigmentosa, and so on.

Symptomatic generalized dystonia may be secondary to a neoplastic or vascular process, trauma, encephalitis, or hypoxic or metabolic encephalopathy. Secondary dystonia in children is often caused by perinatal asphyxia (Menkes). Vascular cerebral malformations and neoplastic conditions can present with localized or generalized dystonia that may mimic the idyopathic type.

Dystonia can also be related to an acute brain infection or trauma, or can be secondary to toxic agents such as manganese or carbon monoxide, or drug ingestion such as neuroleptics, phenytoin, phenobarbital, anthistamines, and so on.

Psychogenic dystonia is also a consideration in a small percentage of children but some clinical characteristics such as bizarre movements, gait inconsistency, and decreased movement when the child is distracted, may help the correct diagnosis.

In summary, dystonia can be etiologically distinguished into primary, or idiopathic, and secondary, or symptomatic. The idiopathic group is characterized by disorders with dystonic postures as the only abnormality and with absence of other neurological symptomatology. Symptomatic dystonias, which are associated with hereditary or acquired disorders, usually present with a multitude of symptoms including dementia, seizures, spasticity, hyperreflexia, ataxia, retinitis pigmentosa, and so on.

Clinical Features

Idiopathic torsion dystonia is a familial or sporadic disorder with various modes of inheritance: autosomal dominant, autosomal recessive, or X-linked recessive. Generalized dystonia is the most common form observed in children. The age of presentation varies between 6 and 12 years in children who have a normal developmental history.

The first symptoms can present with intermittent involuntary posturing of the foot with plantar flexion and inversion while the child walks, but not during rest or when he is running or walking backwards. With progression of the disease, the motor abnormalities became persistent and may spread to involve contiguous areas, such as the pelvic girdle muscles, shoulders, and spinal and neck muscles, often interfering with daily activities. Almost all children for whom the dystonia begins in the legs progress to have generalized dystonia within one to five years (Robertson et al.). Dystonia of the tongue and pharyngeal and laryngeal muscles may cause dysarthria and dysphagia. Paroxysmal dyspnea has also been described (Menkes). The dystonic movements disappear during sleep and are exacerbated by stress, fatigue, and excitement.

The neurological examination in idiopathic torsion dystonia does not reveal any abnormality except for the dystonic posture and movements. The intellectual function is normal.

Dopa-responsive dystonia, which affects children in the first decade of life, needs to be differentiated from idiopathic torsion dystonia because of its characteristic diurnal fluctuations and excellent response to levodopa treatment.

Myoclonic dystonia is an inherited condition characterized by torsion dystonia in association with myoclonic jerks.

Treatment

The treatment of torsion dystonia is based on the use of anticholinergic agents such as trihexyphenidyl (Artane), which is given in a dose that starts at 2 to 4 mg/day and is gradually increased up to 60 to 80 mg/day until the maximum benefit or intolerable side effects are encountered (Menkes). Baclofen has been beneficial in some patients. Intratheral baclofen has been used in selective cases of severe intractable torsion dystonia. Levodopa appears to be effective in patients with late-onset dystonia. Botulinum toxin can be utilized in the treatment of facial dystonia, but not in the generalized form. In intractable cases, surgery may represent an option, particularly unilateral or bilateral pallidotomy.

Tic Disorders

Vignette

An 8-year-old boy was referred to an allergist after the teacher noticed that he was sniffing, coughing, and clearing his throat with unusual frequency. The mother admitted that at home he seemed very nervous, often blinking, grimacing, grunting, or shoulder shrugging, especially while watching television. These symptoms probably started at age 6. On examination he was a very bright boy, with occasional squeezing of his eyelids and nasal twitches. The neurological examination was unremarkable. Past medical and developmental history were normal.

Summary An 8-year-old boy with history of involuntary movements (motor tics) and involuntary making of sounds (phonic tics) since age 6. The neurological and medical history are normal.

Localization, Differential Diagnosis, and Diagnosis

Tics, characterized by involuntary, sudden, purposeless, repetitive, stereotyped, motor movements or vocalizations, are the most common involuntary movement disorders of childhood (Erenberg). Tic disorders vary in severity from a transient tic disorder to Tourette's syndrome (TS). Transient tic disorder, which is common in children, has a duration of less than one year. Chronic tic disorder, characterized by motor or vocal tics but not both, has a duration longer than a year.

The boy described in the vignette has experienced both motor and vocal tics for over a year, therefore he strongly represents a case of Tourette's syndrome. Diagnostic criteria for Tourette's syndrome, according to the DSM-IV-TR, include

- Onset before 18 years of age.
- Presence of multiple motor tics and one or more vocal tics.
- Recurrence of the tics many times a day, nearly every day, or intermittently throughout a period of more than one year.
- Etiology not related to the use of medications or other medical conditions.

Tics can be motor or vocal, simple or complex. Simple motor tics usually affect only one muscle and can be represented by eye blinking, eye movement, nose twitching, shoulder shrugging, mouth opening, and so on. Complex motor tics can include more complex movement, often in sequence, such as jumping, twisting, spitting, touching, smelling, rubbing, and copropraxia (obscene gestures). Simple vocal tics are represented by various noises or sounds, such as throat clearing, snorting, sniffing, coughing, or barking. Complex vocal tics include words, phrases, echolalia, and coprolalia (obscene words or phrases). Patients describe an "involuntary urge" like tingling or itching to perform the movement or make the sound. The Tourette's syndrome classification study group has defined these feelings as sensory tics: uncomfortable sensations that can be focal, localized, or generalized, and are relieved by the movement of the affected body part.

TS usually manifests in the first decade of life and has a male predominance. Motor and vocal tics are precipitated by stress, fatigue, and emotional excitement, and can be temporarily suppressed, for example, when the child is in school. Typically they increase when the child is relaxing, for example, when watching television. Tourette patients tend to have obsessive compulsive behaviors in over half the cases. Other disorders associated with Tourette syndrome include attention deficit–hyperactivity disorder, mood disorder, depression, antisocial behavior, anxiety disorder, dyslexia, and so on. The long-term prognosis of TS is favorable with spontaneous remission or marked improvement of the symptoms in over half of the cases.

Other movement disorders need to be distinguished from tics and enter in the differential diagnosis of the patient in the vignette. Hyperkinetic movement disorders that need to be differentiated from tics include myoclonus, dystonia, chorea, akathisia, tardive dyskinesia, stereotypes and psychogenic movement disorders.

Myoclonus is defined as a brief, sudden, shock-like movement caused by an abrupt contraction of a muscle or a group of muscles. It can be focal, multifocal, segmental, or generalized, and can be physiological, e.g., associated with epilepsy or secondary to hypoxia or metabolic, or toxic disorders.

Dystonia manifests with prolonged muscle contractions causing repetitive movements or abnormal postures. Dystonic tics, such as twisting, pulling, or squeezing, usually are preceded by an urge and are responsible for abnormal twisting or posturing that only last as long as the tic.

Chorea is characterized by involuntary, irregular, rapid, purposeless movements that cannot be suppressed but can be incorporated by the patient in a semipurposeful movement and is not preceded by an urge to make the movement.

Akathisia is defined as motor restlessness that cannot be suppressed and does not have an urge to make the movement, and varies in severity from jumpiness and fidgetiness to inability to sit or stand still.

Tardive dyskinesia, which typically occurs in patients treated with neuroleptics, includes a variety of involuntary movements that can be choreoathetoid and dystonic, and preferentially involve the oral-buccal and lingual region.

Stereotypes are involuntary stereotyped movements, such as arm flapping and hand waving, that can occur during stress or excitement, and can decrease if the child is distracted.

Tics can be secondary to acute and chronic insult causing cerebral dysfunction, such as trauma, cerebrovascular accident, encephalitis, and so on, or can be secondary to metabolic disorders such as hypoglycemia, toxic agents such as carbon monoxide, or drug ingestion such as neuroleptics, lithium, levodopa, and so on.

Hereditary neurodegenerative disorders can also be associated with tics, in particular neuroacanthocytosis, Huntington's disease, Hallervorden-Spatz disease, and so on.

Treatment

The medical treatment of tic disorder is particularly important when tics affect the quality of life and create a disabling psychosocial situation.

Alpha agonist agents, such as clonidine and guanadine, are now the first line of treatment and may be particularly useful in children with hyperactivity. Neuroleptic drugs, such as pimozide, haloperidol, and fluphenazine, have been widely used for TS. Pimozide is less sedative than haloperidol but may cause prolonged QT interval. Haloperidol can have several adverse effects, such as acute dystonic reactions, school phobia, depression, and parkinsonism. Atypical neuroleptics (risperidone, olanzapine, and ziprasidone) have fewer motor adverse effects and are also used. Botulinum toxin has been considered for patients with disabling intractable tics.

Alternative approaches include behavioral treatments such as relaxation techniques, biofeedback, and hypnosis.

References

Huntington's Disease

Brett, E.M. Paediatric Neurology, ed. 2. New York: Churchill Livingstone, 223–262, 1991.

Fenichel, G.M. Clinical Pediatric Neurology, ed. 3. Philadelphia: W.B. Saunders, 293–309, 1997.

Lyon, G. et al. Neurology of Hereditary and Metabolic Diseases of Children, ed. 2. New York: McGraw Hill, 199–219, 1996

Menkes, J. Heredodegenerative Diseases. In: Menkes, J.H. and Sarnat, H.B. (Eds.). Child Neurology, ed. 6. Philadelphia: Lippincott Williams & Wilkins, 171–239, 2000.

Robertson, M.M. et al. Movement and Allied Disorders in Childhood. New York: John Wiley and Sons, 1995.

Sydenham's Chorea

Allan, W.C. Acute hemichorea in 14-year-old boy. Semin. Neurol. 3:164–169, 1996.

Fenichel, G.M. Movement disorders. In: Clinical Pediatric Neurology: A Sign and Symptoms Approach, ed. 3. Philadelphia: W.B. Saunders, 292–309, 1997.

Menkes, J.H. and Sarnat, H.B. Child Neurology, ed. 6. Philadelphia: Lippincott Williams & Wilkins, 652–657, 2000.

O'Brien, C.F. Sydenham chorea. Neurobase MedLink, Arbor, 1993–2000

Robertson, M.M. and Eapen, V. Movement and Allied Disorders in Childhood. New York: John Wiley and Sons, 1995.

Dystonia Musculorum Deformans

Eapen V, and Robertson, M.M. Movement and Allied Disorders in Childhood. New York: John Wiley and Sons, 105–147, 1995.

Menkes, J.H. and Sarnat, H.B. Child Neurology, ed. 6. Philadelphia: Lippincott Williams & Wilkins, 177–181, 2000.

Tsui, J.K.C. Idiophatic torsion dystonia. Neurobase MedLink, Arbor, 1993–2000.

Tic Disorders

Erenberg, G. The clinical neurology of Tourette syndrome. CNS Spectrum 4:36–53, 1999.

Kurlan, R. Handbook of Tourette's Syndrome and Related Tic and Behavioral Disorders. New York: Marcel Dekker, 1993.

Marcus, D. and Kurlan, R. Tic and its disorders. In: Neurol. Clin. 19:735–758, 2001.

Singer H.S. Tics, stereotypes and other movement disorders. American Academy of Neurology, 53rd Annual Meeting, Philadelphia, May 5–11, 2001.

24
Pediatric Neurometabolic Disorders

Early Infantile Neurometabolic Disorders

Neurometabolic disorders occurring during early infancy affect children in the first year of life. Some clinical features can help identify these syndromes and include

- Progressive encephalopathy with psychosensory-motor regression with signs such as lack of interest in the surroundings, poor head control, and loss of milestones such as inability to roll over or sit without support.
- Hypotonia, developmental delay.
- Neurological signs: Abnormal startle response, tonic spasms, opistotonus, evidence of peripheral neuropathy, chorea, athetosis, dystonia, and so on.
- Ocular findings: Cherry red spot, macular degeneration, optic atrophy, cataracts, and so on.
- Involvement of other organs: Hepatomegaly, splenomegaly, kidney dysfunction, failure to thrive due to unexplained nausea and vomiting, dysmorphic features, and skin, air, and skeletal abnormalities.
- Siblings or relatives with a similar or unexplained neurological syndrome.

GM₂ Gangliosidosis: Tay-Sachs Disease

Vignette

An 8-month-old boy had a normal developmental history till the age of 4 months, when he started becoming increasingly restless, irritable, and over-sensitive to sounds. During the evaluation he was unable to sit, transfer objects from hand to hand, did not babble, and had an exaggerated extension response to unexpected sound. There was a red spot in his macular area on funduscopic examination. Increased DTR and bilateral Babinski's signs were present but no organomegaly. His paternal cousin became blind and bedridden and died at 24 months of uncontrolled seizures.

Summary An 8-month-old baby with developmental regression starting at 4 months, hypersensitivity to sounds, red spot in the macular area, and no organomegaly. The history indicates a paternal cousin who become blind, bedridden, and died of uncontrolled seizures.

Differential Diagnosis

First, it is important to determine in which category the disorder described in the vignette belongs.

The vignette indicates several clinical features:

- Developmental delay and regression presenting in a child who does not have major congenital abnormalities.
- Progressive neurological deterioration with focal findings represented by hyperreflexia and bilateral Babinski's signs.
- Abnormal startle response.
- Ocular abnormalities consisting of red spot in the macular area (cherry red spot).
- No evidence of hepatosplenomegaly or other organomegaly.
- A paternal cousin with blindness and uncontrolled seizures who was bedridden and died at 24 months.

These characteristic clinical findings should raise the suspicion of an hereditary neurometabolic disorder that started during early infancy. In order to narrow the differential diagnosis it is important to consider if the central

217

or peripheral nervous system is involved, if there is any evidence of organomegaly, and if preferentially the white matter or gray matter is affected. The vignette describes a case of progressive neurological deterioration with ocular findings but without clinical evidence of extraneurological involvement. Following are the disorders to be considered:

• Tay-Sachs disease.
• Krabbe's disease.
• Canavan-Van Bogaert-Bertrand disease.

Tay-Sachs disease (the best tentative diagnosis) is part of the GM$_2$ gangliosidoses.

The GM$_2$ gangliosidoses are characterized by the accumulation of GM$_2$ ganglioside, due to lysosomal enzymes deficiency. The hydrolysis of gangliosides is determined by

• Hexosaminidase A (which carries two subunits, alpha and beta).
• Hexosaminidase B (which carries two beta subunits).
• The GM$_2$ activator protein.

Tay-Sachs disease is a hereditary autosomal recessive disorder caused by hexosaminidase A alpha subunit deficiency. The abnormal gene is linked to chromosome 15.

The clinical features are characterized by progressive neurological deterioration that appears after the first few months. Children became listless, irritable, and oversensitive, and experience a characteristic startle response to auditory and also visual and tactile stimuli. The startle response is represented by a sudden extension of the arms and legs, often accompanied by clonic jerks. Repetition of the sound causes repetitive response without adaptation as opposed to a normal startle reaction of infants that rapidly shows adaptation. As the disease progresses the child becomes unable to sit, roll, or vocalize. Hypotonia and corticospinal signs are also present.

A cherry red spot of the macula can be observed in more than 90 percent of cases (Lyon et al.). The finding of a cherry red spot in the macula is characteristic but not specific for Tay-Sachs disease and can also be identified in other disorders (see below).

The neurological symptoms also include progressive blindness and the occurrence of seizures that consist of generalized, myoclonic, or gelastic convulsions.

After 2 to 3 years the children became demented, decerebrate, and blind. Death occurs by the age of 5 to 6 years.

Diagnosis

The diagnosis is based on demonstration of deficiency of hexosaminidase A with normal or elevated activity of hexosaminidase B in white blood cells or serum. Prenatal diagnosis is obtained by measuring hexosaminidase A and B in amniotic fluid. There is no treatment available.

Krabbe's and Canavan's diseases are the other hereditary metabolic diseases without clinically evident extraneurological involvement (Lyon et al.). Krabbe's disease is characterized by onset before 6 months of age with restless irritability, increased tone, tonic spasms, opisthotonic recurvation of the trunk and neck, and recurrent fever without evidence of infection. Only rarely does auditory stimulation induce a startle response, as in Tay-Sachs disease, and signs of peripheral nerve involvement are manifested early in the disease (Lyon et al.).

Canavan disease is characterized by hypotonia, tonic spasms, psychomotor regression, progressive head enlargement, and blindness. Tonic spasms are precipitated by tactile and auditory stimuli, but the typical startle response of Tay-Sachs patients that does not attenuate with stimulus repetition, is not a feature.

Summary of GM$_2$ gangliosidoses
• GM$_2$ Gangliosidosis: Hexosaminidase A (subunits: alpha beta) and Hexosaminidase B (subunits: beta beta).
  • Disorders due to deficiency in hexosaminidase alpha subunit, affecting hexosaminidase A (alpha, beta).
    • Tay-Sachs disease.
    • Later onset variant of GM$_2$ gangliosidosis.
  • Disorders due to deficiency of beta subunit, affecting both hexosaminidase A and B.
    • Sanhoff disease.
      • Early infant.
      • Juvenile.
  • GM$_2$ activator deficiency.
• Disorders in which cherry red spots in the macula can be observed.
  • Storage diseases.
    • GM$_2$ gangliosidosis.
    • GM$_1$ gangliosidosis.
    • Niemann-Pick disease.
    • Metachromatic leukodystrophy.
    • Farber's lipogranulomatosis.
    • Sialidoses.
    • Cherry red spot–myoclonus syndrome.
  • Vascular and traumatic disorders.
    • Central retinal artery occlusion.
    • Intramacular hemorrhage.
    • Retinal trauma.

Leukodystrophies

The leukodystrophies are hereditary disorders of the white matter presenting with a variety of manifestations that reflect involvement of the long motor corticospinal and corticobulbar tract, cerebellum, optic nerve, geniculocalcarine structures, and peripheral nervous system (demyelinating neuropathy). Main disorders include

- Krabbe's disease.
- Metachromatic leukodystrophy.
- Juvenile X-linked adrenoleukodystrophy.
- Pelizaeus-Merzbacher disease.
- Sudanophilic leukodystrophies.

Krabbe's Disease

Vignette

A 6-month-old baby boy started experiencing list-lessness, irritability, bouts of inconsolable crying, and regression of previously acquired motor skills associated with episodes of extensor spasm precipitated by feeding and touching. His history was significant for recurrent vomiting, feeding difficulties, and unexplained fever. On examination the child was extremely irritable. Tone was increased and deep tendon reflexes could not be elicited. Optic atrophy was noted but no organomegaly deformities or dysmorphic features.

Summary A 6-month-old baby with neurological regression and history of vomiting, poor feeding, and unexplained fever, and neurological signs suggestive of central and peripheral nerve involvment, such as extensor spasm, stimulus sensitive, hypertonia, and absent deep tendon reflexes. Important findings include no organomegaly deformities or dysmorphic features.

Localization and Differential Diagnosis

The signs point to a neurometabolic disorder of early infancy. The combination of irritability, developmental regression, extensor spasms, and peripheral neuropathy may indicate the possibility of Krabbe's disease (globoid cell leukodystrophy).

Tay-Sachs disease, which also presents during early infancy and is characterized by an exaggerated abnormal startle reaction to auditory and other stimuli, can be excluded clinically by the signs of peripheral neuropathy, and the absence of a cherry red spot in the macula.

The infantile form of Batten disease, which also shows progressive psychomotor regression and visual dysfunction, does not have signs of peripheral nerve involvement.

Other disorders to be distinguished are the infantile forms of Niemann-Pick and Gaucher's diseases, but they can be differentiated by the presence of organomegaly (hepatomegaly and splenomegaly), cherry red spot, and no evidence of peripheral neuropathy.

Pelizaeus-Merzbacher disease, another infantile leukodystrophy, differs from Krabbe's disease by the abnormal eye movements and progressive significant cerebellar and pyramidal signs.

Metachromatic leukodystrophy that clinically carries some resemblance to Krabbe's disease usually manifests during the late infantile period.

Clinical Features

Globoid cell leukodystrophy, or Krabbe's disease, is a hereditary disorder transmitted with an autosomal recessive pattern of inheritance and due to deficiency of the lysosomal enzyme galactocerebrosidase. The clinical manifestations are usually characteristic of the early infantile period with vomiting and poor feeding. Other less common variants are the late infantile, juvenile, and adult forms.

In the early infantile form, the symptoms usually appear before 6 months of age with increased irritability, apathy, bouts of inconsolable crying, failure to thrive due to recurrent vomiting, increased tone, and tonic spasms precipitated by external stimuli and feeding, in combination with signs of peripheral nerve dysfunction. Ocular abnormalities include optic atrophy and blindness, and rarely a cherry red spot. Seizures are not common. Tonic spasms precede permanent opisthotonus characterized by flexion of the arms, wrists, and fingers and marked extension of the legs. In the end, the infant becomes blind, decerebrate, and in a chronic vegetative state.

The early infantile form of Krabbe's disease has been divided into three stages:

- Stage 1: Usually starts around 3 months of age, is characterized by increased irritability and listlesness, episodes of severe crying, unexplained fever and vomiting, psychomotor regression, and tonic spasm.
- Stage 2: A state of permanent opisthotonus develops, characterized by flexion of the arms, wrists, and fingers and marked extension of the legs. Seizures can be frequent and optic atrophy and blindness occur.
- Stage 3: During this stage, the child is decerebrate and hypotonic. Death usually occurs at a mean age of 1.2 years (Kolodny).

The late infantile form, which usually starts after the second year of life is less common and is characterized by progressive spastic quadriparesis, ataxia, marked visual dysfunction with optic atrophy and cortical blindness, seizures, and signs of peripheral nerve involvement.

The juvenile variant, presenting in the second decade of life, and the adult form, occurring in the third or fourth decade of life, have features that include gait disturbances, progressive spastic weakness, pes cavus, and signs of peripheral neuropathy with normal cognition in 50 percent of cases.

Diagnosis

The evaluation of a child suspected of having Krabbe's disease should include CSF sudies, which usually demonstrate marked increase in the protein content. Nerve conduction studies may show a demyelinating neuropathy with marked decreased conduction velocities. MRI of the brain indicates diffuse demyelination of the white matter.

The diagnosis is confirmed by the assessment of activity of galactosylceramide beta-galactosidase in leukocytes or cultured fibroblasts.

Treatment

Treatment is limited and bone marrow transplantation has been performed in selected cases.

Late Infantile Neurometabolic Disorders

The late infantile progressive neurometabolic disorders that usually appear after the first year of life are characterized by loss of prior acquired motor skills due to involvement of the corticospinal tract, cerebellum, and extrapyramidal and peripheral nervous system.

The presentation of the disorders that belong to this group varies and includes;

- Progressive gait dysfunction due to involvement of the central and peripheral nervous systems.
- Progressive cerebellar ataxia in combination with involuntary movements, such as choreoathetosis or dystonia.
- Recurrent episodes of confusion or coma.
- Seizures, myoclonus, and blindness.
- Psychomotor regression, dysmorphic features, and skeletal anomalies.

Metachromatic Leukodystrophy

Vignette

A 3-year-old girl had experienced gait difficulties with unsteadiness and frequent falls since the age of 20 months. One year later, she was only able to stand with support and was unable to walk, often refusing to try because of pain in her legs. Her speech had become slurred, she had some problems swallowing and was very irritable and sometimes apathetic and unaware of her surrounding. On examination the girl responded only to some very simple commands, had a dysarthric speech, general-ized spasticity, and bilateral Babinski's signs. Ankle jerks were absent. Bilateral optic atrophy was noted.

Summary A 3-year-old girl with gait difficulties, dysarthria, dysphagia, and behavioral and cognitive problems. The neurological examination shows signs of involvement of the central and peripheral nervous systems (spasticity, bilateral Babinski's signs, absent ankle jerk). The age of onset is late infantile. Several clinical features should suggest the possibility of a hereditary metabolic disease:

- Progressive difficulty in walking due to involvement of the central and/or peripheral motor system.
- Developmental regression with loss of prior acquired motor skills.
- Ophthalmologic abnormalities (visual loss, bilateral optic atrophy).

Differential Diagnosis

Among the hereditary metabolic disorders that cause spastic weakness and/or peripheral neuropathy in combination with mental regression and optic atrophy, metachromatic leukodystrophy (MLD), particularly the late infantile variant, which is the most common form, deserves serious consideration.

In the differential diagnosis of the vignette, late-onset Krabbe's disease needs to be considered because it can create some diagnostic problems. In the late infantile form of this disorder, the signs of CNS involvement predominate, with progressive spastic weakness, ataxia, optic atrophy, cortical blindness, and cognitive dysfunction. The peripheral nerve involvement is usually milder, particularly compared with the CNS manifestations and is rarely the presenting symptom (Dumitru et al.).

Adrenoleukodystrophy can be differentiated because it is an X-linked disorder that affects only males starting during childhood and characterized by progressive neurological deterioration, optic atrophy, cortical blindness, dementia, spasticity and signs of adrenal insufficiency.

Neuroaxonal dystrophy is a rare disorder characterized by developmental regression, progressive weakness, hypotonia, cortical spinal tract involvement, and hyporeflexia. Therefore, it can create a diagnostic problem in distinction from MLD. In neuroaxonal dystrophy, EMG study shows findings consistent with denervation but motor and sensory conduction velocities are normal. CSF is also normal. MRI of the brain demonstrates evidence of cerebellar atrophy. The most valuable diagnostic test of neuroaxonal dystrophy is the finding of typical neuroaxonal spheroid aggregates in the distal part of peripheral nerves or at the neuromuscular junction after nerve biopsy.

Multiple sulfatase deficiency is an autosomal recessive

hereditary disorder that may simulate the early infantile form of MLD but has some distinctive clinical features, such as severe cognitive impairment since the early stages, dysmorphic features, skeletal anomalies, and organomegaly (Lyon et al.).

Early-onset Strumpell-Lorrain familial spastic paraplegia and other rare forms of familial paraplegia can also be distinguished by the fact that peripheral nerves are not affected and CSF examination is normal (Lyon).

Clinical Features

Metachromatic leukodystrophy is a hereditary disorder transmitted with an autosomal recessive pattern of inheritance characterized by the accumulation of metachromatic material in the central and peripheral nervous systems and visceral organs. It is caused by deficient activity of the enzyme arylsulfatase A or, rarely, to a defect of a nonenzymatic protein activator SAP 1 (in such case, arylsulfatase levels are normal) (Lyon et al.). There are three variants of this disorder: the late infantile form, which is the most common, the juvenile form, and the adult form.

The late infantile form has its onset in the second year of life, usually with walking difficulties. Hagberg, as reported by Luijten, divided the disease into four stages from stage 1 of progressive gait difficulties with unsteadiness, pain, hypotonia, and mental and speech deterioration, to stage 4 characterized by a vegetative state. The combination of progressive central nervous system dysfunction characterized by pyramidal involvement and spasticity with signs of peripheral nerve dysfunction with hyporeflexia is very important for the diagnosis of MLD and is also a common presentation.

Cognitive and visual impairment are not noted in the early stages but become evident as the disease progresses. Seizures are not a prominent manifestation. Later on, progressive mental deterioration, spasticity and dysarthria occur. Ocular abnormalities may demonstrate optic atrophy. In the late stage, the child is bedridden, blind, tetraplegic, and in a vegetative state.

The juvenile form manifests after the fourth year of life with behavioral and emotional abnormalities associated with progressive spastic paralysis and usually without signs of peripheral nerve involvement.

The adult form presents in the second decade of life with marked psychiatric symptoms and progressive cognitive impairment.

Diagnosis

The diagnosis is based on demonstrating decreased or absent arylsulfatase A (ASA) activity in serum, urine, leukocytes, cultured skin fibroblasts, or amniotic fluid cells. Rarely in symptomatic patients, arylsulfatase A activity is normal and there is deficiency of the activator

protein SAP1. Additional diagnostic procedures include CSF studies that show an elevated protein content (>100 mg/dl). MRI imaging demonstrates hyperintense signal in the periventricular and central white matter on T_2-weighted images.

Nerve conduction velocities are decreased, particularly in the late infantile variant. Sural nerve biopsy may demonstrate metachromatic material in Schwann cells and macrophages (Luijten).

The gene for ASA is linked to chromosome 22 (Lyon).

Treatment

The treatment is symptomatic. Selected cases may benefit from bone marrow transplantation.

Neuronal Ceroid Lipofuscinosis

Vignette

A 5-year-old girl became clumsy, apathetic, and irritable, and had sleep difficulties beginning at age 18 months. She then experienced two generalized tonic-clonic seizures that granted a neurological evaluation with undetermined diagnosis. Several months later she was reevaluated because of increased incoordination and difficulty walking, severe intractable seizures, irregular myoclonic jerks, staring spells and visual difficulties. On examination she responded to voice and could follow very simple commands. The ophthalmoscopic examination revealed optic atrophy and pigmentary changes of the macular area. Deep tendon reflexes were increased and bilateral Babinski's sign was noted. Gait was ataxic and very unsteady.

Summary A 5-year-old girl with progressive mental deterioration, seizures, myoclonus, and visual loss starting at age 18 months. The neurological examination indicates mental deterioration, optic atrophy, and increased reflexes with Babinski's sign and ataxia.

Localization and Differential Diagnosis

This is a disorder occurring in the late infantile period and characterized by involvement of the central nervous system and primarily affecting the gray matter, as suggested by personality changes, seizures, and cognitive impairment. Several characteristics should help categorize this vignette into late infantile hereditary metabolic disorders: progressive mental regression, seizures, myoclonus, ophthalmologic abnormalities, and progressive ataxia.

In the differential diagnosis, great consideration needs to be given to neuronal ceroid lipofuscinosis, which has been distinguished into the classic infantile, late infantile, and juvenile variants.

The late infantile form (Jansky-Bielschowski disease) is a hereditary disorder transmitted with an autosomal recessive pattern of inheritance and onset of manifestations between the ages of 2 and 4 (Lyon et al.). Clinical features include seizures of different types: generalized, tonic-clonic, atonic, and myoclonic, and often refractory to treatment. Stimulus-sensitive myoclonus also occurs. Ataxia and progressive mental deterioration are important clinical characteristics as well as progressive visual loss that leads to blindness. Ocular abnormalities consist of optic atrophy, macular degeneration, and hyperpigmentation. The polymyoclonia is characterized by irregular and asymmetrical myoclonic jerks, evoked by proprioceptive stimuli, voluntary movement, or emotional excitement (Lyon et al.).

Diagnostic tests include a careful ophthalmoscopic examination to identify the characteristic atrophy and pigmentary changes. The electroretinogram shows loss of responses. The EEG may demonstrate occipital spikes induced by low-frequency photic stimulation (Lyon et al.). MRI may demonstrate diffuse brain and cerebellar atrophy. Skin or conjunctival biopsy may show intralysosomal inclusions in mesenchymal cells.

Late infantile neuronal ceroid lipofuscinosis needs to be distinguished from other disorders such as severe idiopathic epilepsy, Lennox-Gastaut syndrome, late infantile GM$_2$ gangliosidosis, and so on (Lyon et al.).

Treatment

Treatment is not available.

Childhood-Onset Neurometabolic Disorders

The childhood-onset neurometabolic disorders, which cover the period between the fourth year and adolescence, can include those disorders that present early but allow survival until later years or those typical of childhood onset. A variety of presentations and symptomatologies may occur, such as progressive signs of central nervous system involvement with spasticity and hyperreflexia associated with peripheral neuropathy, progressive ataxia with sensory loss, recurrent stroke-like episodes, extrapyramidal symptoms and ataxia, progressive dementia, and so on.

Adrenoleukodystrophy

Vignette

An 8-year-old boy started becoming moody, apathetic, irritable, and less interested in school and sports, often experiencing violent tantrums that required psychiatric evaluation with a final diagnosis of attention deficit disorder with hyperactivity. Later on, he seemed clumsy and unsteady and was noted to have slurred speech and poor vision. His previous history was unremarkable except for unexplained episodes of vomiting and diarrhea since the age of 4 and excessively tanned skin since than. On examination he was inattentive, poorly cooperative, and clearly dysarthric with gross constriction of the visual fields. DTR were hyperactive with bilateral Babinski's signs. Gait was ataxic. On inspection he had very dark areolae and gums. A maternal uncle died at the age of 10 of an unexplained neurological disorder.

Summary An 8-year-old boy with progressive neurological disorder involving visual, pyramidal, and cerebellar systems associated with extraneurological symptoms, which include hyperpigmentation (excessively tan skin and very dark areolae and gums) and unexplained episodes of vomiting and diarrhea.

Localization and Differential Diagnosis

The case described in the vignette suggests a degenerative disorder of childhood characterized by psychomotor regression with loss of previously acquired functions. A primary involvement of the white matter is indicated by the symptoms of spasticity, cerebellar pathway involvement, and visual dysfunction. Dementia and seizures tend to occur later (Golden).

Some clues in the vignette should point to the most likely diagnosis. These are the presence of nonneurological symptoms. Hyperpigmentation of areolae and gums, excessively tan skin, diarrhea, and vomiting are all indicative of adrenal insufficiency. The history of a maternal uncle who had died at 10 of a neurological disorder suggests an X-linked transmission.

In summary, the case presented in the vignette localizes to the white matter and indicates a progressive hereditary X-linked degenerative disorder involving the nervous system and adrenal glands in childhood.

Childhood cerebral adrenoleukodystrophy (ALD), characterized by progressive demyelination of the central nervous system associated with adrenal cortical insufficiency, is clearly an important first consideration in the differential diagnosis in this child who presents with progressive neurological deterioration with behavioral abnormalities; disturbances of gait, in coordination, and visual abnormalities; and melanodermia.

Mental retardation and Addison's disease are often combined in the X-linked disorder glycerol kinase deficiency (Moser). Addison's disease can manifest with neurological symptoms due to hypoglycemic episodes in addisonian crises or when electrolyte abnormalities cause the picture of cerebral pontine myelinolisis (Moser). In the differential diagnosis, we also need to consider infections, such as encephalitis, neoplastic processes, and demyelinating disorders.

Clinical Features

X-linked adrenoleukodystrophy is a hereditary disorder that affects only males and is caused by accumulation of very-long-chain fatty acids in tissues and plasma. The incidence is 1 in 20,000 male births (Lyon et al.). Affected patients experience impaired ability to oxidize very-long-chain fatty acids, especially hexacosanoic acid, because of deficiency of peroxisomal acyl coenzyme A synthetase (Fenichel).

The childhood cerebral form manifests between the ages of 4 and 8 years in a previously healthy child. Initial presentation may include behavior abnormalities with irritability, restlessness, apathy, and lack of interest in school activities that may be diagnosed as signs of hyperactivity or attention deficit disorders.

Other findings include progressive cognitive impairment leading to dementia, and visual abnormalities such as homonymous hemianopia, loss of visual recognition, cortical blindness, and, less frequently, optic atrophy. Hearing loss can also represent an early feature and is of central origin. Corticospinal tract involvement and cerebellar ataxia are responsible for the gait dysfunction. One third of patients have focal or generalized seizures (Aubourg). The disease is relentlessly progressive and affected children can reach a vegetative state within a few years.

Signs and symptoms of adrenal insufficiency can vary from fatigue, vomiting, and skin pigmentation to typical Addison's disease and may precede the neurological syndrome.

Other clinical phenotypes include

- Adolescent cerebral ALD: Similar to the childhood variant with a later onset, after the first decade of life.
- Adult form of cerebral ALD: Can manifest with prominent psychiatric features that may simulate schizophrenia, psychosis, or even Kluver-Bucy syndrome (Aubourg). Patients also have signs of spinal cord involvement.
- Adrenomyeloneuropathy: Manifests in the second decade of life with features of progressive myelopathy such as spastic weakness mainly involving the lower extremities, impaired vibration, and sphincteric distur-

bance, associated with signs of adrenal insufficiency. A mild peripheral neuropathy is also present.
- Addison's disease: A minority of patients have clinical evidence of primary adrenal insufficiency but lack neurological symptoms, which may eventually develop later.
- Symptomatic ALD heterozygotes: Some women who are heterozygous for ALD may demonstrate signs of adrenomyeloneuropathy that may simulate multiple sclerosis with progressive spastic paraparesis and, rarely, signs of adrenal dysfunction.
- Asymptomatic: Cases that, in spite of the significant laboratory findings of highly elevated, saturated, very-long-chain fatty acid levels, are clinically asymptomatic.

Diagnosis

The diagnosis is based on the presence of abnormally high levels of saturated, very-long-chain fatty acids in plasma, erythrocytes, leukocytes, or cultured fibroblasts. Prenatal diagnosis is possible using VLCFA assays in amniocytes or cultures of chorionic villus.

MRI of the brain shows significant demyelination, particularly in the bilateral parietooccipital region with a caudorostral progression.

Adrenal insufficiency can be demonstrated by abnormally increased levels of ACTH in plasma and abnormal cortisol response to ACTH stimulation (Lott in Berg).

Treatment

Two forms of therapy are recommended: dietary therapy with VLCFA restriction combined with the oral administration of a mixture of glyceryl trioleate and glyceryl trierucate, and bone marrow transplantation.

References

Tay-Sachs Disease

Fenichel, G.M. Clinical Pediatric Neurology, ed. 3. Philadelphia: W.B.Saunders, 118–152, 1997.

Kivlin, J.D. et al. The cherry red spot in Tay-Sachs and other storage diseases. Ann. Neurol. 17:356–360, 1985.

Lyon, G. et al. Neurology of Hereditary Metabolic Diseases of Children, ed. 2. New York: McGraw-Hill, 45–123, 1996.

Schneck, L. et al. The startle response and serum enzyme profile in early detection of Tay-Sachs disease. J. Pediatr. 65:749–756, 1964.

Krabbe's Disease

Brett, E. Pediatric Neurology, ed. 2. New York: Churchill Livingstone, 141–200, 1991.

Fenichel, G.M. Clinical Pediatric Neurology, ed. 3. Philadelphia: W.B. Saunders, 118–152, 1997.

Kaye, EM. Globoid cell leukodystrophy. MedLink, Arbor, 1993–2000.

Kolodny, E.H. Globoid leukodystrophy. In: Moser, W.H. (Ed.). Handbook of Clinical Neurology, Vol. 22: Neurodystrophies and neurolipidoses. New York: Elsevier, 1996.

Lyon, G. et al. Neurology of Hereditary Metabolic Diseases of Children, ed. 2. New York: McGraw-Hill, 45–123, 1996.

Metachromatic Leukodystrophy

Berg, B.O. Principles of Child Neurology. New York: McGraw-Hill, 522–530, 1996.

Dumitru, D. Electrodiagnostic Medicine, ed. 2. Philadelphia: Hanley and Belfus, 2002.

Luijten, J.A.F.M. Metachromatic leukodystrophy. in: de Jong, J. (Ed.). Handbook of Clinical Neurology, Vol. 16: Hereditary neuropathies and spinocerebellar atrophies. New York: Elsevier, 123–129, 1991.

Lyon, G. et al. Neurology of Hereditary Metabolic Diseases of Children, ed. 2. New York: McGraw-Hill, 124–176, 1996.

Menkes, J.H. Heredodegenerative diseases. In: Menkes, J. and Sarnat, H.B. (Eds.). Child Neurology, ed. 6. New York: Lippincott Williams & Wilkins, 171–239, 2000.

Philippart, M. Metachromatic leukodystrophy. In: Moser, W.H. (Ed.). Handbook of Clinical Neurology, Vol. 22: Neurodystrophies and neurolipidoses. New York: Elsevier, 163–185, 1996.

Neuronal Ceroid Lipofuscinosis

Brett, E.M. Pediatric Neurology, ed. 2. New York: Churchill Livingstone, 146–153, 1991.

Fenichel, G.M. Clinical Pediatric Neurology, ed. 3. Philadelphia: W. B. Saunders, 118–152, 1997.

Goebel, H.H. The neuronal ceroid lipofuscinosis. Semin. Pediatr. Neurol. 3:270–278, 1996.

Lyon, G et al. Neurology of Hereditary Metabolic Diseases of Children, ed. 2. New York: McGraw-Hill, 124–176, 1996.

Adrenoleukodystrophy

Aubourg, P. X-linked adrenoleukodystrophy. In: Moser, H.W. (Ed.). Handbook of Clinical Neurology, Vol. 22: Neurodystrophies and neurolipidoses. New York: Elsevier, 447–483, 1996.

Battaglia, A. et al. Adrenoleurodystrophy: Neurophysiological aspects. J. Neurol. Neurosurg. Psychiatry 44:781–785, 1981.

Berg, B.O. Principles of Child Neurology. New York: McGraw-Hill, 1241–1244, 1996.

Case Records of the Massachusetts General Hospital. Case 18. N. Engl. J. Med. 1037–1045, 1979.

Fenichel, G.M. Clinical Pediatric Neurology, ed. 3. Philadelphia: W.B. Saunders, 1997.

Gartner, J. Clinical and genetic aspects of X-linked adrenoleukodystrophy. Neuropediatrics 29:3–13, 1998.

Golden, G.S. Textbook of Pediatric Neurology. New York: Plenum, 195–292, 1987.

Lyon, G. et al. Neurology of hereditary metabolic diseases of children, ed. 2. New York: McGraw-Hill, 248–251, 1996.

Moser, H.W. Adrenoleukodystrophy. MedLink, Arbor, 1993–2000.

Schaumburg, H. et al. Adrenoleukodystrophy: A clinical and pathological study of 17 cases. Arch. Neurol. 32:577–591, 1975.

25
Pediatric Infections

Subacute Sclerosing Panencephalitis

Vignette

An 8-year-old, previously healthy boy started becoming forgetful, apathetic, and irritable after coming back from visiting his grandmother in Mexico. His schoolwork deteriorated and he was soon sent to the school guidance counselor. Several months later he experienced episodes of head nodding, flinging movements of the extremities, and even some falls, without loss of consciousness. His intellectual function continued to deteriorate to the point that he had stopped speaking and was also unable to walk without assistance. On examination the boy had normal vital signs and head circumference. Cranial nerves were normal except for retinal degeneration and optic disc pallor on the right. Some brief, uncontrolled, repetitive movements of the fingers and shoulders occurring every 20 seconds were observed. DTR were brisk with extensor plantar responses. He could only walk holding to furniture. His family history, including two siblings, was unremarkable. He had a history of uncomplicated measles at 15 months and varicella at 3 years.

Summary An 8-year-old boy with progressive changes in mental status, episodes of falling down without loss of consciousness, jerking movements (myoclonic jerks), gait disturbances (ataxia), and visual abnormalities (retinal degeneration and optic atrophy). The examination shows signs of corticospinal tract and possible cerebellar involvement. The medical history given is limited to uncomplicated measles at 15 months and varicella at 3 years.

Differential Diagnosis

The differential diagnosis includes disorders associated with progressive encephalopathies of childhood. A distinction should be made between genetic disorders, such as disorders of the white matter, gray matter, and lisosomal enzyme, and acquired disorders, such as chronic infections, for example, meningitis, encephalitis, and particularly HIV and subacute sclerosing panencephalitis (SSPE).

Among the progressive encephalopathies of childhood and adolescence, there are many disorders characterized by progressive diffuse central nervous system dysfunction, such as mitochondrial disorders (MERFF and MELAS), late-onset form of GM_2 gangliosidosis, late-onset Krabbe's disease, metachromatic leukodystrophy, and adrenoleukodystrophy.

Myoclonus can be a prominent feature of several hereditary disorders, such as mitochondrial disorders (MERFF), Lafora disease, sialidosis, and so on. Myoclonus epilepsy with ragged red fibers (MERFF) is characterized by myoclonus, generalized seizures, cognitive impairment, but also other features such as sensorineural hearing loss, myopathy, optic atrophy, short stature, lactic acidosis, and the appearance of ragged red fibers on muscle biopsy.

Lafora disease, characterized by typical polyglucosan cytoplasmic inclusions in the neurons and other organs, is a hereditary autosomal recessive disorder manifesting with polymyoclonus, mental deterioration, and occipital seizures.

Sialidosis, particularly type I, is characterized by prominent myoclonus and seizures, but also blindness, optic atrophy, cerebellar ataxia, and a macular cherry red spot.

Chronic progressive acquired disorders to be considered are the chronic infections, particularly chronic meningitis, chronic progressive viral infections especially HIV encephalopathy, progressive rubella panencephalitis, and subacute sclerosing panencephalitis.

Chronic meningitis, particularly tuberculous, is characterized by behavior and personality changes, headache, altered consciousness, low-grade fever, anorexia, cranial neuropathies, and even signs of hydrocephalus.

AIDS encephalopathy is characterized by a slowly progressive cognitive decline, loss of prior acquired milestones, motor involvement with corticospinal and corticobulbar signs, microcephaly, and ataxia. Seizures or myoclonus are uncommon (Menkes).

Progressive rubella panencephalitis is a rare disorder characterized by progressive cognitive impairment combined with pyramidal and extrapyramidal signs, ataxia, and myoclonic seizures that occur 3 to 10 years after a congenital or acquired rubella infection.

Subacute sclerosing panencephalitis, which represents a slow viral infection attributed to the measles virus, should rank high on the list of differential diagnoses and is, indeed, the correct and best tentative diagnosis of the vignette presented. The clinical features of the vignette as well as the history of uncomplicated measles at 15 months both point to this diagnosis.

Clinical Features

SSPE represents a chronic progressive disorder primarily affecting children, generally males, in the first decade of life and caused by a persistent infection of the CNS by a mutated form of measles virus. Measles virus infection in children younger than 1 year has been epidemiologically indicated to be one of the risk factors of SSPE (Sawaishi).

Clinical manifestations, which occur in children with a prior history of measles infection and complete resolution of symptoms, consist of progressive cognitive and behavioral abnormalities, hyperactivity, and poor school performance, signs that are included in the first stage of SSPE. Seizures can occur in any stage.

Myoclonus appears in the second stage with unilateral or bilateral muscle contractions involving the head, axial muscles, and extremities, without affecting consciousness. Myoclonic jerks have a regular periodicity that varies between 4 and 20 seconds, and disappear during sleep. Myoclonus in SSPE is considered nonepileptic and instead the result of a massive extrapyramidal discharge (Dyken).

As the disease progresses, the myoclonic spasms increase in severity and may become multifocal (Gascon). Additional neurological symptoms include extrapyramidal and corticospinal tract signs, increasing dementia, visual loss, and so on.

Stage IV is characterized by mutism and a vegetative state.

Diagnosis

The laboratory findings demonstrate elevation of measles-specific antibodies in both the serum and CSF.

The typical electroencephalographic periodic pattern consists of high-voltage (300 to 1500 µV), repetitive, polyphasic sharp and slow wave discharges ranging from 0.5 to 2 seconds in duration, usually recurring every 4 to 15 seconds (Niedermeyer).

Treatment

There is no effective treatment for SSPE, but it can be prevented by measles immunization. Oral isoprinosine and intraventricular interferon-alpha have shown some promising results.

Gradenigo's Syndrome

Vignette

A 12-year-old boy started complaining of severe burning pain in his right eye. The neurological examination revealed paresis of the right lateral gaze, absent right corneal reflex, and mild right facial weakness. He was afebrile and neck was supple. There was a history of right ear pain for a week.

Summary A 12-year-old boy with right eye and right ear pain presenting with a right fifth, sixth, and seventh nerve paralysis.

Differential Diagnosis

The differential diagnosis includes infectious, neoplastic, and traumatic disorders.

Considering infectious processes first, inflammation of the petrous apex due to complicated otitis media or mastoiditis may result in Gradenigo's syndrome, characterized by facial pain and a combination of trigeminal abducens and facial nerve involvement.

Ramsay Hunt syndrome (geniculate herpes zoster), characterized by severe ear pain, vesicular eruption, and involvement of the seventh and sometimes the fifth and other cranial nerves, also enters the differential diagnosis.

Neoplastic disorders involving the petrous bone and closed head trauma need also to be considered.

Neonatal Meningitis

Vignette

A 10-day-old boy became irritable, restless and lethargic. He nursed poorly and vomited twice. In the emergency room he experienced some focal twitches of his left side. He was drowsy, with a tem-

*perature of 100.5°F. The neurological examination
revealed bulging fontanelle and brisk reflexes. Neck
was supple and the funduscopic and cranial nerve
examinations were normal. The baby was the product of a full-term, uncomplicated pregnancy and
delivery.*

Summary A 10-day-old baby with altered level of consciousness, poor feeding, irritability, fever, vomiting,
bulging fontanelle, and a possible focal seizure.

Localization

This infant presented the following clinical features:

- Systemic signs represented by fever and poor feeding.
- Signs of increased intracranial pressure indicated by
  vomiting and bulging fontanelle.
- Signs of cerebral dysfunction characterized by lethargy
  and possible focal seizures.

Differential Diagnosis

Several disorders need to be considered in order to formulate a differential diagnosis, including

- Infectious processes, such as bacterial meningitides, vi-
  ral meningoencephalitides, and systemic infections.
- Brain tumors and vascular malformations.
- Cerebral hemorrhages (subarachnoid, intraventricular).
- Hypoxic-ischemic encephalopathy.
- Metabolic disorders.
- Trauma.

Considering the infections first, great consideration
needs to be given to neonatal meningitis. The major organisms involved are *Escherichia coli* and group b streptococci and represent two thirds of all causes of neonatal
meningitis in North America (Shrier et al.). Clinical manifestations include fever, irritability, poor feeding, vomiting, altered level of consciousness, seizures, bulging
fontanelle, and so on. Nuchal rigidity is not a reliable sign
and is present in less than 25 percent of patients (Seay).

Another consideration in the differential diagnosis is
viral encephalitis, in particular due to herpes simplex virus infection, which is usually due to vertical transmission
of the virus from the mother perinatally. Herpes simplex
encephalitis can manifest in neonates even in the first
week of extrauterine life but is usually later in the second
or third week, with symptoms consisting of irritability,
seizures, fever, poor feeding, drowsiness, respiratory
compromise, jaundice, and trombocytopenia. Seizures,
focal or generalized, often untractable, can be a prominent symptom. Vesicular skin manifestations can be observed, but not in all cases. CSF demonstrates lymphocytic pleocytosis, increased proteins and red blood cells,
often with xanthochromia and hypoglycorrhachia. Prompt
treatment with acyclovir or vidarabine is essential in order
to reduce the mortality.

Neonatal enteroviral infections are also an important
consideration in the differential diagnosis of the child described because they can manifest during the first week
of life with fever, irritability, altered consciousness, and
flaccid weakness associated with systemic involvement
indicative of neonatal sepsis. A more favorable picture of
aseptic meningitis can also occur. Because of the decline
in neonatal bacterial meningitis, enteroviruses have became the most common cause of meningitis in neonates
older than 7 days and are currently responsible for one
third of all cases of neonatal meningitis (Seay). Diagnostic data include isolation of the virus from blood or CSF,
feces, and oropharyngeal swabbing. The PCR technique
demonstrates sensitivity and specificity for the detection
of virus-specific DNA.

In the differential diagnosis of this case, we also need
to include space-occupying lesions, such as congenital
brain tumors and vascular malformations, that may simulate a CNS infection with symptoms of irritability, altered consciousness, focal or generalized seizures, vomiting, signs of increased intracranial pressure, and so on.

Cerebrovascular disorders such as neonatal cerebral
infarction due to coagulopathies, hypoxia-ischemia,
trauma, infections, and so on, can present during the first
few days of life with altered level of consciousness, seizures, and hypotonia. Intraventricular hemorrhages are
usually a consideration in the premature infant and tend
to manifest early in the first day of life with lethargy,
seizures, coma, and so on.

A neurometabolic disorder also needs to be ruled out
in a neonate presenting with seizures, vomiting, poor
feeding, and altered level of consciousness. Some clues
to this diagnosis include the presence of ocular movement
abnormalities, irregular breathing, hypothermia, organomegaly, dysmorphic features, a neurometabolic disorder
in a sibling, and so on.

Clinical Features

The agents responsible for the majority of neonatal bacterial meningitis include group b streptococci and *Escherichia coli.* Symptoms may manifest early after the delivery, during the first week, or may have a late onset.

Clinical signs are usually nonspecific and characterized
by irritability, feeding difficulties, vomiting, fever, altered
level of consciousness, organomegaly, jaundice, seizures,
and bulging fontanelle. Meningeal signs are rarely present. Complications include hydrocephalus and acute cerebral infarction. Cranial nerve involvement can also occur, particularly affecting the third, fourth, and sixth
cranial nerves.

Diagnosis

The diagnosis is based on CSF studies that may demonstrate a neutrophilic pleocytosis, increased protein level,

and hypoglycorrhachia. Gram stain and bacterial cultures are important confirmatory tests. Neuroimaging studies, particularly MRI of the brain, are useful in showing possible cerebral complications and demonstrating cerebral edema, infarction, or hemorrhage.

Treatment

The treatment is based on the possible organism involved, with the use of the appropriate antimicrobial therapy.

References

Subacute Sclerosing Panencephalitis

Brett, E.M. Pediatric Neurology. New York: Churchill Livingstone, 633–638, 1991.

Dluglos, D.J. et al. In: Bodensteiner, J.B. (Ed.). Seminars in Pediatric Neurology. 6(3):164–167, 1999.

Dyken, P.R. Subacute sclerosing panencephalitis. In: Berg, O. (Ed.). Principles of Child Neurology. New York: McGraw-Hill, 859–868, 1996.

Fenichel, G.M. Clinical Pediatric Neurology, ed. 3. Philadelphia: W.B. Saunders, 146, 1997.

Gascon, G.G. Subacute sclerosing panencephalitis. Semin. Pediatr. Neurol. 3:260–269, 1996.

Lyon, G. et al. Neurology of Hereditary Metabolic Diseases of Children, ed. 2. New York: McGraw-Hill, 1996.

Menkes, J.H. Textbook of Child Neurology, ed. 4. Philadelphia: Lea and Febiger, 1990.

Niedermeyer, E. and Lopes Da Silva, F. Electroencephalography, ed. 2. Munich: Urban and Schwarzenberg, 265–266, 1987.

Sawaishi, Y. et al. SSPE following neonatal measles infection. Pediatr. Neurol. 20:63–65, 1999.

Gradenigo's Syndrome

Brazis, P.W. et al. Localization in clinical neurology, ed. 2. Boston: Little Brown, 189–202, 1990.

Glaser, J.S. Neuroophthalmology, ed. 2. Philadelphia: J.B. Lippincott, 259, 1989.

Menkes, J.H. Textbook of Child Neurology, ed. 4. Philadelphia: Lea and Febiger 454, 1990.

Neonatal Meningitis

Adler, S.P. Central nervous system infection. In: Pellock, J.M. and Myer, E.C. (Eds.). Neurologic Emergencies in Infancy and Childhood, ed. 2. Boston: Butterworth-Heinemann, 220–241, 1993.

Seay, A.R. Miscellaneous neurologic disorders of childhood. Neonatal meningitis. Neurobase MedLink, Arbor 1993–2000.

Shrier, L.A. et al. Bacterial and fungal infections of the central nervous system. In: Berg B.O. (Ed.). Principles of Child Neurology. New York: McGraw-Hill, 764–766, 1996.

Weil, M.L. et al. Infections of the nervous system. In: Menkes, J.H. and Sarnat, H.B. (Eds.). Child Neurology, ed. 6. Philadelphia: Lippincott Williams & Wilkins, 467–626, 2000.

Index